Culture in Rehabilitation: From Competency to Proficiency

EDITED BY

Matin Royeen, PhD

International and Diversity Programs Consultant
Glen Carbon, Illinois

AND

Jeffrey L. Crabtree, OTD, OTR, FAOTA

Associate Professor, Department of Occupational Therapy
School of Health and Rehabilitation Sciences
Indiana University, Indiana

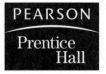

PEARSON
Prentice
Hall

Upper Saddle River, New Jersey 07458

Library of Congress Cataloging-in-Publication Data

Culture in rehabilitation : from competency to proficiency /
[edited by] Matin Royeen, and Jeffrey L. Crabtree.
     p. ; cm.
  Includes bibliographical references.
  ISBN 0–13–090072–9
  1. Rehabilitation.   2. Cultural awareness.
  [DNLM: 1. Rehabilitation.   2. Attitude of Health Personnel.
3. Cultural Diversity.   WB 320 C968 2006]   I. Royeen, Matin
II. Crabtree, Jeffrey L.
  RM930.C84 2006
  362'.0425—dc22

                      2005008363

Publisher: Julie Levin Alexander
Executive Editor: Mark Cohen
Associate Editor: Melissa Kerian
Editorial Assistant: Jaquay Felix
Production Editor: Bruce Hobart, Pine Tree Composition
Director of Manufacturing and Production: Bruce Johnson
Managing Editor for Production: Patrick Walsh
Manufacturing Manager: Ilene Sanford
Manufacturing Buyer: Pat Brown
Cover Design Coordinator: Christopher Weigand
Cover Design and Illustration: Michael Ginsburg
Director of Marketing: Karen Allman
Marketing Coordinator: Michael Sirinides
Channel Marketing Manager: Rachele Strober
Interior Design and Composition: Pine Tree Composition
Printing and Binding: Courier Companies Inc.

Pearson Education LTD.
Pearson Education Australia PTY, Limited
Pearson Education Singapore, Pte. Ltd.
Pearson Education North Asia Ltd.
Pearson Education Canada, Ltd.

Pearson Educación de Mexico, S.A. de C.V.
Pearson Education—Japan
Pearson Education Malaysia, Pte. Ltd.
Pearson Education, Upper Saddle River,
  New Jersey

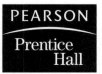

10 9 8 7 6 5 4 3 2 1
ISBN 0-13-090072-9

Contents

Contributors   xi
Acknowledgments   xiii
Reviewers   xiv

1   Cultural Proficiency in Rehabilitation: An Introduction   1
Jeffrey L. Crabtree, Matin Royeen, and Jean Benton

   Introduction   2
   The Purpose of Rehabilitation   3
   Why Cultural Proficiency in Rehabilitation?   4
   Cultural Proficiency   4
   Overview of Predominant Mainstream American Values   6
   Cultural Characteristics   9
   Organization of This Book   10
   Summary   15
   References   15

2   Rehabilitation and Discrimination   17
Awilda R. Haskins

   Introduction   18
   Real Discrimination   18
   Perceived Discrimination   18
   Attitudinal Racism   19
   Institutional Discrimination   19
   Overt Discrimination   19
   Covert Bias   20
   The "-isms"   20
   Racism: Discrimination Against People of Different Races or Ethnic Origins   20
   Heterosexism and Homophobia: Discrimination Against People
      of Different Lifestyles   22
   Ageism: Discrimination Against the Very Young or the Very Old   23
   Sexism: Discrimination Against Women   25
   Discrimination Against the Poor   26
   Discrimination Against the Homeless   27
   Discrimination Against People with HIV Infection   28
   Summary   29
   Questions   30
   Case Study   30
   References   31

iii

3   Communication in Multicultural Settings   37
     Hye-Kyeung Seung and Sandra Bond

        Introduction   38
        Communication   38
        Barriers to Effective Communication   43
        Summary   49
        Case Study 1   50
        Case Study 2   50
        Case Study 3   51
        Case Study 4   52
        Questions   56
        References   57

4   Ethics of Culture in Rehabilitation   59
     Jeffrey L. Crabtree

        Introduction   60
        Individualism and Collectivism: Assumptions of Rehabilitation Practitioners   61
        Ethical Principles and Assumptions Underlying Rehabilitation   63
        Case Study 1   64
        Case Study 2   66
        Case Study 3   68
        Ethical Decision Making in Rehabilitation   70
        Summary   70
        Questions   71
        References   71

5   European Americans   74
     Shannon Munro Cohen

        Introduction   75
        Poland   77
        Croatia   79
        Hungary   81
        Romania   83
        Greece   84
        Italy   86
        Germany   88
        Ireland   89
        United Kingdom   91
        France   93
        Cross-Cultural Communication in the United States   95
        Summary   96
        Questions   96

Working with Interpreters   96
Suggestions for When an Interpreter Is Not Available   97
Case Study 1   97
Case Study 2   98
Case Study 3   98
Suggested Reading   98
References   101
Appendix   102

6   African Americans   103
Shirley Blanchard and Cynthia Jenkins

Introduction   104
Background   105
Concepts of Time and Space   107
Language, Patterns of Interaction, and Communication   108
Patterns of African American Families   110
Health Beliefs and Practices   112
Accessibility to Health Care   115
Health Disparity   115
Culture of African American Eating Habits   116
Mental Illness   118
Disability in the African American Culture   120
Summary   122
Questions   122
Case Study   123
References   126

7   Native Americans   131
Matin Royeen and Jeffrey L. Crabtree

Introduction   132
Rehabilitative Assumptions and Native American Cultures   132
The First Americans: A Brief History   133
The Sacred Land of Native Americans   134
Characteristics of Native American Cultures   135
The Importance of Sport   137
The Native American Arts   138
Health, Healing, and Rehabilitation   139
Traditional Native American Healing   140
Ceremonies and Rituals   141
An Integrative Approach to Practice   142
Case Study   145
Summary   146
Questions   146
References   147

8 Asian Americans   151
Asha Asher

Introduction   152
Chinese   156
Asian Indians   159
Japanese   163
Filipinos   166
Vietnamese   169
Koreans   172
Summary   174
Case Study   176
Questions   176
References   177

9 Arab Americans   181
S. Omar Ahmad, Naser Z. Alsharif, and Matin Royeen

Introduction   182
Rehabilitative Care of Arab-American Patients   182
Background   183
Immigration Patterns   184
Case Study 1   186
Values and Beliefs of Traditional Arab Culture   188
Islamic Law Regulating Patterns of Life   189
Case Study 2   192
History of Middle Eastern Countries   194
Summary   200
Questions   201
References   201

10 Understanding Judaism and Jewish Americans   203
Marcy Coppelman Goldsmith

Introduction   204
Arrival in the United States   204
Jewish Language and Communication   205
Judaism and Its Sects   206
Sects of Judaism   212
Family Structure and Issues of Aging   213
Health Beliefs and Practices   214
Health Risk Factors   215
Summary   215
Questions   216
Case Study   216
References   217

11   The Smorgasbord of the Hispanic Cultures   218
Toni Thompson and Eduardo Blasquez

Introduction   219
Use of the Term "Hispanic"   219
Immigration Patterns   219
Population Demographics   222
Population Distribution   223
Diversities   223
Diversity in Immigration   224
Cultural Differences   224
Language   225
The Influence of Socioeconomic Differences   225
Cultural Values, Cultural Stereotypes   226
High-Contact and Low-Contact Patterns of Communication   226
Tradition-Based Culture   227
Indirect Patterns of Communication   227
The Hispanic "No"   228
The Hispanic "Yes"   228
"Carinos" (Small Gifts)   228
"Palanca"   229
Concepts of Time   229
"Machismo"   229
Last Names   230
Health Care Options: Hot-Cold Model   230
Food and Nutrition   230
Medical Conditions Unique to the Hispanic Cultures   231
Alternative Health Care Options   232
Intervention Techniques and Strategies   233
Intervention Strategies Specific to Therapy   235
Summary   236
Case Study   237
Questions   237
Suggested Readings   238
References   240

12   Pacific Island Peoples and Rehabilitation   242
Katherine T. Ratliffe

Introduction   243
Cultural Proficiency   244
The Pacific Islands   244
Cultural Practices   255
Working with People from the Pacific Islands   269
Summary   271
Annotated Bibliography of Useful References   271

Questions   272
References   272

13   Cross-Cultural Meaning of Disability   274
Ronnie Linda Leavitt

Introduction   275
Acculturation   276
Cultural Beliefs About Disability   276
Cultural Response to the Presence of Disability at the Individual Level   281
Cultural Response to the Presence of Disability at the Societal Level   284
Issues Needing Our Attention to Foster the Development
    of a Culturally Competent Rehabilitation Professional   287
Case Study   288
Summary   289
Questions   290
References   290

14   Poverty in the United States: Making Ends Meet   293
Shannon Munro Cohen

Introduction   294
Socioeconomic Class   294
Social Problems and Poverty   296
Welfare Reform   300
Hunger   301
Health Care Needs   302
Rehabilitation Programs and Legislation   303
Rehabilitation Issues and the Role of Health Care Providers   304
Case Study 1   305
Case Study 2   306
Case Study 3   306
Summary   307
Questions   307
References   308
Appendix   311

15   Gender & Culture   312
L. Margaret Drake

Introduction   313
Infancy   314
Childhood   317
Adolescence   321
Young Adulthood   324

Middle Adulthood   327
Older Adulthood   331
The Wise Elderly   333
Case Study   335
Gender and Immigration   336
Summary   337
Questions   337
References   338

16   Age as Culture in Rehabilitation   342

Tana L. Hadlock and Jeffrey L. Crabtree

Introduction   343
Generational Cohort Theory   346
Cohort Values   347
Overarching Considerations About Aging as Culture   350
Ethical Considerations Across Age Cultures   350
Continuity of Aging   352
Adaptive Capacity   352
Summary   354
Questions   354
Case Study   355
References   355

17   Understanding Sexual Minorities   357

Suzann Robins

Introduction   358
Defining Terms   358
Taking a Medical History   363
The Need for Understanding   364
Teenage Identity Is Difficult for Everyone   365
An Aging Population   366
The Search for Community   368
Stages of Coming Out   370
Cultural Complications   371
Moving Beyond Acceptance   371
Guidelines   372
Summary   372
Case Study   373
Questions   373
References   374

Index   377

Contributors

S. Omar Ahmad, OTD, Ph.D.
Assistant Professor
Occupational Therapy Education
University of Kansas Medical Center
Kansas City, Kansas

Naser Z. Alsharif, Pharm.D., Ph.D.
Associate Professor
Associate Director, Web-Based Pharmacy Pathway
Creighton University
Department of Pharmacy Sciences
Omaha, Nebraska

Asha Asher, M.A. (OT), Med (SP. ED).
Occupational Therapy Coordinator
Sycamore Community Schools
Cincinnati, Ohio

Jean Benton, Ph.D.
Associate Professor
College of Education
Southeast Missouri State University
Cape Girardeau, Missouri

Sandra Bond, M.S., CCC-SLP
San Luis Obispo County Office of Education
San Luis Obispo, California

Shirley A. Blanchard, Ph.D., ABDA, OTR/L
Primary Appointment: Associate Professor
Department of Occupational Therapy
Secondary Appointment: Associate Professor
Department of Medicine
Creighton University Medical Center
Founder Healthy Church Project
Creighton University
Omaha, Nebraska

Jeffrey L. Crabtree, OTD, OTR, FAOTA
Associate Professor
Department of Occupational Therapy
School of Health and Rehabilitation Sciences
Indiana University, Indiana

Shannon Munro Cohen, APRN, BC, FNP-C
Family Nurse Practitioner
Department of Veterans Affairs Medical Center
Salem, Virginia

L. Margaret Drake, Ph.D., OTR-L, ATR-BC, LPAT, FAOTA
Professor of Occupational Therapy
University of Mississippi Medical Center
Jackson, Mississippi

Marcy Coppelman Goldsmith, Ph.D. OTR/L BCP
Senior Staff Therapist
Occupational Therapy Associates-Wakefield
Wakefield, Massachusetts
Lecturer, Tufts University
Medford, Massachusetts

Tana L. Hadlock, M.A., OTR
Instructional Faculty
Yamaguchi Health and Welfare College
Ube City, Japan

Awilda R. Haskins, Ed.D., PT
Associate Professor
Department of Physical Therapy
Florida International University
Miami, Florida

Cynthia Jenkins, Ph.D., LMHP
Counseling Psychologist
Director of Catherine House
Omaha Opportunities Industrialization Center, Inc.
Omaha, Nebraska

Ronnie Linda Leavitt, Ph.D., MPH, PT
Associate Professor
University of Connecticut
Storrs, Connecticut

Katherine T. Ratliffe, Ph.D., PT
Assistant Professor
Center on Disability Studies
University of Hawaii at Manoa
Honolulu, Hawaii

Suzann Robins, M.A.
Adjunct Professor of Psychology
East Orange, New Jersey

Matin Royeen, Ph.D.
International and Diversity Programs Consultant
Glen Carbon, Illinois

Hye-Kyeung Seung, Ph.D.
Assistant Professor
Department of Communicative Disorders
University of Florida—Gainesville
Gainesville, Florida

Toni Thompson, M.A., OTR/L, BCP
Senior Pediatric Occupational Therapist
Shriners Hospitals for Children
Tampa, Florida

Acknowledgments

Diane Monsivais, CRRN, MSN

Clinical Instructor at University of Texas at El Paso, School of Nursing

The editors appreciate Diane Monsivais's help in editing the book during the final phase of this project.

Reviewers

Carol J. Bancroft, PT
Instructional Director
Allied Health/Science Department
Delaware Technical and Community College—
    Wilmington Campus
Wilmington, Delaware

Chris Barrett, PT, M.Ed.
Program Director
Physical Therapist Assistant Program
Lake Area Technical Institute
Watertown, South Dakota

Sharon A. Bryant, Ph.D.
Associate Professor
Decker School of Nursing
Binghamton University
Binghamton, New York

Gwendolyn Gray, M.A.
Assistant Professor and Program Director
Occupational Therapy
Tuskegee University
Tuskegee, Alabama

Dyhalma Izarry, Ph.D., OTR/L, FAOTA
Professor and Chairperson
Occupational Therapy Program
University of Puerto Rico
San Juan, Puerto Rico

Jill Laroussini, RN, M.S.N.
Instructor
College of Nursing and Allied Health Professions
University of Louisiana at Lafayette
Lafayette, Louisiana

Jaime Phillip Muñoz, M.S., OTR, FAOTA
Instructor
Occupational Therapy Department
Duquesne University
Pittsburgh, Pennsylvania

Janet Nagayda, M.S., OTR
Associate Professor
Department of Occupational Therapy
Saginaw Valley State University
University Center, Michigan

Linda J. Netzel, M.A., OTR
Professor
Occupational Therapy Assistant Program
Macomb Community College
Clinton Township, Michigan

Michael Spitz, M.S.A., PTA, CSCS
Professor
Physical Therapist Assistant Program
Delta College
University Center, Michigan

1

Cultural Proficiency in Rehabilitation: An Introduction

Jeffrey L. Crabtree, Matin Royeen, and Jean Benton

Key Words

culture	competence	beliefs
ethnicity	norms	values

Objectives

1. Understand and identify reasons why it is important to work toward cultural proficiency in rehabilitation.
2. Understand and explain the role and impact of culture on the individual.
3. Understand and explain the implications for the rehabilitation of the individual's culture.
4. Understand the theoretical, ethical, and practical reasons for culturally competent rehabilitation.

Introduction

This chapter serves as an introduction both to the concept of cultural proficiency in rehabilitation and to the contents of the book. This book is about how culture unavoidably plays a critical role in the practice and theory of rehabilitation. To explore the concept of cultural proficiency in rehabilitation, we need to make explicit our belief about why it is important to work toward cultural proficiency and what the role and the impact of culture are on the individual, and to provide theoretical, ethical, and practical reasons for culturally proficient rehabilitation, especially for those professionals working in various settings with diverse clients.

Before exploring these issues, it is important to disclose our assumptions about rehabilitation: First, the goal of Western rehabilitation is not only to help restore function, but, as Jennings (1995) has said, but also to help reshape the patient's *self*. "For good therapeutic as well as ethical reasons, rehabilitation must be individually oriented because the patient must be treated as a subject, an active participant and partner in the process of his or her own recovery" (p. S27). Second, as Jennings (1995) also asserted, "the formulation of the treatment goals . . . cannot really be divorced from the broader process of redefining the patient's good in light of societal conceptions of what constitutes the good life" (p. S27). Third, most rehabilitation practitioners are oriented to mainstream Western beliefs about what constitutes "the good life." Finally, people from diverse cultures and people with chronic disease, advanced age, and/or disabilities are likely to define "the good life" in ways other than those common to Western beliefs.

In the United States, we live in a culturally pluralistic society. Our cultural diversity is reflected in both health care practitioners and patients who represent different segments of populations in different health care institutions. Such diversity provides both opportunities and challenges for rehabilitation workers for effective service delivery to those clients representing different cultural backgrounds. The opportunities afford the rehabilitations professional to learn a new set of cultural skills and to provide valuable services to these clients. Challenges occur when rehabilitation professionals lack the necessary skills to provide culturally based effective services to these clients who have diverse cultural backgrounds. For an effective delivery of rehabilitation services, rehabilitation professionals can no longer afford to rely merely on a Western-based model of a health delivery system.

In the Western world, the concept of culture has undergone transformation in the past two hundred years. According to Jandt (1995), the terms *culture* and *Western civilization* were used synonymously in the nineteenth century in order to reflect the superiority of Western culture over the non-Western world. Currently, there are numerous authors from different disciplines who do not adhere to the belief that Western culture is superior to non-Western cultures and who define culture in very broad terms. Hall (1959, 1969, 1976) refers to culture as dynamic and learned symbolic communication. Culture is the total body of tradition passed from one generation to another according to Murphy (1986) and Prosser (1978). Collier and Thomas (1988) define culture as a system of symbols and norms used by individuals as part of their cultural identity. Samovar and Porter (1997) consider culture to be the cumulative deposit of shared meanings and values, and they emphasize characteristics of culture and their importance to intercultural communication.

Anderson and Fenichel (1989) propose culture to be an evolving framework through which human actions (both similarities and differences) are checked. Geertz (1976) emphasizes the activity of actual life, and Schneider (1976) refers to normal elements of life as important ingredients of culture.

For the purpose of this book, we use the abstract term *culture* to refer to the sum of the experiences, values, beliefs, ideals, judgments, and attitudes that shape and give continuous form to each individual. Babies are born into a culture. As they grow and mature, they take on the values, beliefs, and the like of that culture. While living in that culture, people are afforded opportunities to experience and express those beliefs, ideals, and values throughout their daily lives. Culture is at once ideological, emphasizing beliefs, values, ideals, and thoughts, and also is material, social, linguistic, relational, and, most important, is ever-changing and transformative. The process of cultural change and evolution adds to, deletes from, and alters the store of shared information in an ongoing process. Within any culture are many forms of diverse and competing beliefs, experiences, and values. Even people from different geographical regions of the United States display different cultural values, beliefs, and attitudes. Individuals may see one culture as restrictive, another as liberating, and still others as interesting, primitive, enlightened, or the like. The possible number of interpretations and assessment of culture is as numerous as there are people.

We use the term cultural awareness to describe one's ability to understand, appreciate, and acknowledge the similarities and differences between two cultures involved. Cultural awareness deals with gaining the necessary knowledge and developing new attitudes toward clients' cultural belief system. We use the term cultural competence to mean applying the benefits of cultural awareness during practice in a most effective and culturally meaningful way with desirable rehabilitation results.

The Purpose of Rehabilitation

An appreciation of the importance of culture to the rehabilitation process comes from exploring the deep and significant purpose of rehabilitation. A common purpose, and one that is often offered to patients and family members, is that rehabilitation is a process of helping people function in their daily lives or of helping them become independent in some particular activity. Although often important to the patient and rewarding to the rehabilitation practitioner, function and independence pale in light of the deep and lasting purpose of helping people reconstruct or redesign their personal "good life." Jennings (1995) asserted that, within the context of institutionalized rehabilitation of individuals, the purpose of rehabilitation takes on a significance that transcends the more specific medical values and goals that apply in acute health care. For example, a stroke may leave a person with speech, motor, and cognitive disabilities that pose significant challenges to the patient, family, and rehabilitation practitioners. And certainly rehabilitation practitioners must do what they can to help the person with a stroke to overcome these challenges. However, as Jennings stated,

It is the restoration of the [individual's] power of living well, living meaningfully, that rehabilitation essentially seeks. What does it mean to live well? What is the good in the good life? These are questions that require social and cultural answers as well as individual, personal ones. (1995, p. S26)

Why Cultural Proficiency in Rehabilitation?

The most critical issue in culturally proficient rehabilitation is to recognize that individuals receiving rehabilitation services are part of a multifaceted system of shared beliefs, meanings, values, and the like, that are expressed through those individuals' beliefs about things like independence, health, and function (Helman, 1994; Keesing, 1981). To put it another way, to know individuals' personal wishes, beliefs, preferences, choices, expectations, values, and so on is to know something of their culture. This book discusses and explores culture as an abstraction in the hope that by gaining understanding of different cultures, the rehabilitation practitioner can come close to understanding the beliefs and values of the individual and thereby can deal effectively with the specific culture in which the individual patient lives.

To provide effective rehabilitation services, the rehabilitation practitioner must understand the patient's personal and cultural belief systems regarding illness and health. It is very important to remember that each member of the rehabilitation team brings a set of personal values from his or her own culture and values acquired during the professional acculturation process that serves as a basis for intervention. Without exploration of the patient's cultural values, motivations, and expectation of the outcomes, and without examination of the practitioner's assumptions, the rehabilitation practitioner will have difficulty providing effective services for the patient. Otherwise, the gap between the rehabilitation professional's and the patient's values will serve as an obstacle to effective treatment. An example includes what can happen when a practitioner, assuming that independence is the "gold standard" of rehabilitation, treats a person from the Philippines who, because of his age, expects his family to help with virtually all of his daily living activities. Not understanding the culture and values of this patient, the rehabilitation practitioner may well consider him to be a poor rehabilitation candidate and his family to be uncooperative.

At best, the potential lack of agreement on basic values, beliefs, or attitudes complicates the issues that must be addressed for successful outcomes and confounds the rehabilitation practitioners' efforts to provide competent and effective rehabilitation services. At worst, conflicts between ethnic and cultural beliefs, values, and attitudes undermine the best intentions of rehabilitation practitioners and the efforts of clients to lead lives that for them are consistent with their ethnic and cultural beliefs and values.

Cultural Proficiency

It is useful to examine how cultural proficiency differs from other constructs like cultural blindness and cultural sensitivity. One way to do this is to explore a continuum of responses to cultural diversity articulated by the late Bob Hallowell (personal communica-

Overt Cultural Destructiveness	Covert Cultural Destructiveness	Cultural Blindness	Cultural Sensitivity	Cultural Competence	Cultural Proficiency	Institutionalized Cultural Proficiency

FIGURE 1.1 Cultural Behavior Continuum.
(Hallowell, R. (2001). Personal communication.)

tion) that range from covert destructive behaviors to institutionalized cultural proficiency. Specifically, these responses to cultural diversity include: overt cultural destructiveness, covert cultural destructiveness, cultural blindness, cultural sensitivity, cultural competence, cultural proficiency, and institutionalized cultural proficiency. Later, we will also discuss in more detail why rehabilitation practitioners must be aware of their responses and of interactions with their patients in order to maximize their effectiveness.

The characteristics of overt *cultural destructive behaviors* include intentional and militant actions to destroy and eradicate a particular culture or group and the values it represents. Examples of large-scale cultural destructiveness include the efforts of regimes or groups like the Third Reich in Germany, the Hutu and Tutsi in central Africa, and the Europeans in the New World of the seventeenth century. In each case, members of one group intentionally killed thousands, or even millions, of people in the name of cultural beliefs and values. *Covert cultural destructiveness*, on the other hand, is a term that can be used to describe subtle, nonlethal actions and behaviors that limit access to social and economic resources, and that prevent individuals or a group of people from practicing cultural-specific rituals and ceremonies and from speaking their native language. In the United States, the public policy at the turn of the seventeenth and eighteenth centuries was meant to assimilate Native Americans into the European culture by sending their children away to boarding schools and teaching them European values and lifestyles (Herring, 1992). In cases of *cultural blindness*, people do not recognize or validate cultural values and differences of other ethnic or cultural groups. Those differences, regardless of their potential value to the observer, do not exist. This reaction to cultural diversity is unconscious, not willful, and is not meant to deny others their own culture or any benefits of the dominant culture. What many people call *cultural sensitivity* indicates an understanding or appreciation of others' differences, values, beliefs, and the like. However, as used in this continuum, cultural sensitivity at its worst is superficial and condescending, and at its best falls short of any meaningful effort on the part of a person of one culture to examine and understand a person of another culture.

We use the term *cultural competence* to describe two important points. The first is the notion of self-examination in relation to one's own culture, values, beliefs, and experiences of people from different ethnic groups and cultures. The second is the ability to apply those relevant cultural concepts in everyday practice to patients of different cultural backgrounds. In this context, cultural competence embodies both the necessary theoretical values and the practical application of those values in everyday practice. Cultural proficiency is an ongoing, evolving process. We acknowledge that the so-called culturally proficient person could never completely understand a different culture or could not know what it was like to have been born in a different ethnic group. Becoming culturally proficient is *process*, not outcome; the person who strives for cultural proficiency never reaches that goal; however, by continually striving to gain an understanding and appreciation of others' beliefs, values, and experiences, the person can successfully apply what is learned in his or her daily life. At best, people who strive for cultural proficiency change their way of thinking about other people and their different cultures on the basis of this self-examination. *Institutionalized cultural proficiency* describes the circumstance in which an organization, a hospital, or a rehabilitation clinic incorporates standards that call for culturally proficient behaviors resulting from self-examination and for efforts to understand and appreciate the beliefs and values of different cultures.

Presumably, rehabilitation practitioners never engage in overt or covert culturally destructive relationships with their patients. However, there may be little understanding of why it might be important to engage in culturally proficient relationships with their patients.

Overview of Predominant Mainstream American Values

As mentioned earlier, every culture represents a system of learned values or social principles that determine what is good, right, or just in a society. It is through these values that people define their relationships both to members of immediate groups and to members of society in general. These values are unconsciously expressed by a majority of members in a society through norms. Since cultures are dynamic, these norms change and evolve over time. However, the fundamental boundaries of the culture do not change, and the structure of any culture resists major alterations. The contemporary American society adheres to a set of European-dominant mainstream normative values. Understanding these mainstream cultural norms can provide a useful frame of reference for the reader. A brief discussion of some mainstream American values will follow. These American norms can be used as a baseline for cultural comparison by the rehabilitation practitioner during interactions with patients representing different cultures. Lynch and Hanson (1992), Pederson, Lonner and Draguns (1976), and Spector (1996) discuss the following values that characterize American society today.

Scientific Orientation

Mainstream Americans in general have accepted scientific methods and scientific reasoning as the way to understand the physical world, and they believe that everything in the physical world should have a logical, understandable basis. Many peoples of other cultures do not necessarily accept scientific explanations and are likely to be guided in their beliefs and understanding of behavior by religious mysticism, tradition, or other nonanalytical bases. Within the mainstream American culture, there is a scientific explanation and diagnosis of disease invading the human body. By contrast, many other cultural groups explain the causes of illness as an imbalance or a lack of harmony between the individual and the environment. For example, among Latinos, maintaining the balance between hot and cold is important for maintaining good health (Downes, 1994).

Control of the Natural Environment

Mainstream Americans usually think of nature as something that can be altered, conquered, and controlled for their comfort and convenience. Modern advances in technology and sciences make it easier for people to explore nature, predict hazardous conditions, and avoid danger to life and property. In contrast to mainstream Americans attitudes toward nature, peoples from many other cultures accept nature as a force greater than humans and as something to which people must adapt rather than something they can change or control. For example, living in harmony with nature is the most important hallmark of the Native American and Alaskan native cultures. The land (mother and earth) is considered sacred to the tribal groups who continue to teach respect for the land to the younger generations through rituals and various ceremonies (Lynch & Hanson, 1992).

Progress and Change

Change and progress are the necessary natural ingredients for social/economic mobility in American life. Americans are preoccupied with the here and now and seek immediate results and gratification for future security and prosperity. Thus, to most mainstream Americans, changes in jobs, ownership of automobiles, and ownership of homes are necessary for upward mobility in life. On the other hand, people of other cultural backgrounds tend to look to their traditions as a guide to the future and are not as much preoccupied with change and progress.

Materialism

Mainstream Americans usually look for measurable results of their efforts so that they can decide whether they are making forward progress. They often stress material comfort and convenience, whereas many cultural groups of non-Western origin strive for spiritual and aesthetic values that stress the inner experience of a person rather than any tangible result. Mainstream Americans will often judge another culture by its material progress and thus will neglect to consider other possible aspects of that culture, such as quality of life.

Individualism

As discussed earlier, the dominant American culture emphasizes the individual. Each individual, for the most part, is responsible for making the decisions that affect his or her life. In other cultural groups, decisions are often made by a family, clan, group, or someone in authority. Mainstream Americans think that individuals should take control of their own lives, develop their own potentialities, use their own initiative to move ahead, and compete with others to "get ahead." Members of other cultural groups are likely to regard their individual role in life as a part of the greater family circle.

Moralistic Orientation

Mainstream Americans tend to have a missionary spirit to win other people over to their way of thinking and are likely to judge others in terms of mainstream American cultural values. Therefore, it is not unusual for mainstream Americans to expect other ethnic groups to adopt those mainstream beliefs, values, and ways of doing things.

Time Orientation

Americans are generally very time conscience, treating time as a material thing that should be used and manipulated to the best advantage. People who waste time or do not make good use of their time are considered lazy and unmotivated. A by-product of time consciousness is punctuality. Americans set a specific time for meetings, conferences, parties, dates, and so on, and others are expected to arrive at that time. In business and social situations, anyone who arrives after that time is considered late, and someone who arrives more than about fifteen minutes after the specific hour is expected to offer an apology for being late. Mainstream Americans often have difficulty with people from cultures in which time is less important and in which people are not expected to arrive at a set hour. It is interesting to note that in the United States, there is a saying that "Time is money," whereas in Arabic there is a saying that "Hurry is of the devil."

Doing Rather than Being

Because Americans are motivated by a desire to achieve and get ahead, there tends to be a sharp distinction between work and play, between being productive and leisure. Americans are serious at work and want to get down to business, rather than spend time on unrelated matters. As a result, mainstream Americans often have difficulties functioning with other cultural groups whose members will take time to establish a social relationship before the transaction of business.

Egalitarianism

Although there are many differences in social, economic, and educational levels in the United States, there is a theme of equality that runs through social relationships, in part because mainstream Americans do not accept a fixed position in society and believe that one can achieve and succeed in life. Socially, although sometimes superficial, there is generally an attempt to equalize the relationship and to avoid calling attention to rank and authority as a way of exercising power over someone. Mainstream Americans call each other by first names much sooner and more often than people in most other cultures. Arguably, there is a general belief among Americans that people in our society have equal rights, equal social obligations, and equal opportunities to develop their own potential. However, realistically, there are many people in American society who are privileged because of wealth, ethnicity, education, and other characteristics and many others for whom the notions of equal rights and opportunities are only a hope or dream.

Role of Woman

There is a strong feminist movement, or women's liberation movement, in the United States that aims to ensure that women have responsibilities and opportunities equal to those of men. Although there are still many aspects of society in which women have not yet achieved equality, women play a much more public and visible role in the mainstream culture than in many other ethnic and cultural groups. What some cultures consider the proper role for women is considered by many Americans to be sexist or treatment examples of male chauvinism.

Friendliness and Openness

To a mainstream American, a friend can be anyone from a mere acquaintance to a lifelong intimate, and the friendships may depend on a particular activity. Americans have friendships that revolve around work, political activity, volunteer activity, special interest, and so on. Americans often have different friends for each kind of activity—friends who are rarely all together at a given time and who may never meet each other. An American may have many friendships on a casual, occasional basis but only a very few deep, meaningful relationships that last throughout life. People from non-Western cultural backgrounds sometimes see these cultural relationships as a reluctance of Americans to become deeply involved with others. In some circumstances in which a person in another culture would turn to a friend for help or support, we may turn to a professional, such as a counselor, rather than burdening friends with our problems. Americans live in a very mobile society and therefore not only can form friendships but also can give them up much more easily with less stress than for people of many other cultural backgrounds.

Cultural Characteristics

As stated earlier, culture is a dynamic, fluid concept. People are not simply members of the dominant culture, but they can also be bicultural, members of a counterculture, of subcultures, and of any number of combinations and permutations of the possibilities. In addition, there exist many processes involved in being and becoming members of given cultures. These include the processes of acculturation, enculturation, and assimilation. It is interesting to note that terms such as *counterculture* and *subculture* were likely coined by members of the more powerful, dominant, culture and are likely to have connotations for many of those who are labeled as being part of a counterculture or a subculture. Given this power differential, countercultures and subcultures are terms for cultures within the dominant culture. For example, various health care professions such as occupational therapy, physical therapy, nursing, etc. form subcultures of unique values, experiences, beliefs, norms, and the like. When people decide to become rehabilitation practitioners, for example, they must learn a new vocabulary and the history of their chosen profession, and they must acquire a way of thinking and viewing people in light of their new language. Religions, fraternities, labor unions, and service organizations exemplify subcultures within a dominant culture.

Countercultures, according to Loutaunau and Sobo, (1997) "entail alternative lifestyles for those who cannot conform to or actively oppose widely accepted social norms" (p. 11). Within health care and in considering Western biomedicine as part of the dominant culture in the United States, Christian Science could be an example of a counterculture in which people understand the etiology of disease very differently from the view of the dominant culture and may choose very different approaches to curing those diseases. For example, "Christian Scientists respect the work of the medical profession, but choose prayer as treatment for themselves and their children rather than medicine because they have experienced prayer's effectiveness many times in their lives" (Young, n. d.).

It is not uncommon for many people to be bicultural. That is, they function equally well in their traditional culture and in the dominant culture. In these cases, individuals may voluntarily give up certain values, beliefs, and traditions of either their traditional or the adopted culture. One example is that of the many Mexicans and Mexican-Americans who live along the U.S.-Mexico border. As in the case of the border between El Paso, Texas, and Ciudad Juárez, Mexico, there are about 6 million crossings each year. Many individuals living in this region have family on both sides of the border and take advantage of resources on either side, depending on their needs. They speak both English and Spanish, and engage with ease in both the American and the Mexican cultures.

The **enculturation** of someone into the dominant culture generally occurs during the socialization process of growing up in a culture from birth, with parents of the dominant culture. During that powerful process, children generally learn and adopt the beliefs, values, and norms of the culture in which they are reared, and they have many opportunities throughout the maturation process to "practice," experience, and express those beliefs, values, and norms. **Acculturation,** on the other hand, according to some (Locke, 1992), is a process of newcomers' adopting their own values and attitudes to those of the dominant culture. An example of acculturation is the experience of many younger immigrants who come to the United States with their families and who gradually adjust well to the new American culture. These young people still maintain some of their own cultural values while acquiring the new ones (Downes, 1994). **Assimilation** involves giving up the old cultural values in favor of the new cultural features of the dominant culture. This is similar to the example of the "melting pot" in which it is assumed that immigrants would assimilate and form one culture in the United States (Downes, 1994).

Organization of This Book

The purpose of each chapter is to help the reader develop what we are calling "cultural proficiency" from the perspective of a given ethnic or cultural group. What do we mean by cultural proficiency? We mean that the rehabilitation practitioner not only will develop awareness and sensitivity to different cultural and ethnic beliefs, values, and attitudes about rehabilitation, but, as Green and Leigh (1989) put it, but also will "learn about the cultural context of a presenting problem and to integrate that knowledge into a professional assessment, diagnosis, and intervention" (p. 8). Further, working toward cultural competence means that practitioners provide services "in ways that are acceptable and useful to [clients] because [those services] are congruent with the recipient's cultural background and expectations" (p. 8).

To accomplish this purpose, the book includes a discussion of a broad range of ethnic and cultural groups; therefore, the discussion is necessarily general and sometimes simplistic. The authors use case studies in each chapter to help the reader understand and appreciate the dynamics and complexities of ethnic and cultural groups. We hope that readers will take it upon themselves to use this book as a springboard for more detailed and specific research about the cultural and ethnic groups with which they work.

The book is divided into three sections. One need not read the chapters in the order presented in order to receive the benefit of the book. The first section includes Chapters 1 through 4, which explore the concept of culture in the rehabilitation context and which examine the need for cultural competence in rehabilitation from three perspectives: communication, ethics, and discrimination.

Chapter 1. Cultural Competence in Rehabilitation: An Introduction

In the first chapter, the authors explore definitions of culture and the dynamics of mulitculturalism in contemporary American society. The authors present a global view of what culture is and how it dominates the individual's belief system, values, and views in all spheres of life activities. The chapter offers an overview of the meaning of culture, the way that American mainstream culture evolved, and its implications for rehabilitation.

Chapter 2: Rehabilitation and Discrimination

Chapter 2 explores discrimination, unequal health care access sometimes found in rehabilitation, and types of discrimination and bias that can occur in health care in general and in rehabilitation settings in particular. Although this literature review does not include every possible ethnic and cultural group, the reader interested in becoming culturally proficient will be able to see the implications that this chapter has for any group of people who have ethnic or cultural backgrounds, beliefs, and values different from the mainstream culture.

Chapter 3: Communication in Multicultural Settings

This chapter examines the complexities and pitfalls of communication in a multicultural, pluralistic setting. Here the authors attempt to strip cultural differences from communication skills in order to identify common communication pitfalls found in virtually any rehabilitation setting and to provide effective communication techniques useful in most any setting.

Chapter 4: Ethics of Culture in Rehabilitation

In Chapter 4 the author explores the core differences between the constructs of individualism and collectivism. The author shows how collectivism embodies the values and beliefs of many nonmainstream cultures and ethnic groups and how collectivism includes notions of cooperation and deference to the family, whereas individualism generally embodies those values and beliefs we typically associate with mainstream European-America culture and includes notions of individual self-actualization even when such efforts are not supported by the family. The implications for understanding these core differences and the ethical dilemmas and decision making in rehabilitation are discussed.

Section two introduces themes of ethnic diversity and includes a general description and an overview of the experiences, values, and beliefs of eight broad ethnic groups.

Chapter 5: European Americans

Chapter 5 offers a snapshot of the values and beliefs of most of the European cultures whose value systems constitute the core American culture. The chapter includes many of the characteristics of the European Americans along with migration patterns to the United States. The author shows how division between cultures in the United States has blurred, because many European immigrants have adopted the beliefs, values, and customs of this country, and also shows how understanding the roots of our blended society and relationships to health care beliefs and rehabilitation presents a challenge to the health care provider. A brief overview of several European countries is presented in this chapter in order to give the reader a better understanding of the basis of current health beliefs and behaviors.

Chapter 6: African Americans

The author discusses the culture, including health belief systems and practices, of this varied and dynamic group of peoples often called African Americans. This chapter emphasizes the need for a basic understanding of and familiarity with culturally sanctioned experiences, practices, and beliefs that may be of importance to African Americans. The author shows how mainstream practitioners should also be aware of both the differences between themselves and their African American clients and of the similarities in beliefs, experiences, and health practices. With added insight, the practitioner may develop an understanding of the client's needs, fears, and strengths that will aid in facilitating communication and developing appropriate treatments that support the healing process.

Chapter 7: Native Americans

In this chapter the authors offer a brief history of the indigenous peoples of North America prior to and during the time that Europeans explored, colonized, and eventually conquered these people. In addition, the authors briefly discuss characteristics of Native American cultures including health beliefs and practices, as well as other information that will help rehabilitation professionals understand the unique Native American cultures. Finally, they offer a strategy for maximizing a culturally competent approach to delivering rehabilitation services.

Chapter 8: Asian Americans

This chapter explores the diverse and dynamic group of peoples referred to as Asian Americans. This group's long and established histories and cultures which range from rural-agricultural to technical-industrial, and economies that extend from dire impoverishment to the world's foremost exporter and creditor, with governments that range from democracies to totalitarian regimes. The author discusses some of the common beliefs and attitudes that can be attributed to this group, discusses, in more detail, some characteristics and belief systems of specific Asian groups, and explores the implications of these cultural characteristics for rehabilitation.

Chapter 9: Arab Americans

The authors of this chapter provide an overview of the Arab culture and the implications for rehabilitation of the beliefs and values of Arabian people. In addition, the authors discuss some diverse cultural features of the people originating from this part of the world, and the authors provide general information about some countries in the region. Because this region is very culturally diverse, the authors offer specific rehabilitation cases dealing with Arab American patients and present specific recommendations for the rehabilitation practitioner working with the Arab American patient.

Chapter 10: Understanding Judaism and Jewish Americans

In this chapter, the author discusses Judaism both as a cultural force and as a religion. The author shows us that throughout history, the Jewish community has been small and close-knit for both internal and external reasons. Religious principles and social values formed the internal ties, whereas the political environment shaped the external ones. The author explains that because Jews were not given full rights as citizens and in turn not given full access to health care and other services, they established an infrastructure of businesses and health care services by and for the Jewish people regardless of the country of origin. This chapter describes the religion, customs, and value systems of Judaism, and also the implications for rehabilitation of these beliefs and values.

Chapter 11: The Smorgasbord of the Hispanic Cultures

The authors of this chapter describe what many call Hispanic cultures—a group of cultures that encompass a vast number of people with a history of migrations into the United States over the past five hundred years. The authors discuss the cultural characteristics of specific groups of people from Central and South America. In addition, the authors explore how each of these groups tends to express its values, beliefs, and customs, and they discuss implications for rehabilitation practitioners of these cultural expressions.

Chapter 12: Pacific Island Peoples and Rehabilitation

This chapter describes the geography, history, and cultural values of Pacific Islanders and highlights their many different communication styles and time orientations likely foreign to most mainstream rehabilitation professionals. To do so, the chapter follows the stories of four individuals, each from a different cultural background in the Pacific Islands and also in different life circumstances. The author explores ways of delivering rehabilitation services in a culturally competent manner.

Section three, the last section, explores themes of cultural diversity (Chapters 13–17), focusing on cultural constructs of gender, age, disability, poverty, class, and sexuality. The section also discusses the implications for rehabilitation practitioners of these cultural constructs.

Chapter 13: Cross-Cultural Meaning of Disability

This chapter discusses the impact of disability on people and also examines the meaning of disability from a cross-cultural perspective. Specifically, beliefs and behaviors associated with disability, attitudes toward people with disabilities (PWD), the macro (societal and community) and micro (individual and family) level responses to the presence of disability, and some strategies to increase cultural competence will be addressed. The underlying goal of the chapter is to add to the cultural knowledge base of rehabilitation clinicians, while acknowledging at all times the need to consider both **intercultural** diversity and **intracultural** diversity. Information and examples given within the chapter may be extrapolated to other cultures.

Chapter 14: Poverty in the United States: Making Ends Meet

Even though the United States is considered one of the richest countries in the world, it has a large number of homeless individuals and many more people who live in poverty. Although social class is less distinct in this country, it deserves an introduction in the context of poverty in the United States. This chapter begins with a review of the socioeconomic classes: upper, middle, and lower class. In each class, there are additional distinctions between levels as well. Briefly addressed are problems of urban versus rural poverty; hunger; violence; homelessness; the effect of poverty on women, children, and the elderly; and the needs of immigrants to this country. In addition, recent changes in legislation and the health and rehabilitation needs of this group are outlined.

Chapter 15: Gender and Culture

The author of this chapter treats gender as both biological and learned. The biological aspect has to do with genetics, and primary and secondary sex characteristics. The learned part of gender includes the individual's gender identity and gender role. In this chapter, the author explores how gender identity has to do with how one identifies oneself as male, female, or androgynous and with how gender role is what one thinks of when presenting oneself to the public, such as family members or workers. These gender roles are discussed within Maslow's hierarchy of needs. The author explores gender role implications for rehabilitation practitioners.

Chapter 16: Age as Culture in Rehabilitation

This chapter proposes a construct of age, or age groups, as subcultures in themselves, apart from ethnic, racial, or gender diversity factors, and explores the considerations necessary for rehabilitation professionals in providing effective and ethical services for persons who are members of different age-culture groups. Also, the chapter explores assumptions about rehabilitation providers and mainstream Western recipients as members of particular age-cohort "cultures." It examines cohort theory and ethical concerns peculiar to rehabilitation practice with older recipients. Finally, the chapter discusses continuity theory as a way of explaining the life, treatment, and goals of older persons who seek our services.

Chapter 17: Understanding Sexual Minorities

In this chapter the author defines some terminology related to sexual minorities and identifies some problems and issues that gays, lesbians, and others of different lifestyles experience in our society. The author discusses how many people, including health care professionals, remain prejudiced toward anyone who does not fit within a predetermined narrow, "normal" range of sexual behavior. Also, the author offers to rehabilitation practitioners suggestions and guidelines for working successfully with this population.

Summary

Although all of the chapters in this book explore more fully the idea of cultural proficiency, it is important to reiterate some ways of behaving here. Cultural proficiency is achieved not only by learning facts about other cultures but also by suspending one's own cultural perspectives and biases. In so doing, we are more likely to appreciate others' perspectives. Suspending personal points of view and "trying on" those of others can lead to greater understanding and acceptance. Respecting the attitudes and beliefs of others, even if they contradict our personal beliefs, can lead to greater empathy. And finally, adapting professional practice to accommodate the values and beliefs of others will lead to more culturally proficient care. These steps are not always easy: they take practice, but they pay great dividends in culturally proficient services.

References

Anderson, P. & Fenichel, E. (1989). *Serving culturally diverse families of infants and toddlers with disabilities.* Washington, DC: National Center for Clinical Infants Program.

Collier, M. & Thomas, M. (1988). Cultural identity: An interpretive perspective. *International and Intercultural Communication Annual, 12,* 99–120.

Downes, N. (1994). *Ethnic Americans.* Dubuque, IW: Kendall/Hunt Publishing Company.

Geertz, C. (1976). Notes toward a theory of culture. In K. Basso and H. Selby (Eds.), *Meaning in anthropology.* Albuquerque: University of New Mexico Press.

Green, J. W. & Leigh, J. W. (1989). Teaching ethnographic methods to social service workers. *Practicing Anthropology, 11,* 8–10.

Hall, E. (1959). *The silent language.* New York: Doubleday.

Hall, E. (1969). *The hidden dimension.* New York: Anchor.

Hall, E. (1976). *Beyond culture.* New York: Anchor.

Helman, C. G. (1994). *Culture, health and illness* (3rd ed.). Oxford: Butterworth-Heinmann.

Herring, E. (1992). Seeking a new paradigm: Counseling Native Americans. *Journal of Multicultural Counseling and Development 20*(1): 35–43.

Hallowell, R. (2001). Personal communication.

Jandt, F. (1995). *Intercultural communication.* Thousand Oaks, CA: Sage Publications.

Jennings, B. (1995). Healing the self: The moral meaning of relationships in rehabilitation. *American Journal of Physical Medicine & Rehabilitation, 72,* S25–S28.

Keesing, R. M. (1981). *Cultural anthropology: A contemporary perspective.* New York: Holt, Rinehart & Winston.

Locke, D. (1992). *Increasing multicultural understanding: A comprehensive model.* Newbury Park, CA: Sage.

Loutaunau, M. O. & Sobo, E. J. (1997). *The cultural context of health, illness, and medicine.* Westport, CT: Bergin & Garvey.

Lynch, E. & Hanson, W. (1992). *Developing cross-cultural competence.* Baltimore: Paul Brookes Publishing.

Murphy, R. (1986). *Culture and social anthropology: An overture* (2nd ed.) Upper Saddle River, NJ: Prentice Hall.

Peat, M. (1997). *Community based rehabilitation.* London: W. B. Saunders Company.

Pedersen, P., Lonner, W., & Draguns, J. (Eds). (1976). *Counseling across cultures.* Honolulu: East West Center Press.

Prosser, M. (1978). *The cultural dialogue: An introduction to intercultural communication.* Boston: Houghton Mifflin.

Samovar, L. & Porter, R. (1997). *Intercultural communication.* New York: Wadsworth.

Schneider, D. (1976). *Notes toward a theory of culture.* In K. Basso and H. Selby (Eds.), *Meaning in anthropology.* Albuquerque: University of New Mexico.

Spector, R. (1996). *Cultural diversity in health and illness.* Stamford, CT: Appleton & Lang.

Young, L. (no date). The Church of Christ, Scientist (Christian Science). http://www.religioustolerance.org/cr_sci.htm. Retrieved 9/27/2004.

2

Rehabilitation and Discrimination

Awilda R. Haskins

Key Words

rehabilitation	racisim	disparities
discrimination	ageism	research

Learning Objectives

1. Develop an awareness of the many forms that discriminatory practice can take.
2. Identify the effects of discrimination on health care services and the way that they may affect outcomes.
3. Explore personal biases and the way that they may influence the care provided.

Introduction

The common assumption is that in the United States, the richest country in the world, no one has to die unnecessarily from illness or disease. If one does not have employer-subsidized or private health insurance, there are plenty of government-sponsored programs (Medicare, Medicaid, Aid for Dependent Children, Public Health clinics, tax-supported public hospitals, charity clinics) that will provide free or subsidized health care to anyone. Yet, there are many factors that conspire to hinder access to health care, even to those with insurance, public or private. The most insidious of these hindrances is discrimination.

The United States is one of the most culturally diverse countries in the world. The heritage of most Americans is that their ancestors fled poverty or oppression and sought prosperity and freedom for themselves and their heirs. Yet discrimination (real or perceived, attitudinal or institutional, overt or covert) has an adverse impact on the health status of the population. That is, discrimination results in many persons who are living in the United States suffering the effects of preventable or treatable illness and disease.

Real Discrimination

Discrimination is often real. Feelings of territorialism, as well as the need to protect one's own culture and heritage, are natural to the human condition. In certain countries, rival groups that are virtually indistinguishable from each other tattoo or scar themselves so that they can distinguish their friends from their enemies.

Appreciation of diversity and valuing differences is a learned response. In a country as diverse as is the United States, appreciating diversity is necessary for survival, both physically and economically. The manifestation of racial and ethnic discrimination can be recognized in urban youth gang violence, our modern version of "tribal wars." The disruption to the population and to the economy is obvious.

Rehabilitation professionals, as members of a larger society, bring their own prejudices and biases with them to the clinical setting. These prejudices and biases may result in discrimination against clients that is based on their race or ethnicity, religion, sexual preference, age, gender, or socioeconomic status. Discrimination can result in services not being provided or in disparate treatment, whereby the services provided are not the same in quality or quantity regardless of race, ethnicity, sexual preference, age, gender, or socioeconomic status. The result is an adverse impact on the health and well-being of the population.

Perceived Discrimination

Perceived discrimination affects individuals and groups as much as does real racism. Perceived discrimination occurs when the individual fears prejudicial treatment by another person, even though the other person is not in actuality inclined to intolerance. Fearing discrimination against homosexuals, a gay man may delay seeking treatment for a gastrointestinal disorder that resulted from anal intercourse. Not even having seen the physician yet, the gay man assumes that the physician will be disapproving, blaming, or even condemning of his lifestyle. Fearing discrimination by her peers, a lesbian rehabilitation professional may feel compelled to hide from her coworkers the grief of losing her partner of many years.

Attitudinal Racism

Attitudinal racism arises when persons who hold stereotypical beliefs about a group of people exhibit behavior toward those people on the basis of the stereotype. Believing all old people to be hard of hearing, senile, or dim-witted, a rehabilitation professional might treat an elder as a child, calling him "honey" or "Pops." Elderly persons treated disrespectfully may rebel and demonstrate hostility and noncompliance with therapeutic regimens. Conversely, an older person may start to believe that the attitudes being shown are based in reality and so may begin to lose her self-respect and feelings of self-worth. In either case, the attitude of the biased rehabilitation professional has resulted in a poor outcome for the elderly person.

Institutional Discrimination

Institutional discrimination occurs when the practices or policies of the institution create an inequity or an unfair situation for one group. Until passage of the Americans with Disabilities Act in 1990, most of our public and private institutions discriminated legally against persons with disabilities by allowing workplaces, meeting areas, restaurants, restroom facilities, and most forms of public transportation to be inaccessible to persons with impaired mobility. Yet, even in rehabilitation hospitals, the restrooms may be designed so that a person in a wheelchair, although able to enter the stall, needs to bend over to reach the toilet paper, a feat difficult if not impossible for someone with no trunk control. Hallways may be cluttered with equipment or file cabinets, making independent turning of a wheelchair difficult. A hospital policy that prohibits a partner of the same gender from visiting his loved one in the intensive care unit because he is not a blood relative is another example of institutional discrimination.

Overt Discrimination

Overt discrimination is open and unmistakable. In a true story reported widely in the media, a black man questioned a Miami Beach, Florida, restaurant owner about why his bill had a 15% tip already added to the bill, whereas the white people at the next table had no such charge on their bill. The owner replied, "Because black people don't tip well." But for the owner's public apology, the resulting furor almost put the restaurant out of business.

In rehabilitation, some home health providers refuse to go into certain neighborhoods because they hold negative stereotypical beliefs about the minority population that inhabits that neighborhood. In the clinical setting, therapists may be unwilling to treat a homeless client who smells bad or who looks "scary." Non-Hispanic white rehabilitation professionals may use condescending or disrespectful language or nonverbal communications with black, Hispanic, Asian, or Native American clients.

In this day and age, most people do not intentionally exhibit overt bias, the exceptions making juicy material for the media, particularly when it is a celebrity or politician making what is considered to be a politically incorrect blunder. Instead, most rehabilitation professionals exhibit covert bias.

Covert Bias

Biased attitudes are deeply engrained, and most will manifest themselves covertly rather than overtly. Covert bias occurs when the attitudes or beliefs of a person toward another person or group have a negative impact on that other person, although the stated cause of the negative effect has nothing to do with any apparent prejudice or bias. A highly qualified and competent female therapist may be passed over for a promotion. The stated reason may be that she lacks experience, when in reality she has considerable experience. She did, however, recently miss a year of work to stay home with a new baby. It matters not that the therapist kept current by reading and home study, or that her management skills may be superior to those of the person who was granted promotion. The bias against women in the workforce and against career interruptions to raise families has manifested itself covertly and has resulted in the loss of advancement in the career. Until recently, many upwardly mobile women voluntarily abstained from marriage and/or having children.

The "-isms"

Discrimination includes the "-isms" that affect persons of different races and ethnicities (racism), lifestyle preferences (heterosexism), ages (ageism), physical or mental abilities (ableism), and genders (sexism), as well as discrimination against the poor, the homeless, and those who are HIV infected. In the rehabilitation setting, discrimination is a pernicious cancer that erodes the trust that people have in the system and that leaves many persons living in the United States suffering the effects of preventable or treatable illness and disease.

The remainder of this chapter will discuss discrimination that is due to race and ethnic origins, lifestyle preferences, age, and gender, as well as discrimination against the poor, the homeless, and people with HIV infection. Given that there are but few studies related to discrimination and rehabilitation, the following discussions will focus mainly on health care and discrimination. The reader should keep in mind, though, that the dearth of research by rehabilitation professionals contributes to perpetuating the problems of discrimination in health care.

Racism: Discrimination Against People of Different Races or Ethnic Origins

The literature is replete with reports of disproportionately poor health and poor access to health care among members of minority groups, particularly among African Americans. Members of minority groups, insured or uninsured, are more likely than non-Hispanic white persons to suffer from chronic or fatal illness. According to the Institute of Medicine report, *Unequal Treatment: Confronting Racial And Ethnic Disparities in Healthcare* (Smedley, Stith, & Nelson, 2002), "minorities are less likely than whites to receive needed services, including clinically necessary procedures." Studies that the IOM reviewed found disparities "in a number of disease areas, including cancer, cardiovascular disease, HIV/AIDS, diabetes, and mental illness" and found that these disparities existed, even when controlling for (or holding constant) variations in insurance status, patient income, and other access-related factors.

African Americans have a higher rate of stroke than do other population groups in the United States (Okumabua, Martin, Clayton-Davis, & Pearson, 1997). There is a high prevalence of obesity among African Americans, particularly women, and it is associated with hypertension (Kumnayika, 1997) that can and often does lead to stroke. African American persons represent an increasing percentage of new cases of spinal cord injury that is due to violence (Seelman, 1995), and they experience disproportionately high rates of mortality from homicide, accidents, cancer, cirrhosis, and diabetes (U.S. Commission on Civil Rights, 1999). African American women, in particular, are at higher risk for developing fatal diseases such as lupus, cancer, and diabetes (Sullivan, 1996). Coronary heart disease disproportionately disables the African American population, and in fact it is the leading cause of death among African American persons (Fulwood, 1997; Potts, 1997). The rate of prostate cancer for African American men is twice that of white men (U.S. Commission on Civil Rights, 1999).

Since members of minority groups suffer disproportionately from certain conditions, one might assume, then, that these persons must be receiving a disproportionately large share of rehabilitation and health care services and resources. This is not the case, however. Members of minority groups, insured or uninsured, are less likely than non-Hispanic white persons to receive needed health services, including rehabilitation.

African Americans are less likely than non-Hispanic white persons (of similar health and socioeconomic status and insurance coverage) to receive referrals for rehabilitation, from either a physician or a welfare agency, and are more likely to be discharged early from rehabilitation services (Belgrave, 1998). The percentage of African American persons with hypertension whose conditions are detected, treated, and controlled lags behind that of white persons with hypertension (Kong, 1997). African Americans are less likely than non-Hispanic white persons to undergo cardiac procedures, bypass operations, and organ transplants (Braun, Pietsch, & Blanchette, 2000). Among Medicaid recipients, African Americans were 55% less likely than non-Hispanic white persons to receive antidepressants at the time of diagnosis, and 25% less likely to receive the medication of choice as the initial antidepressant (Melfi, Croghan, Hanna, & Robinson, 2000).

Although at least 15% of the adult Hispanic population in the United States is affected by Type 2 diabetes, Hispanics have been treated with the less desirable intervention of insulin more often than persons from other cultures (Brown & Hanis, 1999). Hispanics with poor or no English proficiency have 22% fewer physician visits than do those whose native language is English (Derose & Baker, 2000).

Members of minority groups are less likely than nonminorities to get regular checkups, immunizations, and cancer screenings (Brooks, 1998). Although they have a higher rate of mortality from breast and cervical cancers, minority women receive less screening than nonminority women (Gotay & Wilson, 1998). Even though members of minority groups bear a disproportionate share of the adverse health effects of cigarette smoking, they are less likely to receive cessation advice from health care providers (Okuyemi, Ahluwahlia, & Harris, 2000).

Members of minority groups are more likely than non-Hispanic white persons (of similar health and socioeconomic status) to have negative first-contact primary care experiences. They are more likely to be seen in hospital clinics than in private offices, to have greater difficulty getting an appointment, and to experience long waits for care (Shi, 1999). In nursing homes, members of minority groups are less likely to receive analgesics for non-malignant pain (Won et al., 1999). Schulman et al. (1999) found that black persons were less likely to be referred for cardiac catheterization than white persons with identical symptoms.

Studies examining the effect of race on health professional interaction with students and patients indicate that racial bias affects the opinion of health professionals. In a study on covert bias in the evaluation of physical therapist students' clinical performance, Haskins, Rose-St. Prix, and Elbaum (1997) found that the black student consistently received lower ratings than did the non-Hispanic white, Hispanic, or Asian American students.

Thus, racism remains a stubborn societal problem and continues to create an unacceptable barrier to health care delivery in the United States. Although there is little research relating racism to rehabilitation, it can be assumed that racism does exist in the rehabilitation setting.

Heterosexism and Homophobia: Discrimination Against People of Different Lifestyles

Heterosexism (the assumption that heterosexuality is the norm) and homophobia (fear of homosexuals) are forms of discrimination. As with other forms of discrimination, heterosexism and homophobia can manifest themselves as real or perceived, attitudinal or institutional, overt or covert. In any fashion, heterosexism and homophobia combine to diminish the health and access to rehabilitation and health care of gay, lesbian, bisexual, transsexual, and transgender individuals.

Homophobia increases the likelihood of mental illness in gay people and affects access to health care (Wells, 1997). Societal attitudes against homosexuality are so strong that many homosexuals deny or struggle with their own sexuality and sexual urges to the detriment of their mental well-being. Internalized homophobia (the acceptance of homophobic beliefs by the homosexual person), stigma, and actual experiences of discrimination and violence are associated with high levels of distress and poor mental health (Meyer, 1995). This finding is particularly true among adolescents. Social isolation and heterosexist attitudes disproportionately affect gay youths, and 30% of adolescent suicides are committed by gay youths (Nelson, 1997).

Homophobia is present in the rehabilitation and medical communities. Fifty-nine percent of gay and lesbian physicians and medical students report experiencing job-related discrimination because of their sexuality (Robb, 1996). Medical students fear ostracism by their peers, report encountering bias among older faculty members (Robb, 1996), and openly gay medical students receive lower residency ranks than students assumed to be heterosexual (Oriel, Madlon-Kay, Govaker, and Mersy, 1996).

Homophobia can interfere with seeking access to rehabilitation and health care services. Lesbians have a higher body mass index than heterosexual females and engage in high-risk behaviors such as smoking, heavy use of alcohol, and unsafe sex. Yet they avoid or delay seeking access to breast cancer screening, Pap tests, and other health care because of difficulty in obtaining health care, difficulty in communicating with the primary care provider, and discomfort in discussing depression. Women with female partners do not receive the regular screening that women with male partners receive, and they tend to rely on their female partners for health advice rather than consulting a health care professional. The prevalence of high-risk behaviors (possibly due to mental stress caused by homophobia and heterosexism), the delays in seeking access to screenings, and the tendency to rely on the partner for advice, place lesbians at high risk for breast, lung, cervical, head and neck, and colon cancers, as well as cardiovascular disease and HIV infection (White & Dull, 1997).

Heterosexism and homophobia can affect health and mental services delivery in a variety of ways (Faria, 1997):

- Hospital policies restrict a partner's visiting in intensive care units, as well as a partner's ability to make decisions for an incapacitated lover.
- Health care personnel exhibit homophobic responses to expressions of affection between homosexual lovers.
- Diagnoses of psychotic disorders or personality disorders are overused or inappropriately diagnosed among gay men and lesbians.
- Some conditions go undiagnosed or untreated (e.g., rectal irritation or rupture, sexually transmitted diseases, gastrointestinal infections secondary to anal intercourse or manipulation).
- Domestic violence and battering go unnoticed.
- Complicated grief reactions are inappropriately treated.

Discrimination against gay, lesbian, bisexual, transgender, and transsexual individuals in the rehabilitation and health care arenas diminishes the trust that these persons have in the system, not only increasing the likelihood that they will delay seeking needed rehabilitation and health care but also increasing the chances that they will seek alternative, and possibly ineffective alternative, therapies and treatments before trying more effective, traditional medical approaches, including rehabilitation services.

Ageism: Discrimination Against the Very Young or the Very Old

Ageism is discrimination based on age. As with other forms of discrimination, ageism can be real or perceived, attitudinal or institutional, overt or covert. Children and old people are most often the targets of ageism in rehabilitation and in our health care delivery system.

Slightly over 6% of children and adolescents in the United States have a disability. The causes (ranked) are (1) diseases of the respiratory system (asthma most common); (2) mental retardation; (3) mental disorders; (4) diseases of the nervous system and sense organs; and (5) speech impairments (Bryan, 1999).

The health of a child depends on the socioeconomic status, employment status, educational level, and insurance status of the parents or caregivers. Often, however, the child's health status depends on membership in a racial or an ethnic minority group.

Minority children are at particularly high risk for chronic and fatal illness. Compared with non-Hispanic white children, African American and American Indian children have a disproportionately high infant mortality rate, and African American children are more likely to be hospitalized for asthma (U.S. Commission on Civil Rights, 1999). Compared with African American children, Hispanic children, particularly those whose parents have little education or whose parents are unemployed, are more likely to be in fair or poor health (Weinick, Weigers, & Cohen, 1998).

Elderly persons experience the effects of negative stereotyping in society. Hearing or visual loses are associated in younger people's minds with senility. An old person who gets lost walking because he or she cannot read street signs because of poor eyesight is assumed to be disoriented. An inappropriate response to a question that is due to a hearing loss is assumed to be a sign of mental confusion.

Old people may also experience the effects of ageism in rehabilitation. Attitudinal bias against treating old people can be encountered among rehabilitation professionals. Concerns about self-respect and appearance are ignored when an old person is sent for rehabilitation without his teeth or without her makeup. Elderly persons are often made to wait for long periods of time when unable to get to the toilet unassisted. Resulting bladder or bowel accidents are treated lightly as humorous incidents, whereas to the old person, these incidents are excruciatingly embarrassing and degrading. Studies have shown that health professionals need education to overcome the negative stereotypes held by society in general. From the beginning of their professional education, students hold unfavorable attitudes toward the elderly and prefer treating younger persons (Reuben, Fullerton, Tschann, & Croughan-Minihane, 1995).

Attitudinal bias is also responsible for the beliefs that some rehabilitation and health professionals hold that little can be done to help the ailments of the elderly. Physicians often tell their elderly patients that losses of appetite or arthritic pain are to be expected in someone of their age. Among nursing home residents, those over the age of 85 (along with racial minorities and those with cognitive impairment) have a greater chance of not receiving analgesics to relieve their pain (Won et al., 1999). Treatment options, such as surgical interventions and drug therapy for cardiovascular disease, have been regarded as futile for the elderly (Scharf, Flamer, & Christophidis, 1996). Few elderly persons with functional psychological problems receive mental health care, with age discrimination being a factor (Depla, 1996). Age discrimination is a factor in the low rate of use of radiation therapy for elderly persons with lung cancer (Smith et al., 1995).

Some rehabilitation professionals do not recognize the elderly as having interest in sexual activities or as being sexually active. Thus, institutional discrimination results in the absence of private rooms for sexual activities in nursing homes, and sexually transmitted diseases in the elderly are often misdiagnosed or mistreated. Mosen, Wenger, Shapiro, Andersen, and Cunningham (1998) found that elderly HIV infected persons are less likely than younger HIV infected persons to receive HIV testing and counseling.

Discrimination against the very young and the very old has no place in the rehabilitation setting. Ageism, combined with racism, conspires to deny both the young and the old of the quality of life that both deserve.

Sexism: Discrimination Against Women

Sexism is discrimination based on gender. Infrequently, sexism works against males. In some female-dominated careers, men may be at a disadvantage in getting positions or promotions. More frequently, however, sexism is used to describe discriminatory practices against women.

In the workforce, including the rehabilitation setting, women experience sexism on the job, often being overlooked for promotions or other forms of career advancement in favor of men. There has also been significant media attention given to disparities in the salaries of women and men doing the same job. Women have traditionally not entered certain fields, such as medicine, business, or engineering, in the same numbers as have men. When they have entered these fields, it has been into areas considered suitable for women, such as pediatric or geriatric medicine or personnel management in business. This tendency is changing, since women have been the primary beneficiaries of affirmative action policies during the end of the twentieth century.

Sexism in health care has been a sinister shadow over women's health. It has affected women's access to certain diagnostic and therapeutic procedures, and it has resulted in less research being done on women's health concerns.

Discrimination against women in health care is real. Female internists report verbal or physical sexual harassment by physician peers (Cook, Griffith, Cohen, Guyatt, & O'Brien, 1995). Women have less access than men to HIV medications (Smith & Kirking, 1999). Women have less access than men to catheterization for coronary bypass surgery, kidney dialysis, and kidney transplants (U.S. Commission on Civil Rights, 1999). Only recently has violence against women been recognized as a health concern (Varkevisser, 1995). Women with HIV infection, despite social support or medical treatments, continue to experience higher levels of health care discrimination, social isolation, and depression than their seronegative counterparts (Lester, Partridge, Chesney, & Cooke, 1995). Concerns about social discrimination have a negative effect on women's participation in prophylactic HIV vaccine research (Jenkins, Temoshok, & Virchsiri, 1995).

Women have historically been excluded from clinical research trials, and insufficient research has been done on the unique health problems of women (U.S. Commission on

Civil Rights, 1999). Jensvold, Hamilton, and Mackey (1994) indicate that a factor in the exclusion of women as subjects in clinical research may be that few or no women scientists participate in the design and conduct of experiments. African American women, in particular, have been absent from clinical trials (Allen, 1994).

The absence of research on women has dire consequences. Rowley (1994) postulates that the infant mortality rate of African American children will not drop until prevention research is conducted. The mortality rate among women with breast cancer in the United States is in excess of 27%.

Black and Hispanic women suffer the "double whammy" of racism and sexism. Very little research has focused on inactivity in women, and what little research has been done, has focused on white women of higher income and education (Ransdell & Wells, 1998). Black and Hispanic women are more likely than women from other groups to die in childbirth (U.S. Commission on Civil Rights, 1999). Black rural women are less likely than white rural women to be screened for cervical cancer (Mueller, Ortega, Parker, Patil, & Askenazi, 1999). Perceived discrimination results in increased job stress and has implications for the health of African American women (Mays, Coleman, & Jackson, 1996).

Sexism in education and health care delivery has severe negative impact on women's health. Discrimination based on gender does a disservice not only to women but also to their offspring and society in general.

Discrimination Against the Poor

As one would expect, poverty affects a person's ability to access the health care system for diagnosis and treatment. Persons of low income are less likely to purchase health insurance than persons of higher income (Saver & Doescher, 2000). Uninsured persons are less likely to have access to health care or to a regular provider, or to be satisfied with the care received (Schoen, Lyons, Rowland, Davis, & Puleo, 1997). The uninsured or persons with public rather than private insurance are more likely to have poor health (Shi, 2000).

Children living in poverty, in particular minority children, exhibit poor or fair health. Black and Hispanic children are less likely than non-Hispanic white children to have insurance and are more likely to have public insurance only, with Hispanic children at a higher risk than black children for remaining uninsured (Weinick et al., 1998). Twenty-two percent of Medicaid-eligible children are uninsured (Selden, Banthin, & Cohen, 1998).

Newacheck, Stoddard, Hughes, and Pearl (1998) found that 13% of children in the United States were uninsured. They found that uninsured children are less likely than insured children to have a usual source of care. Even when uninsured children had a usual source of care, they were less likely to have a regular physician, access to medical care after hours, and families that were satisfied with their care. Uninsured children were more likely than insured children to have gone without needed medical, dental, or other health care, and less likely to have had contact with a physician during the previous year. Children from families living in extreme poverty have lower birth weights, higher infant mortality, higher malnutrition rates, and more frequent hospitalizations (Issler et al., 1996). Poverty was the strongest demographic correlate for psychiatric disorder in a study of rural youths (Costello et al., 1996).

Poor economic conditions also affect access to preventive services. Socioeconomically disadvantaged individuals have inadequate access to HIV testing and counseling (Mosen, Wenger, Shapiro, Andersen, & Cunningham, 1998). Although persons with low income are more likely than higher income persons to be obese and to smoke, physicians are unlikely to discuss diet and smoking cessation with persons of low income (Taira, Safran, Seto, Rogers, & Tarlov, 1997).

Adults, too, have adverse health effects that are due to poverty. Poverty is associated with high diabetes death rates (Brown & Hanis, 1999). Compared with the general population, low-income-housed mothers have higher rates of smoking, and high rates of ulcers, anemia, and asthma (Weinreb, Goldberg, & Perloff, 1998). Poverty is an indirect factor in elder loneliness (Mullins, Elston, & Gutkowski, 1996). Lifelong poverty has been implicated in increased disability among indigent black older adults (Stegbauer, Engle, & Graney, 1995).

In summary, poverty leads to poor health. Persons of low income are likely to be underinsured or to not have insurance. Without adequate insurance, they must go to public clinics. Since they perceive the care of public clinics to be less than satisfactory, they may delay going until their health is poor or until it is too late to receive effective care. Without a regular source of care, those who live in poverty are unlikely to receive preventive care or education about health risks. Although this author was unable to find any research examining the relationship of poverty and access to rehabilitation services, it can be assumed that poverty limits access to rehabilitation services.

Discrimination Against the Homeless

The homeless are everywhere. They stand on corners asking for handouts, most often receiving a shake of the head or an impatient wave to go away. They pace our streets, mumbling to themselves or railing against an imaginary foe. They live under bridges or highway overpasses, and they are victims of crime and are at the mercy of nature's elements. Often, they are invisible to those of us who pass them every day, rushing to our jobs or families, not giving them more than a moment's notice. When we do think about the homeless, it is without fully comprehending who they are, how they got to be homeless, and why they stay homeless. We are just grateful that we are not one of them.

Living on the streets is dangerous to the homeless person's physical and psychological well-being. Homeless men experience stress from the fear of violence and of having their belongings stolen (Murray, 1996). They experience inconsistent enforcement of rules by shelter staff, and they are dehumanized and humiliated by others. Women who are homeless are likely to experience physical and sexual abuse (Harris, 1996). Runaway and homeless youths exhibit aggression, conduct disorders, or other behavioral problems (Booth & Zhang, 1996). Homeless youths are at higher risk of contracting AIDS than their domiciled peers (Pinto et al., 1994). Homeless and substance dependent persons are likely to have threatened suicide (Lambert & Bonner, 1996).

The rehabilitation and health problems of poverty are compounded in the homeless. Compared with persons living in poverty but domiciled, homeless persons have higher rates of substance abuse, are less healthy, and have more mental illness (Stein & Gelberg,

1997). Homeless persons also suffer from high blood pressure, poor vision, peripheral vascular diseases of the feet and legs, and significant skin conditions (Kleinman, Freeman, Perlman, & Gelberg, 1996).

The homeless rely on the charity of others, seeking health care in public or religiously affiliated centers. Yet homeless persons are not likely to receive the care they need for their mental or physical illnesses or for their problems of substance abuse. In a cohort of homeless persons studied in Los Angeles, 50% of the homeless persons studied were substance abusers, and close to 25% suffered from mental illness. Yet, only 50% of the substance abusers had ever received any treatment, and only 60% of those with mental illness had ever received any form of mental health service (Koegel, Sullivan, Burnam, Morton, & Wenzel, 1999).

The problem of treating substance abusers may in fact be worse than these figures estimate. Researchers have found that self-reports of substance abuse are severely underestimated, particularly among those with mental illness (Goldfinger et al., 1996).

It is possible that society may view the homeless as having less potential for successful drug rehabilitation. However, studies have shown that homeless persons addicted to crack cocaine, methamphetamines, and other amphetamines are just as likely as nonhomeless persons to comply with and complete substance abuse programs (Wenzel, Ebner, Koegel, & Gelberg, 1996).

The physical problems of the homeless with mental illness may go undiagnosed, misdiagnosed, or untreated. Wainberg (1999) found that the organic problems, including those of HIV infection, of persons with mental illness are often misdiagnosed as psychiatric symptomatology.

Homeless persons are also unlikely to receive preventive services or to have a regular source of care. Compared with low income, domiciled women, homeless women are less likely to be screened for tuberculosis, more likely to engage in HIV risk behaviors, and more likely to have frequent emergency room visits (Weinreb et al., 1998). Even in communities that offer health care services to the homeless, the homeless are more likely to use the emergency room as a primary care provider (Little & Watson, 1996). Although this author found no research on the provision of rehabilitation services to the homeless, it can be assumed that the homeless are an underserved population as regards rehabilitation services.

Discrimination Against People with HIV Infection

Persons with HIV infection are among the most likely to be victims of discrimination. They have a disease most prevalent in homosexual males, intravenous drug users, prostitutes, and members of minority groups, none of which earn a person "most favored status" in American society. While needing massive amounts of medical attention, persons with HIV infection are likely to be underinsured or uninsured, and not to have access to a regular source of care or one that provides satisfactory care.

In a cohort study of HIV-infected persons receiving care at public clinics, the level of reported access to care was well below that for other chronic disease patients. This low level of access to care is in contrast to the substantial need for care of persons with HIV infection (Cunningham et al., 1998).

Since many HIV-infected individuals are homosexual, homophobia contributes to the lower quantity and quality of care. The biggest influence on attitudes toward persons with AIDS is homosexual intolerance (Johnson, 1995). This type of intolerance is characteristic of a political and traditional conservative philosophy that blames the individual for contracting AIDS and credits God with punishing the individual for the homosexual behavior that led to the disease.

Balogun, Kaplan, Hoeberlein-Miller, Anthony, Lefkowitz, and Hsia (1998) surveyed physical therapist, occupational therapist, diagnostic and medical imaging, health information management, and midwifery students. The authors found that overall, the students had poor knowledge about AIDS and that their knowledge was related to attitudes toward persons with AIDS. They also found that students who had prior health care work experience, midwifery and physical therapist students, students with a desire to work with persons with AIDS, and persons who identified themselves as Catholic, were more likely to have positive attitude toward persons with AIDS than were those with no prior health care work experience, those with no desire to work with persons with AIDS, diagnostic and medical imaging students, and persons who identified themselves as Jewish. A positive attitude was related to willingness to treat persons with AIDS. Radecki, Shapiro, Thrupp, Gandhi, Sangha, & Miller (1999) studied the continuum of premedical students through faculty physicians and found that discomfort with and negative attitudes toward homosexuals affect the treatment of HIV infected persons.

Paquin, Lapierre, and Jordan-Jonescu (1994) found that even though an intervention aimed at improving attitudes of nursing personnel toward persons with AIDS improved attitudes with respect to homosexuality, it did not improve attitudes toward persons with AIDS. The authors found that although nursing personnel wanted to help persons with AIDS, they experienced feelings of shame about not being able to show empathy.

Since many HIV-infected persons are gay members of minority groups, racism, homophobia, and an irrational fear of contracting AIDS result in decreased access to health care (Wainberg, 1999). Montoya, Trevino, and Kreitz (1999) found that regardless of race or ethnicity, a major problem area for access for persons with HIV infection was dental care.

There is also low satisfaction with the care received. African American and Hispanic men perceive their HIV-related care as substandard and geared toward nonminority and middle-class clientele (Siegel & Raveis, 1997).

Women with HIV infection are mostly poor and African American or Hispanic. These women experience many forms of discrimination and oppression based on their minority status, poverty level, sexuality, and gender (Bunting, 1996). In addition to discrimination by medical professionals, they suffer from internal and external stigmatization as drug users or sex workers (Lawless, Kipax, & Crawford, 1996). Because of discrimination, women are hesitant to disclose their HIV status (Moneyham et al., 1996).

Societal attitudes toward persons most likely to become infected with the HIV virus result in discrimination against persons with HIV infection. Decreased access to rehabilitation and health care, substandard rehabilitation and health care except for the middle class, and an unwillingness to treat by the rehabilitation and health professionals, are all manifestations of that discrimination.

Summary

In this chapter we discussed the many forms that prejudice can take in practice and that rehabilitation professionals bring their own prejudices and biases with them to the clinical setting. Prejudices and biases are often in reaction to having clients of diversity in race or ethnicity, religion, sexual preference, age, gender, and/or socioeconomic status. These prejudices can result in real or perceived, attitudinal or institutional, and overt or covert discrimination. Furthermore, this discrimination can result in services not being provided or in disparate treatment, whereby the services provided are not the same in quality or quantity regardless of race, ethnicity, sexual preference, age, gender, or socioeconomic status. Appreciation of diversity and valuing differences in a country as diverse as the United States are necessary for providing effective and culturally competent rehabilitation services.

Questions

1. How willing are you to treat someone infected with the HIV virus? What are some of the considerations in making this determination? Can you design a research question that would examine the existence of discrimination against persons with AIDS in the rehabilitation setting?

2. Describe an instance of discrimination that occurred to you, or to someone you have known, or that you have heard about in the media. From the following list, select which form(s) the discrimination has taken: real, perceived, attitudinal, institutional, overt, covert. What has been the effect of that discrimination on yourself, on your friend, and on society in general?

3. Are you familiar with any rehabilitation services available in your community for the homeless? Can you design a research question that examines whether there is discrimination against the homeless in rehabilitation? What can or should be done to eliminate discrimination against the homeless in health care?

4. Examine your profession's Code of Ethics or equivalent standards. Is there a standard about providing pro bono services? Have you ever done so? Do you know of any practitioner in your field (not someone in a public facility) who has done so? Can you design a research question that would test discrimination against the poor in the rehabilitation setting? What can or should be done about eliminating discrimination against poor people in the delivery of rehabilitation services?

5. Reflect on societal disparities between men and women. How do these carry over into the rehabilitation setting? What research questions could test the presence of sexism in the rehabilitation setting? What can or should be done to eliminate the effects of sexism in rehabilitation?

6. How could heterosexism and homophobia affect the provision of rehabilitation services? Can you design a research question that would test the presence of homopho-

bia in the rehabilitation setting? What can or should be done to eliminate heterosexism and homophobia in the delivery of rehabilitation services?

7. What are some of the ways in which the rehabilitation professional treats very young and very old people in the same way?

8. What can or should be done to eliminate the effects of ageism in the rehabilitation setting?

9. Looking at the effects of racism in health care described earlier, what research questions would you ask to see whether these problems also exist in the rehabilitation setting?

10. What can or should be done to eliminate racial and ethnic disparities in the delivery of rehabilitation services?

Case Study

You are the Director of Rehabilitation at Cherry Hill Crest Memorial Hospital and Regional Medical Center, a large public hospital. The hospital is located not far from downtown Cherry Hill, a medium-sized city in a medium-sized state in the United States. The city's population is 65% white non-Hispanic, 18% African American, 9% Hispanic, 5% Asian, 0.7% American Indian, and 2.3% other (multiracial or unknown).

Your professional staff consists of physical therapists, occupational therapists, speech therapists, rehabilitation counselors, one exercise physiologist, a driver education specialist, and a vocational education specialist. You also have physical therapist assistants, occupational therapy assistants, and several aides and transporters on staff.

The professional staff is 95% white non-Hispanic (one of the rehabilitation counselors and the vocational education specialist are African American, and one of the speech therapists is Asian American). Several of the aides and transporters (about 50%) are African American.

A recent analysis of the utilization of rehabilitation services indicated that middle-class, white non-Hispanic clients were the primary beneficiaries of the services, and that Asian clients were being seen in proportion to their representation in the community. It also indicated that what few African American and Hispanic clients were being treated, were being discharged earlier than white non-Hispanic clients. (American Indians were using their own clinic for rehabilitation services.)

The director of the hospital has asked that you increase utilization of rehabilitation services by African American and Hispanic clients.

Questions

1. What are some of the reasons why utilization of rehabilitation services by African American and Hispanic clients may be low?

2. What are some steps you can take to increase utilization services by African American and Hispanic clients?

3. Assuming that you do increase access of African American and Hispanic clients to your rehabilitation services, what steps should be taken with the staff to ensure that clients of different cultures are treated equitably?

4. Besides discrimination, what other barriers to access may exist for members of minority groups?

5. Is having a racially and an ethnically diverse professional staff important to the provision of rehabilitative services? Why, or why not?

6. Assuming that you wish to increase the diversity of your professional staff, describe some steps you will take to identify successful strategies.

References

Allen, M. (1994). The dilemma for women of color in clinical trails. *Journal of the American Medical Women's Association, 49*(4), 105–109.

Balogun, J. A., Kaplan, M. T., Hoeberlein-Miller, T., Anthony, A., Lefkowitz, R., & Hsia, L. (1998). Knowledge, attitudes, and willingness of junior health care professional students to provide services for patients with Acquired Immunodeficiency Syndrome. *Journal of Physical Therapy Education, 12*(1), 57–64.

Belgrave, F. Z. (1998). *Psychosocial Aspects of Chronic Illness and Disability Among African-Americans.* Westport, CT: Auburn House.

Booth, R. E., & Zhang, Y. (1996). Severe aggression and related conduct problems among runaway and homeless adolescents. *Psychiatric Services, 47*, 75–80.

Braun, K. L., Pietsch, J. H., & Blanchette, P. L. (2000). *Cultural Issues in End-of-Life Decision Making.* Thousand Oaks, CA: Sage Publications, Inc.

Brooks, J. (1998, April). Clinton announces racial and ethnic health disparities initiative. In *Closing the Gap: A Newsletter of the Office of Minority Health,* p. 11.

Brown, S. A., & Hanis, C. L. (1999). Culturally competent diabetes education for Mexican Americans: The Starr County study. *The Diabetes Educator, 25*(2), 226–236.

Bryan, W. V. (1999). *Multicultural Aspects of Disabilities.* Springfield, IL: Charles C. Thomas Publishers, Ltd.

Bunting, S. M. (1996). Sources of stigma associate with women with HIV. *Advances in Nursing Science, 19*(2), 64–73.

Cook, D. J., Griffith, L. E., Cohen, M., Guyatt, G. H., & O'Brien, B. (1995). Discrimination and abuse experienced by general internists in Canada. *Journal of General Internal Medicine, 10*, 565–572.

Costello, E. J., Angold, A., Burns, B. J., Stangl, D. K., Tweed, D. L., Erkanli, A., et al. (1996). The Great Smoky Mountains Study of Youth. Goals, design, methods, and the prevalence of DSM-III-R disorders. *Archives of General Psychiatry, 63*, 1129–1136.

Cunningham, W. E., Hays, R. D., Ettl, M. K., Dixon, W. J., Liu, R. C., Beck, C. K., et al. (1998). The prospective effect of access to medical care on health-related quality-of-life outcomes in patients with symptomatic HIV disease. *Medical Care, 36*(3), 295–306.

Depla, M. F. (1996). Filters in mental health care for the elderly: A literature study of the prevalence of psychiatric problems and the utilization of care by the elderly. *Tijdschrift voor Gerontologie en Geriatrie, 27*(5), 206–214.

Derose, K. P., & Baker, D. W. (2000). Limited English proficiency and Latinos' use of physician services. *Medical Care Research and Review, 57*(1), 76–91.

Faria, G. (1997). The challenges of health care social work with gay men and lesbians. *Social Work in Health Care, 25*(1/2), 65–72.

Fulwood, R. (1997). Setting the agenda for research and education on coronary heart disease. *Journal of Health Care for the Poor and Underserved, 8,* 247–249.

Goldfinger, S. M., Schutt, R. K., Seidman, L. J., Turner, W. M., Penk, W. E., & Tolomiczenko, G. S. (1996). Self-report and observer measures of substance abuse among homeless mentally ill persons in the cross-section and over time. *The Journal of Nervous and Mental Disease, 184*(11), 667–672.

Gotay, C. C., & Wilson, M. E. (1998). Social support and cancer screening in African American, Hispanic, and Native American women. *Cancer Practice, 6*(1), 31–37.

Harris, M. (1996). Treating sexual abuse trauma with dually diagnosed women. *Community Mental Health Journal, 32*(4), 371–385.

Haskins, A. R., Rose-St. Prix, C., & Elbaum, L. (1997). Covert bias in evaluation of physical therapist students' clinical performance. *Physical Therapy, 77,* 155–163.

Issler, R. M., Giugliani, E. R., Kreutz, G. T., Meneses, C. F., Justo, E. B., Kreutz, V. M., et al. (1996). Poverty levels and children's health status: Study of risk factors in an urban population of low socioeconomic level. *Revista de Saude Publica, 30,* 506–511.

Jenkins, R. A., Temoshok, L. R., & Virochsiri, K. (1995). Incentives and disincentives to participate in prophylactic HIV vaccine research. *Journal of Acquired Immune Deficiency Syndromes and Human Retrovirology, 9,* 36–42.

Jensvold, M. F., Hamilton, J. A., & Mackey, B. (1994). Including women in clinical trials: How about the women scientists? *Journal of the American Medical Women's Association, 49*(4), 110–112.

Johnson, S. D. (1995). Model of factors related to tendencies to discriminate against people with AIDS. *Psychological Reports, 76,* 563–572.

Kleinman, L. C., Freeman, H., Perlman, J., & Gelberg, L. (1996). Homing in on the homeless: Assessing the physical health of homeless adults in Los Angeles County using an original method to obtain physical examination data in a survey. *Health Services Research, 31,* 533–549.

Koegel, P., Sullivan, G., Burnam, A., Morton, S. C., & Wenzel, S. (1999). Utilization of mental and substance abuse services among homeless adults in Los Angeles. *Medical Care, 37*(3), 306–317.

Kong, B. W. (1997). Community-based hypertension control programs that work. *Journal of Health Care for the Poor and Underserved, 8,* 409–415.

Kumnayika, S. K. (1997). The impact of obesity on hypertension management in African Americans. *Journal of Health Care for the Poor and Underserved, 8,* 352–364.

Lambert, M. T., & Bonner, J. (1996). Characteristics and six-month outcome of patients who use suicide threats to seek hospital admission. *Psychiatric Services, 47*, 871–873.

Lawless, S., Kippax, S., & Crawford, J. (1996). Dirty, diseased and undeserving: The positioning of HIV positive women. *Social Science and Medicine, 43*, 1371–1377.

Lester, P., Partridge, J. C., Chesney, M. A., & Cooke, M. (1995). The consequences of a positive prenatal HIV antibody test for women. *Journal of Acquired Immune Deficiency Syndromes and Human Retrovirology, 10*, 341–349.

Little, G. F., & Watson, D. P. (1996). The homeless in the emergency department: A patient profile. *Journal of Accident and Emergency Medicine, 13*, 415–417.

Mays, V. M., Coleman, L. M., & Jackson, J. S. (1996). *Journal of Occupational Health Psychology, 1*, 319–329.

Melfi, C. A., Croghan, T. W., Hanna, M. P., & Robinson, R. L. (2000). Racial Variation in Antidepressant Treatment in a Medicaid population. *Journal of Clinical Psychiatry, 61*(1), 16–21.

Meyer, I. H. (1995). Minority stress and mental health in gay men. *Journal of Health and Social Behavior, 36*(1), 38–56.

Moneyham, L., Seals, B., Demi, A., Sowell, R., Cohen, L., & Guillory, J. (1996). Experiences of disclosure in women infected with HIV. *Health Care for Women International, 17*, 209–221.

Montoya, I. D., Trevino, R. A., & Kreitz, D. L. (1999). Access to HIV services by the urban poor. *Journal of Community Health, 24*(5), 331–346.

Mosen, D. M., Wenger N. S., Shapiro, M. F., Andersen, R. M., & Cunningham, W. E. (1998). Is access to medical care associated with receipt of HIV testing and counseling? *Aids Care, 10*(5), 617–628.

Mueller, K. J., Ortega, S. T., Parker, K., Patil, K., & Askenazi, A. (1999). Health status and access to care among rural minorities. *Journal of Health Care for the Poor and Underserved, 10*(2), 230–249.

Mullins, L. C., Elston, C. H., & Gutkowski, S. M. (1996). Social determinants of loneliness among older Americans. *Genetic, Social, and General Psychology Monographs, 122*, 453–473.

Murray, R. B. (1996). Stressors and coping strategies of homeless men. *Journal of Psychosocial Nursing and Mental Health Services, 34*(8), 16–22.

Nelson, J. A. (1997). Gay, lesbian, and bisexual adolescents: Providing esteem-enhancing care to a battered population. *The Nurse Practitioner, 22*(2), 94–109.

Newacheck, P. W., Stoddard, J. J., Hughes, D. C., & Pearl, M. (1998). Health insurance and access to primary care for children. *The New England Journal of Medicine, 338*, 513–519.

Okumabua, J. O., Martin, B., Clayton-Davis, J., & Pearson, C. M. (1997). Stroke belt initiative: The Tennessee experience. *Journal of Health Care for the Poor and Underserved, 8*, 292–299.

Okuyemi, K. S., Ahluwalia, J. S., & Harris, K. J. (2000). Pharmacotherapy of smoking cessation. *Archives of Family Medicine, 9*, 270–281.

Oriel, K. A., Madlon-Kay, D. J., Govaker, D., & Mersy, D. J. (1996). Gay and lesbian physicians in training: Family practice program directors' attitudes and students' perceptions of bias. *Family Medicine, 28*, 720–725.

Paquin, L., Lapierre, S., & Jordan-Jonescu, C. (1994). Attitude of nursing personnel towards patients with AIDS: Impact of an awareness program. *Sante Mentale au Quebec*, *19*(2), 191–209.

Pinto, J. A., Ruff, A. J., Paiva, J. V., Antunes, C. M., Adams, I. K., Halsey, N. A., et al. (1994). HIV risk behavior and medical status of underprivileged youths in Belo Horizonte, Brazil. *The Journal of Adolescent Health*, *15*, 179–185.

Potts, J. L. (1997). Diagnosis and therapeutic intervention in the management of coronary artery disease in African Americans. *Journal of Health Care for the Poor and Underserved*, *8*, 285–291.

Radecki, S., Shapiro, J., Thrupp, L. D., Gandhi, S. M., Sangha, S. S., & Miller, R. B. (1999). Willingness to treat HIV-positive patients at different stages of medical education and experience. *AIDS Patient Care and STDs*, *13*(7), 403–414.

Ransdell, L. B., & Wells, C. L. (1998). Physical activity in urban White, African-American, and Mexican-American women. *Medicine & Science in Sports and Exercise*, *30*(11), 1608–1615.

Reuben, D. B., Fullerton, J. T., Tschann, J. M., & Croughan-Minihane, M. (1995). Attitudes of beginning medical students toward older persons: A five-campus study. *Journal of the American Geriatrics Society*, *43*, 1430–1436.

Robb, N. (1996). Fear of ostracism still silences some gay MDs, students. *Journal of the Canadian Medical Association*, *155*, 972–977.

Rowley, D. L. (1994). Research issues in the study of very low birthweight and preterm delivery among African-American women. *Journal of the National Medical Association*, *86*, 761–764.

Saver, B., & Doescher, M. P. (2000). To buy or not to buy: Factors associated with the purchase of non-group, private health insurance. *Medical Care*, *38*(2), 141–151.

Scharf, S., Flamer, H., & Christophidis, N. (1996). Age as a basis for healthcare rationing: Arguments against ageism. *Drugs and Aging*, *9*, 399–402.

Schoen, C., Lyons, B., Rowland, D., Davis, K., & Puleo, E. (1997). Insurance matters for low-income adults: Results from a five-state survey. *Health Affairs*, *16*(5), 163–171.

Schulman, K. A, Berlin, J. A., Harless, W., Kerner, J. F., Sistrunk, S., Gersh, B. J., et al. (1999). The effect of race and sex on physicians' recommendations for cardiac catheterization. *The New England Journal of Medicine*, *340*, 618–626.

Seelman, K. D. (1995). Physical rehabilitation and violence: Initiatives of the National Institute on Disability and Rehabilitation Research. *Journal of Health Care for the Poor and Underserved*, *6*, 217–232.

Selden, T. M., Banthin, J. S., & Cohen, J. W. (1998). Medicaid's problem children: Eligible but not enrolled. *Health Affairs*, *17*(3), 192–200.

Shi, L. (1999). Experience of primary care by racial and ethnic groups in the United States. *Journal of Medical Care*, *37*, 1068–1077.

Shi, L. (2000). Vulnerable populations and health insurance. *Medical Care Research and Review*, *57*, 110–134.

Siegel, K., & Raveis, V. (1997). Perceptions of access to HIV-related information, care, and services among infected minority men. *Qualitative Health Research*, *7*, 9–31.

Smedley, B. D., Stith, A. Y., & Nelson, R. (Eds). (2002). *Unequal Treatment: Confronting Racial and Ethnic Disparities in Health Care.* Washington, DC: National Academies Press.

Smith, S. R., & Kirking, D. M. (1999). Access and use of medications in HIV disease. *Health Services Research, 34,* 123–144.

Smith, T. J., Penberthy, L., Desch, C. E., Whittemore, M., Newschaffer, C., Hillner, B. E., McClish, D., & Retchin, S. M. (1995). Differences in initial treatment patterns and outcomes in the elderly. *Lung Cancer, 13,* 235–252.

Stegbauer, C. C., Engle, V. F., & Graney, M. J. (1995). Admission health status differences of black and white indigent nursing home residents. *Journal of the American Geriatrics Society, 43,* 1103–1106.

Stein, J. A., & Gelberg, L. (1997). Comparability and representativeness of clinical homeless, community homeless, and domiciled clinic samples: Physical and mental health, substance use, and health services utilization. *Health Psychology, 16,* 155–162.

Taira, D. A., Safran, D. G., Seto, T. B., Rogers, W. H., & Tarlov, A. R. (1997). The relationship between patient income and physician discussion of health risk behaviors. *Journal of the American Medical Association, 278,* 1412–1417.

U.S. Commission on Civil Rights. (1999). *The Health Care Challenge: Acknowledging Disparity, Confronting Discrimination, and Ensuring Equality.* Washington, D.C.: U.S. Commission on Civil Rights.

Varkevisser, C. M. (1995). Women's health in a changing world: A continuous challenge. *Tropical and Geographical Medicine, 47,* 186–192.

Wainberg, M. L. (1999). The Hispanic, gay, lesbian, bisexual, and HIV-infected experience in health care. *Mount Sinai Journal of Medicine, 66*(4), 263–266.

Weinick, R. M., Weigers, M. E., & Cohen, J. W. (1998). Children's health insurance, access to care, and health status: New findings. *Health Affairs, 17*(2), 127–136.

Weinreb, L., Goldberg, R., & Perloff, J. (1998). Health characteristics and medical service use patterns of sheltered homeless and low-income housed mothers. *Journal of General Internal Medicine, 13,* 389–397.

Wells, A. (1997). Homophobia and nursing care. *Nursing Standard, 12*(6), 41–42.

Wenzel, S. L., Ebener, P. A., Koegel, P., & Gelberg, L. (1996). Drug-abusing homeless clients in California's substance abuse treatment system. *Journal of Psychoactive Drugs, 28*(2), 147–159.

White, J. C., & Dull, V. T. (1997). Health risk factors and health-seeking behavior in lesbians. *Journal of Women's Health, 6*(1), 103–134.

Won, A., Lapane, K., Gambassi, G., Bernabei, R., Mor, V., & Lipsitz, L. A. (1999). Correlates and management of nonmalignant pain in the nursing home. *Journal of the American Geriatrics Society, 47,* 936–942.

3

Communication in Multicultural Settings

Hye-Kyeung Seung and Sandra Bond

Key Words

communication

verbal communication

nonverbal communication

communication disorders

communication mismatch

Objectives

1. Define communication, and describe components of communication.
2. Emphasize the impact of culture on communication.
3. Identify and describe cultural rules that may influence communication between rehabilitation practitioners and their clients.
4. Describe communication disorders.
5. Describe communication competency.
6. Provide recommendations on communication mismatch while working with clients.

Introduction

Much of what happens in the rehabilitation process depends on communication. Often clients' understanding of their conditions, their interactions with practitioners, their decisions to work with the team—all factors that ultimately influence the success of intervention—hinge on effective communication. When communication breaks down for any reason, we see behaviors that we often label as "noncompliance," "poor carryover," "disinterest," or "lack of motivation."

Given that communication involves the exchange of ideas between two or more people, the reasons for breakdowns in communication are infinite. However, there are some predictable situations that you, as a rehabilitation practitioner, will almost certainly encounter. In this chapter, we will introduce you to some basic notions about communication, discuss some highly likely areas of communication breakdown in the rehabilitation setting, and offer some suggestions for optimizing communication with different populations.

Communication

In the following section, we will review some key issues about communication. What is communication? What does communication consist of? What aspects of communication are important for conveying thoughts and ideas? What cultural variables are involved in communication?

Definition of Communication

Owen (2001) defines communication as "the process participants use to exchange information and ideas, needs and desires. The process is an active one that involves encoding, transmitting, and decoding the intended message" (p. 11).

Components of Communication

Communication is a social act. In order for communication to occur, there has to be an *exchange* of information, ideas, or emotions between two or more people. Communication includes a *sender*, a person who encodes or produces the *message*, and a *receiver*, someone who decodes or comprehends the message.

For communication to occur,

1. A message has to be conceived.
2. The message has to be encoded (planned).
3. The message has to be executed at the *linguistic* and *motor* levels.
4. The message has to be received (sensed).
5. The message has to be perceived (recognized).
6. The message has to be decoded (interpreted).

Note that interpretation can be influenced by *linguistic variable*s and by *cultural variables*. Linguistic variables can include such factors as an individual's ability to understand and/or express language; experience (linguistic input); developmental maturity of the language system; or stages in acquisition of a second language. Cultural variables involve learned beliefs about how messages are to be interpreted. For instance, an American and a British speaker may both use the same language but could misunderstand each other because of cultural rules. The American may expect and use more direct language (e.g., "Please turn the heater up."), whereas the British speaker may be more indirect (e.g., "My, isn't it cold in here?").

Aspects of Communication

Communication is a complex, multifaceted process with multiple events occurring simultaneously. For the current discussion, we will talk about two broad, yet somewhat artificial, categories of communication: *verbal* and *nonverbal*. Verbal communication involves the sounds and the sentence structures we use. Although verbal aspects of communication are clearly important, they constitute only part of the message. Consider the statement "No." Can you imagine that single word meaning more than one thing? Certainly. It could mean, "You can't be serious," "Absolutely not," or "I don't think so," among many other things. Nonverbal communications such as gestures, facial expressions, body movements, personal space, voice pitch, intonation changes, voice volume, speech rate, and pauses contribute as much, if not more, meaning, than do verbal messages. Recently one of the authors spoke over the telephone with a friend who knows her well. The author, discussing an emotionally laden topic, believed that she was expressing herself in a "neutral," "well-controlled" manner. However, her friend began probing her about the issue. Why? Because she understood the real meaning, not only from the words used but also from voice tones, changes in volume, and rate of speech. Or, using the preceding terminology, she derived more meaning from the nonverbal than from the verbal aspects of the message.

Think about what we all do when we don't speak the language of the community. To a greater or lesser extent, we employ nonverbal communications such as gestures, facial expressions, and drawings. The more we are inclined to make use of these nonverbal aspects of communication, the more successful we are as communicators. Of course, as we will discuss later in this chapter—and as many of you may have already discovered—not all gestures mean the same things to all people.

As a rehabilitation practitioner, it is important for you to be able to observe your clients and understand how they express their needs and wants. Your patient does not always have to use verbal language to communicate. Sometimes you will work with patients who cannot use verbal language or cannot use it well. It is easy to misinterpret messages if you fail to take nonverbal communications into as much account as verbal communications. You, as a clinician, cannot afford to ignore anything that could potentially help your clients express their needs more effectively.

Keep the notion of nonverbal aspects of communication in mind as we explore how and why communication works or doesn't work. Which aspects of communication we use, under what conditions we use them, and with whom we use them are all determined by a complex set of *cultural rules* that vary significantly among different social, ethnic, geographic, political, or religious groups.

Cultural Influence on Communication

Some authors contend that "Culture is communication. Communication is culture" (Hall, 1959, cited in Battle, 1998). Not everyone sees the relationship between language and culture as that intimate; however, there is no doubt that culture significantly impacts communication, especially in the way that people interpret messages. Cultural rules dictate the *pragmatic*, or interactive, aspects of language. Although we recognize the importance of language content (word meanings) and form (structure of sounds, words, and sentences), we need to be aware that these aspects of language cannot be realized without pragmatic rules. The pragmatic aspect of language dictates such things as when someone will speak, what he or she will speak about, with whom, under what conditions, which verbal/nonverbal means he or she will use. There are almost certainly an infinite number of variations in cultural rules, but we will restrict our discussion to variations that seem to be most common to speakers living in the United States. To avoid cultural stereotyping, we will list variations we should all consider without assigning any cultural rules to specific ethnic and/or cultural groups. Interested readers can obtain more specific descriptions for individuals of the following ethnicities from the following authors: African American (Terrell, Battle, & Grantham, 1998; Terrell, Terrell, & Taylor, 1988); Hispanic (Anderson, 1995; Goldstein, 1995; Kayser, 1998; Langdon, 1992; Merino, 1992; Quinn, 1995); Pacific Rim (Cheng, 1998); and Native American (Harris, 1998). Both Paul (1995) and Goldstein (2000) offer general information comparing pragmatic rules used by several ethnic/cultural groups in this country.

Although most of us assume that there is only one way to use the language we have, in fact there are many ways. Here is a list of common variations in cultural rules for language use that can impact communications between rehabilitation practitioners and their clients (Taylor & Payne, 1994).

1. *Topic selection.* This refers to which topics are considered suitable for conversation. Factors may include an individual's belief about how appropriate/inappropriate it is to discuss intimate topics with strangers, whether discussion of body parts and/or body functions is permissible, or who initiates the topic.

2. *Determination of who is allowed to initiate conversations.* For some individuals, this will be defined by authority and/or age. Some cultural rules dictate that certain individuals (i.e., children) can respond to, but cannot initiate, conversations with adults.

3. *Designation of who is to be included when information is dispensed.* In American mainstream culture, we tend to value individual autonomy. As a result, we often speak to individuals privately and often expect them to interpret information and make decisions individually. In other cultures, other people—and often the entire family—expect to be informed about an individual. Individuals may not feel comfortable receiving information and/or acting upon information without the presence of the family.

4. *Narration format.* In mainstream U.S. culture, we use a typical narrative format to talk about events. The narration includes an opening, a body, and a conclusion. We relay information sequentially, with fairly specific detail to time. Speakers from other cultures may provide information in different formats. They may not sequence information in the same way as mainstream speakers, and they may not regard time concepts in the same way.

5. *Perception of authority.* Many mainstream American rehabilitation practitioners strive to establish equality-based partnerships with their clients. Many cultural groups respect and value authority positions more than do mainstream Americans. Implications could involve clients' belief about the rehabilitation providers' respect for their authority or vice versa. For example, use of clients' first names may be permissible in some circles, but many individuals may find this use demeaning. Failure to use honorary titles can also be considered demeaning. On the other hand, if a client regards a rehabilitation practitioner as having a position of authority and respect but if the provider does not see himself or herself in that role, the client may become insecure and confused. An extreme example of this might be when a client has advanced in a rehabilitation program to the point that he or she can maintain given skills without the rehabilitation practitioner. The rehabilitation practitioner regards this outcome as great news and recommends dismissal. The client may regard this as abandonment. Let's look at another example. A rehabilitation practitioner wants to give a client information and instructions, first verbally, then in list form on paper. The clinician picks up the nearest available paper, which is in a spiral notebook, and writes the instructions, tears out the page, and gives it to the client on his or her way out. For a client who has great respect and regard for the formality and protocol of authority, the clinician's well-meant action backfired, and the client may not look at the suggestions. This client would expect information on a letterhead, with a seal, preferably typed, and presented in a formal, businesslike manner.

6. *Definition of appropriate voice volume.* Individuals from many parts of the world regard Americans as too loud. Americans view speakers from some parts of the world as too loud. What constitutes "too loud" is obviously variable but always carries negative connotations. Common interpretation of a loud voice includes aggression, anger, impatience, and lack of refinement.

7. *Use of specific gestures.* As mentioned before, not all gestures mean the same thing to everyone, so be careful and observant. Notice especially pointing-type gestures. In many cultures these are considered rude.

8. *Touch.* Different cultural groups regard touching in different ways. Although touch can be an effective therapeutic tool, violation of touch rules is very offensive.

9. *Personal space.* The amount of space between others and ourselves is defined not only by cultural rules but also by context. Personal space is highly variable, and health care practitioners need to understand the operational rules of their clients. If they are too close, some clients may be uncomfortable. On the other hand, if a client wants to come closer and the rehabilitation provider keeps moving away, the client may feel rejected.

10. *Eye contact.* Although mainstream Americans typically place a high value on eye contact, not everyone does so. In some cultures, it is considered rude to establish direct eye contact, especially with someone in authority.

11. *Use of direct, versus indirect questions.* Rehabilitation practitioners tend to ask direct questions and expect direct answers. For some individuals, this conduct would be considered rude and insensitive.

12. *Silence.* Individuals from different cultures regard and tolerate silence in different ways. Mainstream Americans tend to avoid silence and to fill in silent gaps during interactions. Cultural variations to consider involve what length of silence is permitted and who is permitted to break the silence.

13. *Interruptions.* Different cultural groups vary on their perception of interruptions. Whereas some groups view interruptions as impolite, others regard interruptions as signals of interest or a desire to participate in the conversation.

14. *Organization of information.* Although many cultures value "getting to the point" and brevity in speech, many do not. Often it is expected that a series of speech rituals be observed before presenting new information.

Let's look at a concrete example of cultural rules and impact on communication. Since one of the authors of this chapter is a Korean, some Korean cultural communication rules are summarized in Table 3.1. Keep in mind that Korean culture respects seniority more than anything else.

We have talked about communication and some of its important components. We hope that we have impressed on you the importance of many communication variables people often fail to consider. We've talked about cultural rules that govern the pragmatics of language. A whole series of communication breakdowns can occur when speakers don't use

TABLE 3.1   Examples of Korean Communication Rules

Opening/closing of conversations	Usually the elder initiates the conversation, and the younger person follows the lead.
Interruptions	Interruptions are usually perceived negatively. This is especially true when the younger person interrupts. A single interruption is not regarded negatively, but excessive interruption is.
Turn-taking	Relatively balanced turn-taking in conversation is expected in Korean culture, much like turn-taking in American culture.
Silence	Koreans and Americans typically have a different degree of tolerance with regard to silence or pauses in conversation. Americans tend to fill in pauses faster than Koreans do. This is especially true when there are age differences between speakers. In the Korean culture, the younger speaker is expected to wait patiently until the elder speaks.
Humor	Koreans do not tend to use humor as Americans do in both public and personal communications. At professional conferences, Koreans are noted to present their talks seriously. At an interpersonal level, humor is not considered appropriate until the speaker is well acquainted with the listener.
Amount of speech	Being quiet can be viewed as a merit in Korean culture. For instance, when a man visits his future in-laws, talking too much can give a negative first impression. Korean and other Asian cultures believe that "silence is gold." When the author first came to the United States, she saw people enjoying themselves talking at parties. However, she had a hard time getting involved in conversations. It wasn't just the fact that she was not a native speaker. It seemed that Americans value talking as much as Koreans value silence.

the same communication rules as their listeners use. Heath (1986) refers to this problem as a "communication mismatch." Mismatches create as many, if not more, problems in conveying messages and ideas as do other problems. They tend to be more insidious because they are not as easily recognized. We will discuss communication mismatches and other barriers to effective communication in the rehabilitation setting in the following section.

Barriers to Effective Communication

If rehabilitation practitioners are to become better cross-cultural communicators, they need to recognize elements that will impact communication and to understand how to modify and/or change communication content or style when appropriate. A typical professional will probably be faced with at least one of the following situations that can lead to breakdowns somewhere in the communication cycle. They include the following conditions:

- The client has a communication disorder
- The client is not fluent in the language(s) that the rehabilitation provider speaks.
- The client/family and rehabilitation practitioner speak the same language(s) but experience a communication mismatch.

Let's examine each of these situations in more detail.

Communication Disorders

Definitions of a communication disorder vary, but Taylor and Clarke (1994) describe an individual as having a disorder when communication "deviates sufficiently from the norms, expectations and definitions of his or her language group" (p. 109). For a communication disorder to exist, the individual must show difficulty communicating with others who have the same language background and experiences. When a communication disorder exists, the client lacks the linguistic skills needed for optimum communication. Rehabilitation practitioners work with a variety of people who have conditions that create such pathologies. They include, but are not limited to, *neurogenic trauma* (stroke, traumatic brain injury, and tumors, for example); *degenerative conditions* such as Alzheimer's disease; Amyotrophic Lateral Sclerosis; and Multiple Sclerosis; or *developmental disabilities* such as Down Syndrome, Autism Spectrum Disorder, and Pervasive Developmental Disorders. When a client has a communication disorder, rehabilitation providers have three primary responsibilities. They are as follows:

a. Recognize the symptoms.
b. Refer to a specialist in communication disorders when appropriate. Ask for specific recommendations for establishing optimal communications with the client.
c. Modify communication as appropriate to assist the client with language comprehension and/or production (expression). Although each communication interaction is unique, here are some general suggestions.

- Give clients who have communication impairments more *time* to process your information and to formulate their own response. WAIT. WAIT SILENTLY.
- Be prepared to repeat what you say, but don't do so unless you're sure you need to. Sometimes, repetition interrupts peoples' thought processes.
- Speak face-to-face. Visual cues often assist in understanding.
- Simplify what you say. Break down long instructions into simple ones.
- If you are working with an individual who has trouble speaking, ask questions in a "yes/no" format instead of an open-ended one. For example, instead of saying "What's the matter," you could rephrase the question to be "Are you in pain?" or "Are you worried?"
- Don't interrupt or fill in words for your client unless you are asked to. For individuals struggling to speak, correcting other people's erroneous assumptions about what they are trying to say is both frustrating and exhausting.
- Best suggestion: learn to tolerate silence and give your clients the valuable gift of time.

Common communication disorders, symptoms, and suggestions for optimizing interactions with individuals who have communication disorders are listed in Table 3.2.

Limited English Proficiency

Limited English fluency is a common and predictable reason why you and your client may not be communicating as you would like. There are several variations on this theme and may include any of the following:

a. Your client speaks a language other than English.
b. Your client speaks some English but prefers another language.
c. Your client speaks more than one language and prefers different languages in different contexts.
d. Your client has problems communicating in both English and the other language or languages, either because skills have not been well developed in all languages or because there is *language loss*, a common phenomenon during acquisition of a second language.

In a society as culturally and ethnically diverse and as well-educated and well-traveled as ours, many of our members are bilingual or multilingual. We will use the broad term *bilingualism* to encompass the overall idea of speakers' using more than one language. Many of our members are also monolingual, generally in English, but also in other languages.

Bilingualism or multilingualism can be broadly defined as competency in more than one language. The notion of competency implies something about how useful a speaker's skills are in a given language. As a rehabilitation practitioner, you should be aware that among second-language speakers, competency varies significantly according to context (Kayser, 1995; Langdon & Merino, 1992). For instance, a person who speaks both Spanish and English may feel more comfortable using Spanish to discuss family relations but prefer to use English when discussing the technical terminology involving her medical condition.

TABLE 3.2 Common Communication Disorders, Symptoms, and Suggestions for Optimizing Communication

Disorders	Symptoms	Suggestions for Optimizing Communication
Language problems • understanding (comprehension)	• difficulty following instructions • incomplete understanding of others' speech • inattentive or distracted appearance • understanding of only the beginning or ending of a message • fatigue after listening to others' speech	• Simplify messages. • Be alert for signs of fatigue. • Look for nonverbal signals that indicate problems in comprehending. • Ask confirmation questions. • Repeat and summarize messages frequently. • Use graphs, diagrams, and charts to supplement information whenever possible.
• expression (production)	• use of short, sometimes telegraphic sentences • speech sometimes limited to content words • frequent use of nonspecific words (e.g., "thing," "stuff") • word substitutions	• Give client more time to formulate speech. • Help client by formulating closed-end questions. • Provide realistic feedback of speech that is not understandable.
• social language (pragmatics)	• speech sounding fluent but lacking in meaning	• Try not to interrupt and supply words for the speaker. Supply diagrams, charts, and pictures to help client express needs or answers to question.
Hearing problems • sensori-neural	• increased volume in speech, on television, and over the phone • partial understandings of messages • loud voice volume	• Face your listener when speaking. • Minimize the amount/volume of background noise. • Simplify your message. • Supplement your speaker information with written information when possible.
• conductive	• see above • soft, muffled voice • fluctuation in hearing level	

(continued)

TABLE 3.2 (*continued*)

Disorders	Symptoms	Suggestions for Optimizing Communication
Problems with speech clarity	• speech being difficult to understand • sounds that may be omitted or substituted • speech that may be slurred or muffled • speech that may be harder to understand after prolonged speaking	• Ask yes/no questions or questions that require short answers. • Note effects of fatigue, and allow clients time to rest when fatigue become obvious. • Don't correct speech errors. • Instead, offer appropriate models in a positive context. • Provide honest feedback about your ability to understand. • If unsure about the message, make a best guess, and ask for clarification.
Fluency disruption	• frequent disruption in the normal flow of speech due to repetition, prolongation, and blockage of sounds • speaker possibly being bothered by disruptions • frequent reformulation of speech (false starts) • speech may sound "cluttered" or "jumbled"	• Give client TIME to formulate his or her own speech. *DON'T INTERRUPT.* • Do not offer word choices until client indicates this would be appropriate. • Ask dysfluent clients what they would like listeners to do when they experience speech disruptions.
Voice disorders • organic	• client possibly not being able to produce voice • voice perhaps being strident, hoarse, breathy, or a combination of these parameters • voice perhaps being too loud or too soft • client possibly feeling fatigued easily when he or she speaks • client perhaps complaining of discomfort in the throat • voice perhaps sounding nasal or denasal	• Provide easily accessible forms of communication for clients who have no voice (e.g., note pad and pen). • Monitor for signs of fatigue, and allow client to rest before he or she needs to resume speech. • Modulate the distance between yourself and the client to compensate for variations in loudness.

Disorders	Symptoms	Suggestions for Optimizing Communication
• functional	• see above. • client perhaps talking excessively • client perhaps experiencing an unusually high degree of musculoskeletal tension • client perhaps engaging in behaviors that abuse the vocal apparatus (e.g., yelling, screaming, extended speaking under stress)	• See above

Communicative competency is broadly defined as the ability to convey ideas and messages to others (Hymes, 1974). The term is a bit subjective, but in our experience, there has been a good correlation between speakers' perception of their competencies and listeners' view of competencies. So, if someone tells you that he doesn't understand English, believe him. If someone tells you that she understands "a little bit" of English, respect that. People are pretty accurate judges of their competencies.

When we talk about competency, we are referring to the ability to send and receive messages (*content*). Many people confuse the content, or the essence, of the message, with the *form*. Be careful! The fact that a given speaker has good form (for example, pronunciation or sentence structure) doesn't guarantee competency in terms of understanding or producing complex messages. Likewise, some speakers (particularly those who learned the second language as an adult) may not have mastered pronunciation or sentence structure (*form*) but are highly competent in understanding and expressing complex messages. Therefore, try not to assume anything about how much a speaker understands on the basis of the way he/she sounds. Remember *form versus content*. Don't confuse the two. Content is most linked to competence. What researchers have learned about the process of acquiring competence in more than one language has tremendous application to you, as a rehabilitation practitioner, as you work with bilingual or multilingual speakers. Think about the following facts and the way that they might apply to the people you work with.

- Knowledge of more than one language is a common attribute worldwide. Humans are equipped for this ability.
- Many factors can influence acquisition of a second language. They include circumstances of immigration to the new country, ethnicity, attitude of the new community toward speakers of other languages, gender, religious preference, degree of similarity between the speaker's culture and the new mainstream culture, degree of similarity between first and second languages, the speaker's educational level, interaction between groups in the new language culture, the speaker's desire to preserve the first language, the speaker's attitude toward the new language, and degree of fear using the second language (Battle, 1998; Goldstein, 2000).

- For many speakers, language competency changes according to context (Kayser, 1995). Mr. Romero may have spoken with you in Spanish when you discussed his family, but don't assume that's going to be his choice of languages when you discuss his surgery and recommendations.

- *Language loss* is a common phenomenon, particularly for children who may have spoken one language at home and began acquiring another language in a different context, such as school. As the child acquires the second language, under certain conditions he or she may come to a standstill or even lose skills in the first language. It's important to recognize this phenomenon so that mislabeling doesn't occur and so that rehabilitation practitioners exercise good communication practices with clients who experience language loss. Remember, if your client is in a phase of language loss, he or she may not be completely competent in *either* the first or the second language. In this case, you cannot assume that reverting back to the first language is a solution.

- Many children who are learning two languages may appear delayed (Battle, 1997; Owen, 2001). While any child who has not mastered general developmental speech-language milestones should be monitored, you should remember that the *normal* acquisition process of more than one language is different in quantity and quality from what we, as the mainstream culture, expect to see in terms of language acquisition (Arnberg, 1987; Gutierrez-Clellen, 1996; Patterson, 1998).

What does this mean to you? Actually, it means quite a bit. You don't need to know everything about theories of bilingualism, but you do need to understand the notion of communicative competence. Your clients can often tell you about their own competencies. Competence can shift, on the basis of context. When clients are competent in one language but not in the other, it is appropriate to use a translator. When, for any reason, competence is low in both languages, a translator is of limited use. Although you may still use a translator, you will need to use the communication modification techniques described in the previous section.

Communication Mismatch

Earlier in this chapter we talked about communication mismatches between speakers and listeners. If you recall, we said that this is an especially dangerous area of communication breakdown because people often don't know that communication failed until it is too late. Here, we will explore some common communication mismatches between rehabilitation providers and clients/families. We will assume in these cases that the rehabilitation practitioner and client/family speak the same language(s) and that the client/family does not have a communication disorder.

Reasons for communication mismatches vary. For example, the rehabilitation provider and/or the client could be poor communicators, engaging in behaviors that somehow negatively impact the communication flow. These could include anything from "presumption" errors (when speakers communicate with the assumption that listeners have the background information that they need to follow a topic, when in fact, they do not), to unclear speech, and to poor organization of thoughts and ideas. Sometimes speakers unconsciously use nonverbal forms of communication that change the intended messages. For example, a health care provider could be sincere in asking "What do you need?" in a volume that to her seemed normal but that appeared loud to a client from Southeast Asia. The client may interpret the question as an angry one, as in "What is it this time?" and be afraid to ask for anything. This is just one example of how quickly *intent* can be misinterpreted. Consider for a moment the very serious implications in this simple example. Because optimal communications are so critical to effective health care outcomes, it behooves health care professions to attempt to eliminate "mismatches" whenever possible. Some strategies include the following:

1. Work on simplifying your message. Do this task even if you're presenting old information. You cannot assume that all information has been processed or that your client sees a given situation the same way you do.
2. Work on your delivery. Clients often complain that rehabilitation practitioners go too fast and say too much. Streamline your message. Practice with your family, peers or, community groups like Toastmasters, who help people speak more effectively.
3. Be open to cultural diversity. Although it is important to get a sense of communication styles within a given cultural group, it is even more important to distinguish between *cultural competence* and *cultural stereotyping*. Cultural competence recognizes that each individual is impacted by his or her own life experiences, family experiences, background, country of birth, language, religion, and many other factors. Stereotyping attempts to categorize individuals. Cultural competence is achieved only when we recognize that we cannot afford to make assumptions or generalizations about anyone and that once we begin categorizing individuals, we create the very communication barriers we attempted to avoid.
4. You can develop cultural competence by reading, observing, asking clients/families and community members for suggestions (Davis, Gentry, & Hubbard-Willey, 1998). You will learn more if you ask open-ended questions, like "What can you tell me about how to speak to someone older in your culture?"; "Can you comment on how families might view this problem in this area of the country?"; or "Is there anything I need to know about your father before I try to work with him on leg extension?"

Summary

In this chapter, we have tried to highlight the importance of communication in terms of treatment efficacy for rehabilitation providers. Good communication is not just something that makes treatment and interaction more pleasant for health care professionals and their clients. It is the crux of successful treatment. No matter how much you, as a rehabilitation practitioner know, your knowledge is of no use to an individual or his or her family unless you can communicate that knowledge to them.

We have discussed three contexts in which it is very probable that rehabilitation providers will have difficulty communicating with clients/families. They involved communication disorders, problems with language competence, and problems with cultural competence.

The following four case studies are for the purpose of reflection and/or discussion. There are no absolute "answers," but in Case Study One, we offer some thoughts and/or questions for each case.

Case Study 1

Charlie is a 17-year-old male who sustained a traumatic brain injury four months ago. He speaks only English. He is a junior in high school and a "B/C" student. Before his accident, Charlie was popular in school and had many friends. He played on the soccer team and in the band.

Charlie has not yet returned to school but is receiving rehabilitation services twice weekly on an outpatient basis. His parents are worried because he doesn't seem motivated, seems "down," and isn't nearly as outgoing as he was. Rehabilitation practitioners at the rehabilitation center complain that Charlie is not cooperative, doesn't follow instructions well, and doesn't seem motivated. Charlie answers their questions but doesn't offer much information.

Questions

1. Are any of Charlie's symptoms indicative of a communication disorder? Can you list some?
2. What could you recommend to other rehabilitation practitioners and Charlie's family and friends?

Case Study 2

Mr. and Mrs. Sanchez are from El Salvador. They have lived in the United States for four months. He is an engineer, and she is a homemaker. Mr. Sanchez speaks some English but is more comfortable reading and writing than speaking. He speaks Spanish when possible at work and with his friends, and always at home with his wife and family who do not speak English.

Mr. and Mrs. Sanchez are expecting their third child. They go to a community clinic for a prenatal exam. When asked whether they speak English, Mr. Sanchez says that he speaks " a little bit" but that his wife speaks none. The nurse says she speaks "some" Spanish and that among the three of them, they should be fine.

After routine screens, including an ultrasound and a serum alpha fetoprotein (AFP) screen, Mr. and Mrs. Sanchez return and speak with the same nurse. Test findings indicate the possibility of a serious genetic anomaly that will probably result in severe physical/cognitive impairments. The nurse starts by explaining the findings and then asks the couple whether they have any questions. They say little, ask no questions, and then leave. Here are the conversations that each party had after the Sanchezes left the clinic.

Nurse (N) and her supervisor (S)

S: Did you talk with Mr. and Mrs. Sanchez?

N: Yes.

S: How did they take the news?

N: OK, I guess. They didn't have any questions. Maybe they suspected all along.

S: So, what are they going to do?

N: Nothing, I guess. They didn't ask about options to terminate the pregnancy. But, I'm sure they're Catholic and that would be something they wouldn't consider.

Mr. and Mrs. Sanchez

Mrs. S: So, how serious do you think this is?

Mr. S: I don't know. She sounded a little vague. I'm not sure if it was because her Spanish was not that good or if she wasn't worried about the test results.

Mrs. S: She seemed mad at us. She didn't even ask how we were before she told us the baby would have problems. I wonder how bad they are.

Mr. S: I don't know, but we have to find out from someone. What if it's really serious? Remember my mother's cousin? Their child was born with almost no brain. I would never want us to go through that.

Questions

1. What happened with communications between the nurse and Mr. and Mrs. Sanchez?

2. Did you see any evidence of communication mismatches? If so, describe the problems.

3. What could the rehabilitation practitioner have done to improve communications?

Case Study 3

Mr. "Mike" Cheng is an 86-year-old Chinese man who just sustained a mild stroke. His speech and language skills do not appear to be affected, but he has weakness in his right arm and leg. Mr. Cheng learned Mandarin as a child, but he immigrated to the United States when he was 18 and has spoken English in the community since then.

"Jim" is a 26-year-old physical therapist who is generally the favorite of the clients in the rehabilitation unit where he works. He is friendly, outgoing, enthusiastic, and approachable.

The following conversation takes place one morning as Mr. Cheng goes to his physical therapy session. His wife accompanies him.

Jim: Hi, Mike, how's it going?

Mr. C: I am fine, thank you. How are you?

Jim: Cool. You ready to roll?

Mr. C: What do you have planned to do?

Jim: Just a minute and I'll show you. We're gonna work on joint range of movement.

Mr. C: I don't understand.

Jim: (turns to wife while working with Mr. Cheng's arm) Well, you see after the stroke your husband can move, but not to the extent he used to. So we need to gradually expand how far he can move.

Later, Mr. Cheng has the following conversation with his doctor:

Mr. C: I don't want to go back to physical therapy.

Doctor: Don't worry, PT is painful for everyone. It will get better.

Mr. C: (doesn't say anything).

Doctor: Is there anything else you're concerned about?

Mr. C: I can't work with someone who doesn't respect me.

Questions

1. Why do you think that Mr. Cheng feels he is not respected?

2. What might you recommend to Jim?

Case Study 4

Omar is a 9-year-old boy who has been coming in to see the school nurse every morning for the past week and a half, complaining of intense stomach pain. After "resting" for about an hour, he "feels better" and goes back to class.

Ms. Smith, the school nurse, is concerned. Omar appears to be in real pain, but he's established a predictable pattern. This behavior makes her think that there might be something he's worried about, which could be manifesting as stomach pain. Ms. Smith tries to talk with Omar. Here is their conversation:

Ms. S: I'm worried about your stomachaches. Can we talk about some things?

Omar: OK.

Ms. S: Well, how is everything?

Omar: OK.

Ms. S: How is school going for you?

Omar: Fine.

Ms. S: Any problems?

Omar: (shrugs).

Ms. S: You know, we can talk about this here, and nobody else has to know what we said.

Omar: (silence).

Ms. S: Is there anything you don't like about school?

Omar: No, I like school.

Later, Ms. Smith calls Omar's mother over the phone. Here's their conversation:

Ms. S: Mrs. R, I'm concerned about Omar. As you know, he's been coming in to my office every day with a complaint of stomach pain.

Ms. R: Well, what should we do?

Ms. S: To tell you the truth, I was hoping you could shed some light on the problem because Omar won't talk to me.

Ms. R: But he's been taught to be respectful and answer people.

Ms. S: Well, he's barely answering me, and I can't figure out what the problem is. I was hoping you'd have some ideas. . . .

Ms. R: I'm not sure. . . .

Ms. S: Anything you could contribute would be helpful.

Ms. R: I don't know. Let me think about it.

Ms. S: OK, if you think of something call me between 9:00 AM and 4:00 PM. My number is 555-5555.

Questions

1. Why do you think that Omar gave only short answers?
2. Why do you think that Omar's mother did not say much about Omar over the telephone?
3. What would you recommend to the nurse?

Commentary

Case Study 1

Are any of Charlie's symptoms indicative of a communication disorder? Can you list some?

What would you recommend to rehabilitation practitioners and to Charlie's family and friends?

Let's review Charlie's symptoms.

- "Lack of motivation"—this apparent behavior could easily stem from symptoms of a pragmatic language deficit. See Table 3.2.
- "Lack of cooperation"—problems "cooperating" or carrying out instructions could be related to problems in language comprehension. See Table 3.2.
- "Incomplete response to questions"—Charlie's use of simple, concrete responses could be related to an expressive language disorder. See Table 3.2.

Case Study 2

What happened with communications between the nurse and Mr. and Mrs. Sanchez? Did you see any evidence of communication mismatches? If so, describe it.

What could the rehabilitation practitioner have done to improve communications?

Let's review the communications between the staff at the clinic and Mr. and Mrs. Sanchez. Here are some issues to consider:

- Could both parties be making assumptions about how well they can really communicate with Mr. Sanchez's limited English and the nurse's limited Spanish?
- Why did Mr. and Mrs. Sanchez not ask questions when the nurse reported screening results? Could it be that they
  1. didn't understand the findings,
  2. needed more elaboration, or
  3. didn't understand that the nurse was waiting for them to ask questions so that she would know how much and what kind of specific information to give them?
- What examples of stereotyping occurred during the conversation between the rehabilitation practitioner and the supervisor?
  1. The assumption that all Hispanics are Catholic.
  2. The assumption that no Catholic would consider termination of a pregnancy under any circumstance.
- Why did Mrs. Sanchez think that the rehabilitation practitioner was mad at them?
  1. There could have been a communication mismatch. The practitioner wanted to "get down to business," whereas Mr. and Mrs. Sanchez were probably expecting her to ask about their family and her health before talking about test results.
- To improve communications, the rehabilitation practitioner could consider the following principles:
  1. Avoid stereotyping.
  2. Develop communicative competence by asking community members and/or professionals in schools, universities, or embassies about typical expectations during interactions.

3. Adhere more closely to good practices of counseling, which include repeated probing for clients' questions.

Case Study 3

Why do you think that Mr. Cheng feels he is not respected?

Let's review the dialogue.

- Consider the degree of informality Jim used. Would this be appropriate for everybody?
- Consider Mr. Cheng's very formal response. That should have been a clue to Jim that Mr. Cheng expected a formal response.
- The fact that Jim gave an explanation to Mr. Cheng's wife after Mr. Cheng asked for clarification is bad practice, regardless of cultural background. Talking around a client implies that he or she is not an active participant in the rehabilitation process. Additionally, talking to Mr. Cheng's wife instead of him could have been interpreted as a sign of disrespect in regard to family status.

What might you recommend to Jim?

- Unless invited to use an informal tone or a client's first name, always use formal address with clients. Incidentally, for Spanish-speaking clients, this would include the use of the formal "Usted" form rather than the informal "tu."
- Always speak directly to clients, regardless of your belief about their ability or inability to understand.

Case Study 4

Why do you think that Omar gave only short answers?

- We need to rule out the possibility of a receptive or an expressive language disorder. See Table 3.2.
- There may have been a communication mismatch. Omar may have been taught that children do not speak with adults unless they are specifically asked to, and that when they speak they are to be as brief as possible. The nurse may have been expecting Omar to "open up" with her so that, from a great deal of information, she could identify a possible problem.

- Omar may be afraid of school, especially if his language skills do not allow him to succeed. He may view the nurse as part of the system, rather than as an ally.

Why do you think that Omar's mother did not say much over the telephone?

- Her ability to communicate in English may be limited, especially over the telephone.
- There could be a communication mismatch between the nurse's intent and Mrs. R's interpretation about the purpose of the telephone call. The nurse may have assumed that she and Mrs. R could problem-solve and arrive at some possible solutions in a short telephone conversation. Mrs. R may have believed that the entire family needed to be involved in any discussion.
- There may have been a mismatch in expectations. Mrs. R may have simply wanted the rehabilitation practitioner to tell the family what to do. The practitioner may have automatically assumed that the family expects to be part of the decision-making process.

What would you recommend to the nurse?

- Consider asking the classroom teacher and possibly the speech-language pathologist about Omar's language and communication competencies. This step would be important for two reasons. If Omar is producing very short responses, he may not understand all of the explicit and implicit meanings in the nurse's questions. Or perhaps he does not have the language to formulate more complex responses. Also, low language skills directly impact the ability to learn in class. Problems learning can cause a tremendous amount of stress and anxiety for a child, and such problems frequently manifest with the symptoms Omar has.
- Find out what Omar's family expect from school personnel. Learn what the family expect their involvement to be.
- Provide the parents with information about family rights in the education process.
- Ask about the family's preference for discussing Omar. Find out who will be involved in the discussion, where the meeting should take place, and what kind of information the family would like school personnel to provide.

Questions

1. What is a definition of communication?
2. What are the basic components of communication?
3. What are two examples of the common variations in cultural rules for language?
4. What are five likely barriers to effective communication?
5. Describe three communication disorders.
6. Describe communication competency.
7. What are two recommendations that will reduce communication mismatch while in practice?

References

Anderson, R. T. (1995). Spanish morphological and syntactic development. In H. Kayser (Ed.), *Bilingual speech-language pathology* (pp. 41–74). San Diego, CA: Singular Publishing.

Arnberg, L. (1987). *Raising children bilingually: The preschool years.* Philadelphia, PA: Multilingual Matters.

Battle, D. (1997). Language and communication disorders in culturally and linguistically diverse children. In D. K. Bernstein & E. Tiegerman-Farber (Eds.), *Language and Communication Disorders in Children* (pp. 301–409). Boston, MA: Allyn and Bacon.

Battle, D. (1998). Communication disorders in a multicultural society. In D. E. Battle, *Communication disorders in multicultural populations* (pp. 3–29). Boston, MA: Butterworth-Heinemann.

Cheng, L-R. L. (1998). Asian and Pacific-American Cultures. In D. Battle (Ed.), *Communication disorders in multicultural populations*, 2nd edition (pp. 73–116). Boston, MA: Butterworth-Heinemann.

Davis, P. N., Gentry, B., & Hubbard-Willey, P. (1998). Clinical practice issues. In D. Battle (Ed.), *Communication disorders in multicultural populations*, 2nd edition (pp. 427–452). Boston, MA: Butterworth-Heinemann.

Goldstein, B. (1995). Acquisition of syntactic and phonologic features in Spanish. In H. Kayser (Ed.), *Bilingual speech-language pathology* (pp. 17–40). San Diego, CA: Singular Publishing.

Goldstein, B. (2000). *Cultural and linguistic diversity resource guide for speech-language pathologists.* San Diego, CA: Singular Publishing.

Gutierrez-Clellen, V. (1996). Language diversity: Implications for assessment. In K. N. Cole, P. S. Dale, & D. J. Thal (Eds.), *Assessment of communication and language* (pp. 29–56). Baltimore, MD: Paul Brookes.

Hall, E. T. (1959). *The Silent Language.* New York: Doubleday

Harris, G. A. (1998). American Indian cultures: A lesson in diversity. In D. Battle (Ed.), *Communication disorders in multicultural populations*, 2nd edition (pp. 117–156). Boston, MA: Butterworth-Heinemann.

Heath, S. B. (1986). Taking a cross-cultural look at narratives. *Topics in Language Disorders, 7* (1), 84–94.

Hymes, D. (1974). *Foundations in sociolinguistics.* Philadelphia, PA: University of Pennsylvania Press.

Kayser, H. (1995). Bilingualism, myths, and language impairments. In H. Kayser (Ed.), *Bilingual speech-language pathology* (pp. 185–206). San Diego, CA: Singular Publishing.

Kayser, H. (1998). Hispanic culture and language. In D. Battle (Ed.), *Communication disorders in multicultural populations*, 2nd edition (pp. 157–196). Boston, MA: Butterworth-Heinemann.

Langdon, H. W. (1992). Language, communication, and sociocultural patterns in Hispanic families. In H. W. Langdon & L. Cheng (Eds.), *Hispanic children and adults with communication disorders* (pp. 99–131). Gaithersburg, MD: Aspen Publication.

Langdon, H. W., & Merino, B. (1992). Acquisition and development of a second language in Spanish speakers. In H. W. Langdon & L. Cheng (Eds.), *Hispanic children and adults with communication disorders* (pp. 132–167). Gaithersburg, MD: Aspen Publication.

Merino, B. (1992). Acquisition of syntactic and phonological features in Spanish. In H. W. Langdon & L. Cheng (Eds.), *Hispanic children and adults with communication disorders* (pp. 57–98). Gaithersburg, MD: Aspen Publication.

Owen, R. E. (2001). Language differences: Bidialectism and bilingualism. In R. E. Owen, *Language development: An introduction*, 5th edition, (pp. 408–437). Boston, MA: Allyn and Bacon.

Patterson, J. L. (1998). Expressive vocabulary development and word combinations of Spanish-English bilingual toddlers. *American Journal of Speech Language Pathology, 7* (4), 46–56.

Paul, R. (1995). Child language disorders in a pluralistic society. In R. Paul (1995), *Language disorders from infancy through adolescence: Assessment and intervention* (pp. 151–185). St. Louis, MO: Mosby.

Quinn, R. (1995). "Early intervention? Qué quiere decir éso?"/. . . What does that mean? In H. W. Kayser, *Bilingual speech-language pathology: An Hispanic focus* (pp. 75–94). San Diego, CA: Singular Publishing.

Taylor, O., & Clarke, M. (1994). Culture and communication disorders: A theoretical framework. *Seminars in Speech and Language, 15* (2), 103–113.

Taylor, O., & Payne, K. T. (1994). Language and communication differences. In G. H. Shames, E. H. Wiig, & W. A. Secord (Eds.), *Human communication disorders: An introduction* (pp. 136–173). New York: Macmillan College Publishing Company.

Terrell, F., Terrell, S. L., & Taylor, J. (1988). The self concept of black adolescents with and without African names. *Psychology in the Schools, 25*, 65–70.

Terrell, S. L., Battle, D. E., & Grantham, R. B. (1998). African American Culture. In D. Battle (Ed.), *Communication disorders in multicultural populations*, 2nd edition (pp. 31–72). Boston, MA: Butterworth-Heinenmann.

4

Ethics of Culture in Rehabilitation

Jeffrey L. Crabtree

Key Words

rehabilitation

autonomy

diversity

individualism

collectivism

ethical principles

Objectives

1. Appreciate and understand the ethical assumptions that underpin rehabilitation practice.
2. Identify and understand the basic ethical principles and issues that rehabilitation practitioners face when providing services to ethnically and culturally diverse clients.
3. Identify ways of making ethical decisions that take into account variations among ethnic and cultural groups.

Introduction

In this chapter, I make the following four assumptions: First, although the proportion of culturally diverse rehabilitation practitioners to those from the dominant Western culture is increasing, most rehabilitation practitioners represent the dominant, Western, European-American culture. Second, those who receive rehabilitation services increasingly come from diverse cultures and ethnic backgrounds. Third, common ethical dilemmas found within the interactions of one culture are confounded when rehabilitation practitioners and clients hold different beliefs, values, and attitudes. And fourth, the underlying assumption of rehabilitation practitioners includes the notion that ethical decisions are made by individuals who hold independence and autonomy to be their preeminent values, whether those individuals are clients, family members, or other surrogate decision makers.

Certainly not all rehabilitation practitioners hold typical, dominant Western cultural beliefs that potentially collide with the beliefs, values, and attitudes of their clients. In addition, not all rehabilitation practitioners have opportunities to provide services to clients of different cultures. However, for the purpose of this chapter and in order to highlight the need for cultural competence in rehabilitation, I will explore the ethics of rehabilitation from the perspective of a plurality of beliefs and values. This exploration includes a discussion of the concepts of individualism and collectivism; a discussion of the basic principles of biomedical ethics from the dominant Western cultural perspective, including the principles of beneficence, veracity, justice, and client and professional autonomy; and the implications of following these principles in ever increasingly cultural diverse rehabilitation settings. Finally, the chapter will explore ethical decision making.

Why examine the ethics of cultural and ethnic diversity? One reason is that since cultural beliefs influence how people view their roles and responsibilities and influence their decisions about health care, cultural differences between rehabilitation providers and their clients can lead to miscommunication and an array of conflicts over issues of informed consent, individual autonomy, the role of the family, end of life issues, and the like (Annas & Miller, 1994; Berger, 1998; Blackhall et al., 1995; Carrese & Rhodes, 1995; Culhane-Pera & Vawter, 1998; Fetters, 1998; Gostin, 1995; Helman, 2000; Meleis & Jonsen, 1983; Pellegrino, 1992, to name a few). Another reason is that rehabilitation does not occur in a vacuum. As expressed earlier, rehabilitation practitioners have their own beliefs, values, and principles; they practice in settings that also have institutionalized standards and values, all of which provide an ethical context in which rehabilitation is practiced. The notion of an ethical context operates in any setting in any nation. However, each setting is unique according to the institutional values and those of the practitioners working in that setting.

A review of ethical and value statements of professional organizations that constitute a significant portion of institutionalized rehabilitation in the United States suggests that ethical behavior upholds the rights of individuals over the rights of families or other groups. Although no two rehabilitation organizations use the same ethical theories or have the same standards, they likely share a written or an unwritten commitment to ethical behavior with the individual patient or client first and then with the family and others as appropriate. This procedure is exemplified by the Federal Patient Self-Determination Act of 1990 (PSDA) (1994) and the American Hospital Association's patient's (AHA) bill of rights

(2001). The AHA patient's bill of rights emphasizes the *individual* patient's rights to privacy, to confidentiality, and to making informed medical choices among other rights (2001, Bill of Rights section). The PSDA was passed to assure the *individual's* autonomous decision-making ability despite serious incapacitating illness or disease.

In addition, the ethical principles of professions that in large measure compose the rehabilitation field exemplify the written and unwritten commitment to upholding the rights of the individual. According to the American Psychological Association, to be ethical, practitioners must "respect the rights of *individuals* to privacy, confidentiality, self-determination, and autonomy. . . ." (1992, Principle D section). The American Academy of Physical Medicine and Rehabilitation's (AAPMR) Code of Conduct defines, among other things, the physiatrist's "principled relationships between *individuals*" (1999, Introduction and Overview section). The Codes of Ethics of both the American Occupational Therapy Association (AOTA) (2000, Occupational Therapy Code of Ethics section) and the American Speech-Language, Hearing Association (ASHA) (1994) uphold the *individual's* autonomy, privacy, and confidentiality. Finally, the American Physical Therapy Association (APTA) Guide for Professional Conduct, in its first principle, asserts the "rights and dignity of all *individuals*" (2001, Principle 1 section).

Although the preceding review is not meant to be an exhaustive analysis of the codes of ethics of representative rehabilitation professions, it does suggest that despite virtually universal recognition of the influence that family members and others have on rehabilitation, the predominant Western cultural perspective of ethics, as seen through the lens of representative professional organizations, considers the practitioners' relationship with individual patients and clients to be primary. This moral perspective reflects common beliefs, values, and principles that govern rehabilitation practice and that inform rehabilitation practitioners in general about how to interact with each other, with patients and clients, and with other health care providers.

Individualism and Collectivism: Assumptions of Rehabilitation Practitioners

In this chapter, I assume that all patient-clients are influenced by their culture. Furthermore, their cultural beliefs and values regarding what it means to be an individual in that culture fall along a continuum from stark individualism to collectivism. Finally, within one family, members may hold contradictory beliefs and views that fall somewhere along this continuum. Consequently, the possible variation among clients of different cultures and ethnic groups is immense. However, for the purpose of this chapter, I offer a simplified discussion of the characteristics of individualism and collectivism.

Individualism

In many ways, the notion of individualism, or the emphasis on one's rights as an individual, is the hallmark of the dominant Western culture. As Bronowski and Mazlish maintain, within the Western intellectual tradition, "the unfettered development of individual personality is praised as the ideal" (1960, p. 501). According to Bronowski and Mazlish (1960), this notion of individualism, along with the idea of personal freedom, compose perhaps the two most formative influences on the dominant American culture. Virtually everyone belonging to the dominant American culture assumes their right to personal fulfillment or to realize their individual potential. As Taylor (1991) said, "we can practically *define* the culture of Western liberal society in terms of those who feel the draw to . . . individualism" (p. 75). Addleson (1994) put it succinctly when he wrote the following:

> It is the decisions, actions, and motives of individuals that are important; individuals are judged, rewarded, and punished. Individuals have rights, duties, obligations, and entitlements, they reason and carry on dialogues with each other. Individuals sin, and they get sick. Individuals get promotions and earn wages and honors. Individuals have knowledge and beliefs, and individuals learn and take advantage of opportunities. In these and other ways, individuals are basic units for the philosophical ethics—and for many of the institutionalized ways in which our lives are managed in the United States. (p. 144)

Dworkin (1988) maintains that autonomy, a concept that combines individualism and personal freedom, "has emerged as the central notion in the area of applied moral philosophy, particularly in the [Western] biomedical context" (pp. 4–5). According to Jennings, Callahan, & Caplan (1988), noted medical ethicists, the autonomy paradigm assumes that the individual's self-interests and autonomy precede the need for medical help and are independent of the process of receiving that medical intervention. In other words, the individual is first an autonomous person who, because of enlightened self-interest, chooses to use medical services when needed.

Collectivism

Collectivism, on the other hand, represents the predominant ideal of vast numbers of people who hold beliefs and values about the individual and his or her relationship to the family and community that are different from the predominantly Western notion of the autonomous individual. It is important to acknowledge that collectivism is not a monolithic concept. Rather, collectivism is a complex concept that has broad social and political implications. Many variations and differences exist within the many ethnic groups and cultures that can be considered collectivist in nature. The term *collectivism* is used in this chapter to characterize the idea of individuals who keep the group needs and goals foremost in their minds, not the individual's (Triandis, 1994). Thus, in the broad sense of the word, when a conflict arises between the individual and the group, within the collectivist environment, the individual is expected to give up his or her needs or interests in favor of the group, whether based on kinship, tribal affiliation, employment, and so on.

Within the Western culture, we assume that the rights of the individual trump the rights of the group. We therefore extend those rights to the individual patient, not recognizing that some patients believe that the values of the collective take precedence over those of the individual. It is likely that most Western rehabilitation practitioners have never doubted their right to seek self-actualization or to attain their fullest potential. However, many patients of other cultures may not see that outlook as a possibility, let alone a reality. Many patients from other cultures hold uniformity as their ideal, have a collective identity defined by group membership, and consider conformity to their ideal and group norms as important. While many within the Western culture feel people should not intrude into one's business, keep personal matters private, and value being alone, many patients from collectivist cultures believe that one's business is also the group's business, and solitude and privacy are not necessarily valued. Furthermore, in some cultures the entire group is believed to be affected by an individual's actions, and the entire group is held responsible for that individual's actions.

Although individual clients' underlying beliefs and values related to what it means to be an individual varies, these clients also have much in common. Kagawa-Singer (1997), when writing about people facing a terminal disease, postulated that people, regardless of their culture and ethnicity, have three things in common: the need to face their fears about their disease or disability, the need to be productive or to be able to contribute to their family or community, and the need to be accepted and wanted in their family or community. Even more basic than these common needs is that people of all cultures and ethnic groups likely desire to lead *authentic* lives (Taylor, 1991).

As rehabilitation practitioners, we can support this basic desire, as Taylor (1991) put it, by "recognizing the equal value of different ways of being" (p. 51). Taylor's grounds for recognizing the equality of value among differences bears quoting:

> It is not because [people] are different, but because overriding the difference are some properties, common or complementary, which are of value. They are beings capable of reason, or love, or memory, or dialogical recognition. To come together on a mutual recognition of difference—that is, of the equal value of different identities—requires that we share more than a belief in this principle; we have to share also some standards of value on which the identities concerned check out as equal. There must be some substantive agreement on value, or else the formal principle of equality will be empty and a sham. We can pay lip-service to equal recognition, but we don't really share an understanding of equality unless we share something more. Recognizing difference, like self-choosing, requires a horizon of significance, in this case a shared one. (pp. 51–52)

In the case of rehabilitation clients or patients, the likely overriding common or complementary properties are the search for significance in life, the attempt to define themselves in meaningful ways (Taylor, 1991). These are probably common properties among both the rehabilitation practitioners and their clients or patients. In the rehabilitation setting, I postulate that these properties, seeking significance and meaning in life, provide what Taylor calls a horizon of significance. As will be discussed in the final section, this horizon of significance can provide the basis for ethical dialogue and decision making.

Ethical Principles and Assumptions Underlying Rehabilitation

Individualism, and the concomitant notion of personal freedom, whether reflected in the concepts of functional independence, the right to choose, or other ethical principles, seems to be the unquestioned, unofficial, moral stance in rehabilitation settings. To the extent that this is true, when rehabilitation practitioners uphold these Western values in morally, ethnically, and culturally heterogeneous settings, how can they be confident that they have made the "right" decision on behalf of the client? If, on the other hand, the rehabilitation client makes the decisions (and the rehabilitation practitioner is responsible for the outcome of the treatment/decisions), how can the rehabilitation practitioner know that the client made the "right" decision?

Rehabilitation professionals and others often look to the ethical principles of beneficence, veracity, justice, individual autonomy, and professional autonomy to help guide their decisions. The following is a simplified discussion of these ethical principles with a discussion of dilemmas that apply in ethnically and culturally diverse rehabilitation settings. It is important to note, however, that use of these principles in decision making is limited to the degree that all of the individuals involved agree with the principles.

Beneficence

The principle of beneficence "asserts an obligation to help others further their important and legitimate interests" (Beauchamp & Childress, 2001, p. 166). According to these authors, the principle of positive beneficence and the principle of utility further refine the concept of beneficence. The principles of positive beneficence dictates that one should provide a good or should remove a harm. The principle of utility asserts that one should balance the benefits of one's action against its harm.

Typically, rehabilitation practitioners are genuinely dedicated to doing good and avoiding harm, but they may not have considered this principle in light of cultural diversity and its concomitant variety of beliefs and values among their clients. Rehabilitation practitioners' concepts of what is good and bad, particularly when those practitioners are members of the dominant Western culture or have been acculturated, are likely to coincide with the rehabilitation institution's policies. For example, in the situation in the accompanying box, most rehabilitation practitioners could assume that "doing good" for Mr. Jacinto would include helping him to bathe and dress himself, walk independently, and in general function at the highest level of independence possible—essentially, elements of what many would call "best practice." Rehabilitation practitioners would expect Mr. Jacinto to actively participate in therapy and would expect his family to support and reinforce his therapeutic gains.

Case Study 1

Mr. Jacinto is an 87-year-old man from the Philippine Islands who recently had a stroke resulting in severe left hemiplegia. He has been transferred to a transitional care unit in preparation for his discharge home. Mr. Jacinto and his wife of 60 years live with their eldest daughter; two sons, two other daughters, and several grandchildren live in the same community. The two oldest children were born in the Philippines.

Questions

1. How might Mr. Jacinto actively participate in rehabilitation?
2. What would you do if a family member insisted on helping with Mr. Jacinto's
3. ADL even though you know he can perform them without help?

However, because the Jacinto family have different beliefs about the value of "independence"—how best to help their disabled father and what to expect from rehabilitation—Mr. Jacinto may not seem motivated. Even after explaining to him and his family how important it is to practice getting in and out of bed, or to feed himself, Mrs. Jacinto and her eldest daughter dress and feed the client, help him out of bed, and do a number of other things for him that the rehabilitation practitioners believes is countertherapeutic. This situation poses a serious dilemma for the rehabilitation practitioner. Should she conclude that on the basis of this client's behavior, he is uncooperative and unlikely to benefit from rehabilitation services? If he and his family's behavior, on the other hand, represents confirmation of different beliefs about individual autonomy and the way that families are to respond to disability, is the rehabilitation practitioner justified in altering her goals to exclude independent ambulation, self-feeding and dressing, or other typical goals of rehabilitation?

Veracity

The principle of veracity, or truth telling, includes at least three obligations: not to lie, not to deceive others, and in certain situations, the obligation to disclose information. In addition, veracity refers to the completeness, accuracy, and objectivity with which information is offered (Beauchamp & Childress, 2001). Furthermore, our obligation is not limited to telling the truth about the client's condition, such as having a terminal disease or the client's rehabilitation potential. This obligation extends to availability of services, referral to services, billing and benefit issues, and the like.

Examples of the obligations not to lie and not to deceive in rehabilitation include intentionally deceiving clients for their own benefit and the manipulation of information. Whether one chooses to tell a client the truth or to alter the truth about his or her condition or not, is influenced by one's beliefs about what is good, about duty, and about the outcome of one's decisions. For example, some might feel that their duty to tell the truth subordinates the possible harm that the truth telling might have on the client. Others might prefer to weigh their decision to tell the truth against the likely benefit to the client and to choose the action that favors a happy or positive outcome.

Our obligation to disclose information "usually depends on special relationships between the parties involved. For example, the patient entrusts care to the clinician and thereby obtains a right to information that the clinician would not otherwise be obligated to provide" (Beauchamp & Childress, 2001, p. 284). Many examples in the literature of this obligation pertain to risks inherent in life-threatening procedures or the risks of a decision not to undergo a procedure. Other examples are associated with risks related to lifestyle issues such as smoking, drinking alcohol in excess, drug abuse, leading a sedentary lifestyle, and the like. According to the dominant Western culture, rehabilitation practitioners have an obligation to disclose the risks associated with those choices and the benefits that accrue from making alternative choices.

The notion of truth telling, in the dominant Western culture, extends to the notion of disclosing information even if that information is not needed for decision making. Take the situation in which an elderly Chinese woman, Mrs. Chin, is diagnosed with terminal cancer. She lives with her eldest son and his family, all of whom are Buddhists. The European-American rehabilitation practitioner would likely feel obliged to disclose this information to

Mrs. Chin on the basis of the belief in the Western model of individualism and self-determinism in which the *individual* has "the right to choose, as well as the right to accept or to decline information" (Beauchamp & Childress, 2001, p. 63). However, Chinese and other Asian cultures value "harmony, consensus, and deference to authority" (Fetters, 1998, p. 133). Many in these cultures view the family as the fundamental social unit that deserves respect and that claims responsibility for making decisions for its members. To disclose this diagnosis to Mrs. Chin but not to the family would be unethical in the eyes of this family.

Justice

The principle of justice encompasses broad notions of fairness and desert, that is, the notion that justice is served when one gets one's due and that justice is not served when one does not get one's due. Distributive justice, opposed to criminal justice, for example, derives from the limits of human benevolence and limited supplies of goods (Lamont, 2003). For the purposes of this chapter, I will focus on two aspects of distributive justice put forth by Beauchamp & Childress (2001): Macroallocation, or decisions that "determine the funds to be expended and the goods made available, as well as the methods of distribution" (p. 250) and microallocation, or decisions that "determine who will receive particular scarce resources" (p. 250).

At both the macro- and the microallocation levels of distributive justice, the central moral question seems to be how to balance the good of the individual against the needs of the many. For example, some have suggested that on the macroallocation level, limits should be placed on society's resources available to rehabilitation clients and others, like older adults, who receive a disproportionate amount of the total health care services. Many assert that the good that might come from caring for those with chronic illness or those in need of technical, and often expensive, services such as a rehabilitation is outweighed by the needs of others who, perhaps because they have more years to live or are employable, can contribute more to society. The money spent on one electromyotic prosthesis, some may explain, is more justly used to inoculate thousands of children against measles or other communicable diseases.

At the microallocation level, in the rehabilitation clinic, for example, issues of justice are more likely expressed in terms of how many sessions of what therapy will be reimbursed, who should get the services of the limited rehabilitation practitioners, or how to balance the good that might come from a particular service to an individual against the needs of that person's family.

Case Study 2

Mr. Rodriguez is 68 years old and has recently had his second foot amputated secondary to diabetes. Mr. Rodriguez's mother, Rosa, lives with her son and daughter-in-law. Rosa is in good health but has cataracts. She requires assistance with most of her activities of daily living. After his first amputation, Mr. Rodriguez was unable to do the heavy labor he had done most of his life. Mrs. Carmen Rodriguez is 65 years old and has done domestic work most of her life. She has a few clients for whom she cleans house, but since her husband's recent amputation, she has had to spend more time caring for her husband. Monica, the eldest of five children, lives in the same home. The other children are married and live nearby in the same town.

Questions

1. What would be the likely rationale for recommending nursing home placement for Mr. Rodriguez?
2. How might you ethically justify the wife and other family members providing care for Mr. Rodriguez in the home?

When considering discharge plans for Mr. Rodriguez, rehabilitation practitioners who share the values and beliefs of the dominant Western culture might seek nursing home placement for Mr. Rodriguez. They would likely base this decision, first, on Mr. Rodriguez's severe disability, and second, on the "care-giving cost," especially considering that in addition to caring for Mr. Rodriguez at home, his wife must also care for her mother-in-law. The rehabilitation practitioners were surprised when the entire Rodriguez family disagreed with that plan. Monica, the eldest daughter, explained that they are a traditional Mexican family. They have a strong tradition of caring for their own. Monica's grandmother essentially raised Monica and her sibling, and Monica intends to remain single, live in the family home, and care for her grandmother and parents until they die. Even when the rehabilitation team recommended home health services, the family adamantly refused, saying that they would be able to care for their father and grandmother.

Professional Autonomy

The notion of professional autonomy includes authority over practice as well as broader issues of establishing fees, who can enter the professions, and how practitioners are regulated. Perhaps physicians, especially during the first half of the nineteenth century, represent the best, if not the most excessive, example of professional autonomy. They decided who to treat, with what, and when. They set their own fees, and through admitting privileges, they controlled the flow of patients into hospitals. Through licensing statutes they "controlled entry into the medical profession, disciplinary action against their colleagues, and the delivery of health care services by persons other than physicians" (Center for Biomedical Ethics, 1989, p. 13). In recent years, other health care professions have gained stature and autonomy within the health care professional community and rehabilitation in particular. All of these disciplines experience varying degrees of threats and limits to their professional autonomy.

Most meaningful to the purpose of this book, however, is the effect that professional autonomy has on rehabilitation clients, their family, and other stakeholders, particularly considering growing ethnic and cultural diversity among rehabilitation clients. In the Western culture, the physicians' and the rehabilitation providers' values and beliefs about the meaning of rehabilitation, independence, function, and the like, tend to trump those of the individual client's, at least while the client is in the rehabilitation setting. However, the more autonomy and authority is exercised by the rehabilitation provider, the less autonomy and authority is available to the client and family; the more choices made by the rehabilitation provider, the fewer the choices available to the client. The challenge for professionals working in rehabilitation is to strike a reasonable balance between the two extremes (Howe, 1998; Martin, 1999).

In addition to values and beliefs about doing good, justice, and the like, the predominant Western culture influences our beliefs about appropriate treatment regimen and the way that a day in the hospital is organized. Clients bathe, eat, and move about the rehabilitation hospital according to the hospital's needs and schedule. Medications must be taken at prescribed intervals, and patients must be on time for each treatment or appointment throughout the day. The patient, regardless of his or her culture, who, for example, wants to bathe at irregular times or wants to bathe more frequently than the official schedule allows, might be considered a "demanding patient."

While in acute care situations, a reasonable person abrogates, on a short-term basis, his or her autonomy to the health care professionals (Jennings, Callahan, & Caplan, 1988). In those situations, it makes sense for the emergency room physician, for example, to make the critical decisions about care. But in rehabilitation settings, clients, whether part of the mainstream culture or not, need to fully participate in rebuilding their own lives both in spite of chronic deficits and in light of their cultural values, experiences, and beliefs. When rehabilitation professionals exercise their professional autonomy heavy-handedly, they risk usurping the client's sense of personal authority and purpose, regardless of whether their cultural orientation is individualistic or collectivistic.

Case Study 3

Abdul Naseri is a 38-year-old male who was shot in the left shoulder and wrist during a jewelry store robbery. His glenohumeral and wrist joints were damaged, and he has peripheral nerve damage affecting the use of his left arm and hand. Abdul is a devout Muslim. His rehabilitation was initiated days before Ramadan, a month-long period of fasting during the daylight hours and of eating small meals in the evening.

Questions

1. How might Abdul's religious beliefs conflict with rehabilitation?
2. What are other examples of religious beliefs that might conflict with rehabilitation goals and expectations?

Conflict between religious beliefs about blood transfusions, the requirements of fasting, and other strongly held beliefs and values exemplify possible conflicts between professional autonomy and individual patient autonomy. Take the case of a young Muslim from Jordan who is injured a couple of weeks before the beginning of Ramadan. Despite severe pain resulting from gun-shot wounds, he refuses to take his pain medications during Ramadan. The resulting discomfort complicates his rehabilitation because he does not participate appropriately in therapy, and he does not follow through with his treatment at home. The rehabilitation practitioners are frustrated by his noncompliance and foresee serious physical consequences resulting from Abdul's refusal to comply with his rehabilitation program. Abdul, on the other hand, believes that his pain is due to the will of Allah and that what he considers a brief interruption in rehabilitation despite the possible consequences is a reasonable price to pay for his obedience to the tenets of the Muslim religion.

Client/Patient Autonomy

The broad Western notion of autonomy is often defined in terms of "self-governance, liberty rights, privacy, individual choice, freedom of will, causing one's own behavior, and being one's own person" (Beauchamp & Childress, 2001, p. 58). Personal autonomy, according to these authors, includes the notion of "self-rule that is free from both controlling interferences by others and personal limitations, . . . that prevent meaningful choice" (p. 58). This Western conception of autonomy appears far removed from the daily experiences of people with severe disabilities and those of nondominant cultures and ethnic groups. Ethicists have begun to differentiate between ethical dilemmas of acute and chronic medical care within the dominant Western culture (Agich, 1990; Jennings, Callahan, & Caplan, 1988). Although these efforts have helped to redefine the concept of autonomy and to increase the awareness that "dependence is a nonaccidental feature of the human condition" (Agich, 1990, p. 12), they have not overcome the predominant Western view of the individual and personal autonomy.

The concept of advanced directives exemplifies the Western notion of autonomy and individualism that assumes "that a future orientation toward life and health is universal and that individualism is of uniform importance" (Berger, 1998, p. 127). Some believe that even though family members are in a unique position to support the patient or client, "the locus of decisional authority should remain in the individual patient" (Blustein, 1993). However, advanced directives are written documents precipitated by a serious condition that attempts to foresee the outcome of and disease of injury. For a number of reasons, advanced directives can pose serious dilemmas for people of diverse non-Western cultures.

Following are some reasons why advanced directives pose dilemmas for people of diverse non-Western cultures:

- Many people are oriented to the present.
- Some American Indian cultures believe that negative thoughts of illness raised in conversation conflict with notions of goodness and harmony.
- Many Chinese believe that specific discussions about death or disability can bring about those events.
- Some believe that the family, not the individual, should make decisions about what might happen in the future.
- Disclosure of a diagnosis might remove hope of a cure (Berger, 1998).

In the increasingly diverse rehabilitation practice setting, it is nearly impossible to draw a clear and an unambiguous distinction between the views of individualism and of collectivism. There exist a blurring and a blending of beliefs and values within family members and across groups and specific situations. For example, in one family from American Samoa, the younger members may have taken on many Western values including the notion of individualism, whereas the older family members may have held on to traditional values of collectivism. To complicate matters, perhaps the youngest member of the family, who you might think would be the most acculturated into the dominant Western culture, may feel a strong obligation to care for her grandmother, whereas the other granddaughter and the grandsons may feel that doing so would be too much of a personal sacrifice.

Ethical Decision Making in Rehabilitation

A number of ethical decision-making models exist. In fact, an Internet search of the term "bioethical decision making" will yield dozens of credible sites (mostly educational institutions and centers for research and study in ethics). Most of these sites offer common steps or points to consider when faced with ethical dilemmas. These steps range from identifying the problem, assessing the facts relevant to the problem, identifying the stakeholders who will be affected by the decision, identifying their opinions and the values at stake, identifying potential legal issues, and prioritizing and making the decision.

Although many of these models will lead to identification of client and family members' cultural beliefs and values, some ethicists believe that the "decision-making model" approach to solving ethical dilemmas does not fully meet the needs of those involved in making these decisions (Carter, n. d.; Howe, 1998; Martin, 1999). However, we are likely never to see a consensus among ethicists about the best model for making decisions about difficult ethical dilemmas in rehabilitation. Dealing with flesh-and-blood ethical dilemmas is, at best, a messy business—far more cluttered and confusing than texts and articles on the subject portray.

As rehabilitation providers we can, to paraphrase Taylor (1991), acknowledge and recognize that despite many differences, we and our patients and clients have common and mutual beliefs, concerns, hopes, and fears, which are of value. However, being able to make ethical decisions in ethnically and culturally diverse settings requires that we share what Taylor calls a horizon of significance. In the case of rehabilitation, the horizon of significance is the awareness that our clients or patients all likely seek significance and meaning in life; they wish to lead meaningful lives within the context of their beliefs and values. Using that "horizon of significance" as a backdrop, we can talk with our patients and their family members; and among our colleagues, we can come to recognize and value all parties' different beliefs and values. We can acknowledge that even though there may exist distinct, and sometimes opposing, differences between the provider and the patient, we have a shared value of leading an authentic and a meaningful life.

Summary

This chapter explored the ethical assumptions about what it means to be an individual in individualist and collectivist cultures—assumptions that underpin rehabilitation practice. It reviewed basic ethical principles and some of the ethical issues that rehabilitation practitioners face when providing services to ethnically and culturally diverse clients. Finally, it offered some suggestions about ways of making ethical decisions that both acknowledge and support the beliefs and values of culturally and ethnically diverse rehabilitation patients.

Questions

1. Why is it important to understand the ethics of cultural and ethnic diversity?
2. What are the similarities and the differences between the concepts of individualism and collectivism?
3. What are some examples of how the basic Western principles of biomedical ethics (for example, the principles of beneficence, veracity, justice, and client and professional autonomy) do not automatically apply to patients of other cultures or ethnicity?
4. What are the common steps in ethical decision making, and why are they important?

References

Addelson, K. P. (1994). *Mortal passages: Toward a collectivist moral theory.* New York: Routledge.

Agich, G. J. (1990). Reassessing autonomy in long-term care. *Hastings Center Report, 20*(6), 12–17.

American Academy of Physical Medicine and Rehabilitation. (1999). *American Academy of Physical Medicine and Rehabilitation Code of Conduct.* Retrieved February 2, 2001, from http://www.aapmr.org/about/codea.htm

American Hospital Association. (2001). *A patient's bill of rights.* Retrieved July 19, 2001, from http://www.aha.org/resource/pbillofrights.asp

American Occupational Therapy Association. (2000). *Occupational therapy code of ethics.* Retrieved December 3, 2001, from http://www.aota.org/general/coe.asp

American Physical Therapy Association. (2001). *APTA guide for professional conduct.* Retrieved December 3, 2001, from http://www.apta.org/PT_Practice/ethics_pt/pro_conduct

American Psychological Association (1992). Principle D Respect for people's rights and dignity. In *Ethical principles of psychologists and code of conduct.* Retrieved August 5, 2000, from http://www.apa.org/ethics/code.html

American Speech-Language Hearing Association. (1994). Code of ethics. *American Speech-Language Hearing Association, 36*(March, Suppl. 13), pp. 1–2.

Annas, G. J. & Miller, F. H. (1994). The empire of death: How culture and economics affect informed consent in the U. S., the U. K., and Japan. *American Journal of Law & Medicine, 20*(4), 357–394.

Beauchamp, T. L. & Childress, J. F. (2001). *Principles of biomedical ethics* (5th ed.). New York: Oxford University Press.

Berger, J. T. (1998). Cultural discrimination in mechanism for health decisions: A view from New York. *Journal of Clinical Ethics, 9*(2), 127–131.

Blackhall et al. (1995). Ethnicity and attitudes toward patient autonomy. *Journal of American Medical Association, 274*(10), 820–825.

Blustein, J. (1993). The family in medical decision making. *Hastings Center Report, 23*(3), 6–13.

Bronowski, J. & Mazlish, B. (1960). *The Western intellectual tradition.* New York: Harper & Row.

Carrese, J. A. & Rhodes, L. A. (1995). Western bioethics on the Navajo Reservation. *Journal of American Medical Association, 274*(10), 826–829.

Carter, M. A. (n. d.). Synthetic model of bioethical inquiry. Retrieved November 24, 2001, from http://bu.edu/wcp/Papers/Bioe/BioeCart.htm

Center for Biomedical Ethics. (1989). *Rethinking medical morality: The ethical implications of changes in health care organization, delivery, and financing.* Minneapolis, MN: University of Minnesota.

Culhane-Pera, K. A. & Vawter, D. E. (1998). A study of healthcare professionals' perspectives about a cross-cultural ethical conflict involving a Hmong patient and her family. *The Journal of Clinical Ethics, 9*(2), p. 179.

Dworkin, G. (1988). *The theory and practice of autonomy.* New York: Cambridge University Press.

Federal Patient Self Determination Act of 1990. (1994). 42 USC 1395cc(a) and 1396a(w).

Fetters, M. D. (1998). The family in medical decision making: Japanese perspectives. *The Journal of Clinical Ethics, 9,* 132–145.

Gostin, L. O. (1995). Informed consent, cultural sensitivity and respect for persons. *Journal of American Medical Association, 274*(10), 844–845.

Helman, C. G. (2000). *Culture, health and illness: An introduction for health professionals* (4th ed.). Oxford: Oxford University Press.

Ho, D. Y-F & Chiu, C-Y. (1994). Component ideas of individualism, collectivism, and social organization: An application in the study of Chinese culture. In U. Kim, H. C. Triandis, C. Kagitcibasi, S-C Choi, & G. Yoon (Eds.). *Individualism and collectivism: Theory, method, and applications* (137–156). Thousand Oaks: Sage.

Howe, E. G. (1998). Commentary: "Missing" patients by seeing only their cultures. *Journal of Clinical Ethics, 9*(2), 191–193.

Jennings, B., Callahan, D., & Caplan, A. L. (1988). Ethical challenges of chronic illness. *The Hastings Center Report, 18*(Suppl.), 1–16.

Kagawa-Singer, M. (1997). Addressing issues for early detection and screening in ethnic populations. *Oncology Nursing Forum, 24*(10), 1705–1711.

Lamont, J. (2003). Distributive justice. The Stanford Encyclopedia of philosoypy (Fall 2003) (Ed.). E. N. Zalta (Ed.). Retrieved September 29, 2004, from http://plato.stanford .edu/cgi-bin/encyclopedia/archinfo.cgi?entry=justice-distributive.

MacIntyre, A. (1984). *After virtue* (2nd ed.). Notre Dame, IN: University of Notre Dame Press.

Martin, P. A. (1999). Bioethics and the whole: Pluralism, consensus, and the transmutation of bioethical methods into gold. *Journal of Law, Medicine & Ethics, 27*(4), 316–327.

Meleis, A. I. & Jonsen, A. R. (1983). Ethical crises and cultural differences. *Medicine in Perspective, 138*(6), 889–893.

Pellegrino, E. D. (1992). Is truth telling to the patient a cultural artifact? *Journal of American Medical Association, 268*(13), 1734–1735.

Taylor, C. (1991). *The ethics of authenticity*. Cambridge, MA: Harvard University Press.

Triandis, H. C. (1994). Theoretical and methodological approaches to the study of collectivism and individualism. In U. Kim, H. C. Trandis, C. Kagitcibasi, S. Choi, & G. Yoon (Eds.). *Individualism and collectivism: Theory, method and applications*. Beverly Hills, CA: Sage.

5

European Americans

Shannon Munro Cohen

Key Words

European Americans   emigrate   assimilation
immigration   acculturation

Objectives

1. Describe immigration patterns of people from some European countries to the United States.
2. Provide an overview of the cultures and health belief systems of several European countries.
3. Discuss the health delivery systems of these European countries and some challenges facing those seeking help for rehabilitation.
4. Provide some statistics related to health for infants in some European countries.
5. Present some case studies of individuals of European descent seeking help from the rehabilitation practitioner.

Introduction

Division between cultures in the United States has blurred, as many European immigrants have adopted the beliefs, values, and customs of this country. Many other European Americans continue to embrace their cultural diversity. Understanding the roots of our blended society and relationships to health care beliefs presents a challenge to the health care provider. A brief overview of several European countries is presented in this chapter in order to give the reader a better understanding of the basis of current health beliefs and behaviors.

This chapter, which is based on personal observations, interviews, and review of literature, is not comprehensive. The reader is asked to use this information as a starting point in the exploration of culture, remembering that individuals with differing background and experiences may not conform to the behaviors and beliefs of a larger group. Issues discussed affecting rehabilitation include poverty, the needs of the group versus those of the individual, language barriers, perception and beliefs regarding health care, and privacy and personal space. Unfortunately, the longer that new immigrants stay in this country, the more likely they are to develop unhealthy habits such as poor nutritional choices, obesity, lack of exercise, and increased tobacco and alcohol use.

Immigration

Over one million immigrants were granted legal resident status during 2002, and of these, 15.6% were from Europe (U.S. Department of Immigration). Europeans arrived in the United States in great numbers between 1820 and 1940. In 1850, 92% of immigrants came from European countries. The first immigrants came for economic reasons and the opportunity to settle in the "new land," whereas others arrived later for religious or political reasons. Early immigrants from Europe came primarily from Germany, Ireland, the United Kingdom, and Italy. Immigrants from France, Poland, and Denmark arrived in smaller numbers.

An estimated 33.5 million people living in the United States, 11.7% of the population, were born in another country (United States Census Bureau, 2003). Ethnic minorities represent one-fourth of the population. Thirty million people in the United States speak a language other than English. Information on second- and third-generation European immigrants is unavailable, because changes in census questions no longer clearly reflect the ancestry of many U.S. residents.

Adjustment is difficult for new arrivals beginning life in the United States, often living in older substandard housing and lacking basic health care coverage. Significant language barriers, lack of transferable skills, lack of transportation, loneliness, and sadness remain challenges. Some may arrive well educated but find that their skills and education are not accepted in this country.

Health Care Values and Beliefs

It is often assumed that all persons value autonomy. Therefore, health care providers in the United States encourage self-care and may not think to include family members in patient education. Patient education programs and making informed individual decisions are relatively new concepts in Europe.

With this focus on individualism comes a difference in many cultures regarding decision making. The group leader or family members often make decisions, whereas in the United States, individuals are expected to make their own health care choices. Families may not want the patient to know the diagnosis and/or treatment options. Physicians may contact the patient's family first with "bad news," allowing the family to decide whether the patient can handle the stress of knowing his or her diagnosis. The reasoning for this approach is that families from European countries do not want their loved one to lose hope. Medical treatment in European countries tend to be more paternalistic with the belief that the "doctor knows best." Likewise, group education and support may not be received well by families who choose to trust the health care provider to make decisions in their best interest.

Another difference in values regarding health care involves privacy issues. Muslim women from Bosnia and Croatia, for example, prefer to be examined only by a female and are unaccustomed to having complete physical and gynecologic care. In the United States, visiting hours in hospitals are short, and accommodations are not made for families to stay with their loved one because of space limitations and privacy concerns. In many cultures, families gather to offer support and express their concern when they learn of illness, without regard for the time of day or visitation policies.

Health beliefs also vary tremendously among cultures (Spector, 2004). Increasingly, individuals believe that one needs medication to get well. People from other cultures, such as Italy, may prefer an injection and often treat viral infections and colds with an injection of vitamins and/or medication. After arriving in the United States, many continue to expect medication in this form. Resources may also be limited in many cultures, with only acute care sought. Treatment often begins with herbs and homeopathic remedies.

Individual beliefs regarding the causes of illness and disability vary widely. Some may believe that sin, disobedience, or marital infidelity causes illness, whereas others believe strongly in God's will and feel that they are divinely chosen to be the parents of a child born with a handicapping condition. Superstitions remain in some cultures, particularly among older generations. There may be concern about catching an illness or having an affected child if a pregnant woman sees a person who is blind, for example. Most, however, recognize the effect of environmental factors, maternal substance abuse, and genetics on pregnancy outcomes. It is interesting that all point to the need to assign blame as a means of reconciling and dealing with illness and disability.

The role of people with disability is dependent on available resources and societal beliefs. The disabled person's role in society varies widely among cultures, ranging from institutionalization; neglect; being "hidden" among the family; remaining with and contributing to the family; and marrying, working, and being active in society. More information on health values, beliefs, and practices will be covered in each of the sections on European countries.

Time

Time is definitely different in America. In England, the last hired in a company was the "tea girl." She served tea to everyone at the 11 A.M. break. When I came to the U.S., I asked "who will do elevens? I guess I will since I was the last hired." Everyone laughed. My nickname became "miss elevens" from then on.

Beliefs regarding time vary widely among cultures. Many cultures consider time precious and not to be wasted. Americans tend to be very future-oriented. Work and family time are scheduled around the clock and the calendar. Even children have very full schedules of after-school activities, music lessons, and sports. Meeting times are set, and those who are more than fifteen minutes late are expected to apologize. Health promotion activities frequently offered in the United States may not be well received by members of other cultures who are less future-oriented.

The people of Greece embrace all time orientations. Through storytelling, they keep their history alive in the minds of the people. They are present-oriented to the needs of their family as well as future-oriented as they encourage their children's occupational and educational achievement. Greeks tend to let activities continue to their natural breaking point.

The Polish do not like to make appointments; instead, they prefer to "drop in." Unexpected visitors are welcomed and offered food. The French also are very flexible with time, accepting changes of plan at the last minute. Conversely, train schedules in Germany are precise; thus, people expect punctuality.

The Irish have a strong allegiance to the past that is the focus of stories about their history and ancestors. A fatalistic time orientation leads many to delay seeking treatment for illness that will "run its course." Italians also share the belief of living one day at a time and do not believe in planning too far ahead.

Personal Space and Touch

Personal space, the distance that one feels comfortable speaking to another, varies widely among people and cultures. People of Irish ancestry tend to stand farther apart than people from other cultures and use touch less frequently in communication. The French and Polish prefer to stand close together when talking, and they touch more frequently; kissing is a typical greeting. For the French, smiling is less frequent and viewed with suspicion if there is no "good reason" to do so. Germans value their privacy with strangers, and touch is less frequent than in some other cultures.

Poland

An elderly Polish woman, a recent immigrant, was admitted to an orthopedic ward in the United States following hip surgery. She spoke no English and spent much of the day alone as her grown children worked. The staff was puzzled as she refused to eat during the day but ate voraciously in the evenings when her family arrived to visit. After careful questioning of the family, it was learned that she ate only one meal a day in remembrance of her experiences during the Holocaust. Furthermore, the hospital dietitians had not been notified of her desire for kosher meals.

History and Economics

Poland has struggled for its independence, only recently gaining freedom from communism. The German occupation of Poland during World War II was followed immediately by Soviet rule until 1989. After a republic government replaced communism, the evolving democracy, free enterprise, and the influx of American goods increased prices to levels that the citizens could not afford. Unemployment remains high. In the crowded cities, families live in large, old apartment buildings.

Before World War II, more than 3 million Jews lived in Poland. Over 90% of the Jewish population were killed in the Holocaust, leaving an estimated 8,000 Jews in Poland today. Those who survived emigrated to Israel or the West. Anti-Semitism continues, and in 2002 less than 1,100 declared Judaism as their religion (Wikipedia Encyclopedia, 2002).

Many nationalities were affected by the Holocaust; Poland is now one of the most ethnically homogenous countries in the world (Gozdziak, 1996). The United States has the largest population of Polish immigrants in the world.

Religion

The Roman Catholic Church exerts a great deal of influence in Poland; over 95% of the population are Roman Catholic. There is much overlap between church and state; religious education is part of the school curricula, and church attendance is high. Other religions are present; Jehovah's Witnesses are a growing group in Poland. Condemned by the church and law, abortion is illegal. Access to birth control is expensive, difficult to obtain, and against Catholic beliefs.

Language

Polish is the official language of Poland, with many different dialects. There are surprising numbers of multilingual residents. Education is compulsory and free for all children beginning at age 7. Many children complete secondary school and go on to college or vocational/technical school at no cost.

Family Roles

In the traditional Polish home, the man is the head of the household, although in today's society, work is shared more equally between spouses. As in many societies today, two incomes are needed to cover expenses. Child care is expensive; often grandmothers provide assistance with child rearing. Extended family members often live together. As in many other cultures, fathers desire sons to carry on the family name. Public hugging and kissing and direct eye contact are acceptable.

Health Care

Poland has a socialized medical system in which a primary care physician first sees patients. Patients requiring special care must travel long distances to university-based hospitals. Health care is free but limited; dental care is almost nonexistent. Medical supplies are scarce, equipment is outdated and often poorly maintained, and there are long waits for elective procedures. Women dominate the medical profession in Poland, receiving very low wages.

Midwives frequently deliver babies in hospitals under the supervision of a physician. Family attendance at the birth is discouraged because of the small size of delivery rooms. Pain tolerance is valued. The average length of stay after birth is lengthy, 5 to 7 days for a normal delivery. Premature deliveries and low-birth-weight babies with resultant cerebral palsy are common because of the lack of prenatal care and proper nutrition. Equipment to care for the smallest infants is unavailable. Breastfeeding is strongly advocated. (See the Appendix at the end of the chapter for population, birth rate, infant mortality, life expectancy, and poverty level statistics for the countries discussed in this chapter.)

The Polish believe that stress and diet cause illness. Some older generations believe in the "evil eye" (Szatan) and may rely on folk medicine, seers, praying, and wearing religious medals to protect them from illness. Those seeking medical care assume a passive role. Laws give patients the right to know their diagnosis and treatment choices; however, physicians do not offer explanations. Most patients do not question their diagnosis or treatment options. Debilitating degenerative diseases such as multiple sclerosis are often called by other names so that the patient does not understand what is wrong and will not lose hope (Slowikowski, 2000). Health promotion classes are nonexistent. It is of interest, however, that many physicians still make house calls.

Tay-Sachs disease and Niemann-Pick disease are enzyme disorders common in infants of Jewish origin that cause death in early childhood. Another disorder found in persons of Polish descent is Phenylketonuria (PKU); lack of treatment leads to irreversible mental retardation. Hepatitis A, diphtheria, and tuberculosis are common in Poland and surrounding countries as a result of flooding and overcrowding. Infants receive the BCG vaccine to protect against tuberculosis (TB) at birth, which later affects TB testing results.

As in the United States, the top health problems in Poland are heart disease, diabetes, lung cancer, hypertension, and diet-related illnesses. The elderly are at a "tremendous disadvantage in Poland" as basic necessities increase in price and pensions do not rise to meet the cost. Many elderly people speak of the desire to return to communism because the free market has led to abject poverty (Slowikowski, 2000).

There is little money dedicated to rehabilitation in the public sector. People with severe disabilities and mental illness are institutionalized and are not seen in public. Modifications such as curb cuts and sidewalk wheelchair access are unavailable, and there are no laws governing access or accommodations for people with disabilities. Children with significant disabilities are not mainstreamed into public classrooms.

As in many other cultures, financial resources are limited and restricted to young patients with the best foreseeable outcomes. The elderly and people with diabetes are ineligible for dialysis. Medication chosen for patients is often based on what has been donated in a particular month. Equipment to help the disabled become more self-sufficient is unavailable.

The main rehabilitation issues for Polish immigrants include avoidance of preventative health care, passive role in decision making, and lack of experience seeking out care for the disabled.

Croatia

On immigrants from Bosnia and Croatia: "They have no concept of preventative medicine. To do a Pap smear for cervical cancer was odd and invasive since they do not have symptoms. It was especially difficult when retesting is needed. They make excuses to avoid further appointments . . . willing to live with it out of fear. Others refuse to take the tuberculosis treatment because they do not feel bad." (Inouye, 2000)

History and Economics

Croatia, which was part of Yugoslavia, was governed by communism from the 1940s to 1990. Now the government is an independent parliamentary democracy. Thousands of Serbians fled to Eastern Slavonia during the political upheaval of 1995. Since 1990, Croatia has struggled after the change in government and adoption of free enterprise. Inflation has decreased from 1000% in 1993 to 1.5% today (United States Department of State, 2004). Unemployment remains high for this country, which is roughly the size of the state of West Virginia. Croatia has sheltered more than 600,000 refugees from war (World Factbook, 2004). All men must serve ten months of compulsory military service.

Religion

The people of Croatia are primarily Roman Catholic. Serbians attend the Serbian Orthodox Church. Intermarriage between Muslims and Catholics is strongly discouraged. The Roman Catholic church encourages abstinence before marriage and then the use of natural birth control methods such as the Billings (rhythm) method. Celibacy, however, is uncommon; birth control pills are covered by insurance, and condoms are readily available. Teenage pregnancies and single motherhood are rare. The Catholic church encourages adoption and leads public campaigns against abortion.

Family Roles

The traditional family prevails in this country. Women in Croatia rear children and work outside the home, since most cannot afford to support their family on one income. Few women receive paid maternity leave. As in other countries, there is conflict over role expectations between men and women.

Health Care

Croatia has state-subsidized health care paid for by a portion of each worker's salary. Health care resources are limited, however; hospital wards are crowded with up to eight patients per room with little privacy. Women deliver their babies in the hospital setting and commonly stay three days. Breastfeeding is the norm. Fathers are often present at the delivery.

Displaced persons from ongoing political conflict face many stresses, including the loss of their home and belongings, death or separation from family members, and personal injury. School problems and increased dropout rates have been documented among adolescents with posttraumatic stress disorder (PTSD) (Ajdukovic, 1998). Many adult survivors are also disabled with unresolved psychological issues. Rates of communicable diseases such as diphtheria are high in this country as well.

Illness is believed to result from scientific causes and nature's failure. A holistic view of health prevails, with health education being well received. Leading a healthy lifestyle is the goal of many, including moderate eating; diet full of fruits, vegetables, and fish; moderate exercise; and time for relaxation and hobbies. Smoking is prohibited in public buildings and transport. The top health problems are cardiovascular disease and stroke, followed by cancer.

People with disabilities are mainstreamed into society, but funds to assist them are limited. Often the disabled and elderly are seen on the streets begging; resources are limited to those with state-funded health insurance. Physical therapy, relaxation training, and stress management are available in public and private centers as well as in long-term care facilities and home care. Rehabilitation challenges for the people of Croatia include PTSD for the new immigrant, avoidance of preventative health care, and continued poverty.

Hungary

History and Economics

As in Poland, Hungary has many streets with multiple names; the streets have been renamed, depending on the country's current ruler. In Budapest, one road is referred to as Stalin Avenue, Street of the People's Republic, and Andrassy Ave. Hungary broke free of communism in 1989 after 40 years and has adopted a parliamentary democratic government. Hungarians are guaranteed a minimum wage; however, many live below the poverty level. Most medical care is free; employees receive health care benefits and pensions from contribution plans. There is distinct differentiation between the upper and the lower class.

In the 1800s, Hungarians immigrated to the United States seeking better job opportunities. The second large influx of immigrants sought refuge after World War II. Displaced from their homes, 16,000 people, including former concentration camp survivors, entered the United States. The last wave of immigration consisted of minorities fleeing ethnic cleansing under the communist regime of Kádár and Ceauşescu.

Religion

The majority of the population of Hungary is Roman Catholic, with one-third Protestant. Orthodox and Unitarian church memberships are increasing. Roma, or Gypsies, and Jewish members of society suffer persecution despite laws ensuring civil liberties and human rights. Despite the teachings of the Roman Catholic church, abortion is legal with high termination rates, as was encouraged by the communist regime.

Language

The primary language spoken is Hungarian. Many people also speak German and Russian because of the years of occupation. The communist regime restricted Hungarians to speaking only Russian, so it is a wonder that their own language did not disappear.

Family Roles

Much of Hungary is rural, with one-half of the populace working in agriculture. Farms are returning to private ownership after many years of communal farming. Many workers live in rural communities and travel to cities to work, and most women work outside the home.

Women are encouraged to stay at home with their children through the use of small child care allowances and are paid maternity leave, because motherhood is considered an important social responsibility.

Health Care

Health care is in the midst of upheaval, with the addition of private as well as government-subsidized health care. Residents are unable to afford private health insurance. Health promotion and primary care are new concepts in Hungary. Alcoholism is a significant health problem in this country, as well as cardiovascular disease, lung cancer, tuberculosis, and other communicable diseases such as diphtheria. Recent laws regulate tobacco sales to minors and also target smoking in workplace and public areas.

Unsafe water supplies in this country lead to gastroenteritis, bacterial dysentery, and salmonellosis. BCG vaccine is administered to infants to prevent tuberculosis. Initial tests for AIDS are performed anonymously, provided that the test results are negative. Persons with communicable diseases have no right to confidentiality in Hungary.

Political upheaval not only led to unemployment and homelessness but also increased rates of substance abuse, depression, and suicide. Recent education programs and funding has led to recognition and treatment with antidepressants.

Women are thoroughly screened during pregnancy, including an average of three ultrasound scans. Pregnant women must see the state physician four times to receive their "confinement grant" that allows them to stay at home to care for their child after delivery. Many also visit a private obstetrician at least once in order to assure that they are receiving adequate care.

The length of stay for new mothers is 6 to 7 days. Hospital care is very rigid for the new family, and home births are illegal unless birth is imminent. Childbirth classes are nonexistent. During labor women walk the halls outside the delivery room. Babies are placed in the nursery immediately after birth and are kept in incubators for up to 24 hours to decrease risk of infection. Fathers view their babies in the nursery on a television screen and are seldom present at the delivery. Breastfeeding is encouraged after the initial separation; however, babies are weighed before and after each feeding and supplemented as deemed necessary by the medical staff.

"Rooming in" is offered in a few hospitals, meaning that the babies are all placed on one large bed with several mothers sharing a room. When one infant cries, all the mothers awaken to see whether it is their child. Most mothers do not want this arrangement. Home visits are arranged for the mother within 24 hours after discharge, and visiting nurses may assist with child care.

Modern farm equipment is not available in Hungary and other agricultural countries in Europe. High rates of occupational injury and arthritis result from hard labor, but rehabilitation services are unavailable. Rehabilitation challenges for the people of Hungary include limited experience with rehabilitation services and preventative health care. Their health risks increase as they are exposed to the American way of life of less exercise, unhealthy food choices, and increased tobacco and alcohol consumption.

Romania

History and Economics

Romania is another European country with a history of years of struggle over boundary lines. Romania was freed from communism in 1989 and adopted a democratic constitution in 1991. Until 1856, the gypsies, or Roma, were bought and sold as were African Americans in the United States. During World War II, 500,000 Roma were killed. Inner conflict continues among Romanians, Hungarians, and Gypsies living in the country.

Communist Nicolae Ceauşescu's attempt to eliminate the national debt caused immeasurable hardship on the people of Romania. Food prices, which are exorbitant, are beyond the low wages of the average farm worker. Long food and milk lines are common. Inflation and unemployment remain high, with much labor unrest among workers.

Immigration to the United States occurred between 1870 and 1900. Romanians left their homeland for religious reasons, desire for freedom from communism, and seeking a better life.

Religion and Language

Christianity is the predominant religion; the majority of people belong to the Roman Orthodox Church. Most of the people speak Romanian with English and French taught in the schools as a second language.

Family Roles

Tradition dictates that men make all the important decisions. Women traditionally defer to the man, serving the meal to him first and using the formal address. The husband's mother often lives in the home and is in charge of household responsibilities. Spousal abuse is against the law but remains common. Gypsies (Roma) live with most of their extended family, which is known as a clan. They consider the clan as their immediate family. Families live in houses in rural areas and in older, crowded single family apartments in the cities.

Health Care

Romania has a socialized medical system with little funding. People often travel all day to obtain health care and then wait hours to be seen. Clinics often see several hundred people a day. Severe shortages of health care providers, equipment, and supplies contribute to the health care burden. Hospitals may place two patients in one bed while other patients wait in the hall.

Farm injuries with antiquated equipment are common. Cardiovascular disease and hypertension, cancer, and injuries account for 80% of deaths. Outbreaks of measles, hepatitis A and B, and diphtheria are common because of inadequate vaccinations. Because Romania does not have a consistent, safe drinking water supply, there are resulting high rates of dysentery, gastroenteritis, hepatitis, and cholera. Romanians believe in seeking assistance with acute illness only, relying first on superstitions, rituals, and self-healing. Teas are concocted for various ills. There is strong concern about avoiding chills believed to cause illness. Preventative health care and rehabilitation are virtually nonexistent.

Midwives deliver most babies in this country. Breastfeeding is the only option because formula and milk are often unavailable. For their older children, parents often purchase calcium tablets on the black market. Under the communist government, birth control was illegal, and maternal death rates from illegal abortions were ten times higher than in any other European nation. Kulczycki, Potts, & Rosenfield (1996) found that one-fifth of women were infertile and 86% died from illegal abortions. Legalized abortions continue to exceed live births. Birth control is now legal but remains difficult to obtain because of low wages and short supply.

Many children have been left in state orphanages. Humanitarian efforts have reached out to children left in 700 of these orphanages. Many children die there from malnutrition, AIDS, and hepatitis. Hospital staff, who had the task of intravenously feeding abandoned, malnourished newborn infants, reused needles and other medical supplies. Communist-era use of untested blood led to an outbreak of AIDS among Romanian infants; it is reportedly not a serious problem among adults. As a result, Romania has the highest infant mortality rate in Europe.

Rehabilitation challenges for the people of Romania include their lack of experience with modern health care and rehabilitation, and the need to include the elder family member in decision making.

Greece

History and Economics

Greek migration to the United States peaked between 1900 and 1920 with the failure of the country's main crop, currants. Almost 350,000 young men arrived seeking economic opportunity, hoping to make enough money to support their families and then return to Greece. Another influx of immigrants occurred in the 1960s as quotas were increased. Today, few Greeks migrate to the United States because of improving economic conditions in their country; Greece is an agricultural society with strong shipping and tourism trades. A president heads the parliamentary government.

Language

Greek is commonly spoken, although puristic, or Katharevousa, is the official language. There is also considerable variation in dialects. The head motion for "no" is the head tossed backward. Raising an outstretched hand (the American "stop") or showing the palm of the hand with fingers extended is an insult. Crossing fingers indicates two people in a close, romantic relationship. It is common for Greeks to greet each other with a hug and kiss on both cheeks. Staring is acceptable.

Religion

The Greek Orthodox Church is the religion of 98% of the people. Sunday morning liturgy is a 1½ to 3-hour service with chanting, singing, and use of heavily scented incense. Sundays are a day of rest. Faith is important, especially in the maintenance of health. Many bargain with the saints on behalf of their family; two healing saints, Cosmas and Damian, are frequently called upon. There is a strong belief in miracles even among third-generation Greeks.

Birth control is acceptable and available, but abortion is not. Adoption is rare. Shame and dishonor are brought on the family with unwed pregnancy as well as infertility.

Family Roles

The Greek people are known for their strong family ties and their care of the elderly. Caring for the elderly and less fortunate are said to bring good luck and honor to the family. Greeks value closeness and affection; privacy is not valued. Core values of honor (*philotimo*) and avoidance of family shame (*endropi*) are important.

The husband is considered the head of the household, with the marriage relationship of less importance than the family as a unit. Labor is traditionally divided, with the wife managing the home but occasionally also working in her husband's business.

Children are seldom left with babysitters, and they are often disciplined by teasing and are expected to "toughen up." Adolescents live with their parents until marriage. Prohibition from dating until the last years of schooling remains common. Young women are allowed to attend church-related activities with close supervision; Greek fathers pride themselves on the virtue of their daughters.

The grandmother, *giagia*, and grandfather, *pappou*, are respected family members and often move into the home after the death of the spouse. As in Italian and Catholic tradition, many families adopt *koumbari*, who act as godparents to their children. The ties between the family and *koumbaros* are so strong that they do not intermarry.

Health Care

Two genetic blood disorders, thalassemia and glucose 6 phosphate dehydrogenase (G6PD), are common in Greece. For people with G6PD enzyme deficiency, ingestion of broad (fava) beans and oxidant medications, including aspirin, can cause internal bleeding. Lactose intolerance is also common among Greeks. Cardiovascular and cerebrovascular disease are threats to health, as well as communicable diseases such as hepatitis A and B, tetanus, and typhoid.

Although alcohol is consumed with meals, alcoholism is rare, since high-risk behaviors bring shame on the family. Smoking and obesity, however, are common. Regular physical examination and health promotion activities are viewed as unnecessary.

There is considerable mistrust regarding health care professionals. Health problems are attributed to stress and worry, the devil, spirits, and the envy of others. Illness is thought to be caused by the afflicted person's behavior. Roupas (2000) gave the following example; a man mowed his lawn on a very hot day against the advice of his spouse; consequently, when he had a stroke and became wheelchair bound, it was "his fault."

Others believe that the cause of illness is *matiasma* (evil eye). Protective charms are worn to protect the wearer; ritual prayers and acts are believed to help those afflicted with *matiasma*. Herbal remedies such as the use of garlic and *vendousas* (cupping) may be used for initial self-treatment. Cupping is performed by placing a bottle containing steam against the body. As the bottle cools, impurities are drawn out. Circular bruises are left behind and should not be mistaken for abuse.

Mental illness is viewed with shame in Greek culture. When seeking treatment, the client presents with various somatic complaints to the practitioner. Disfiguring conditions such as cerebral palsy or socially unacceptable addictions are responded to with disdain in Greek society.

Pain is not something to be endured and is shared with family members; restraint is shown with outsiders. Family members surround the sick person, making certain that the person receives the best care. Rehabilitation challenges for the people of Greece include general distrust of health care providers, beliefs about the cause of illness, and the tendency for somatization making it difficult to determine whether symptoms are related to depression or illness.

Italy

History and Economics

Over 5 million Italians immigrated to the United States between 1820 and 1990, with the peak years of 1901 through 1920. Italians came to America seeking a better life. They did not initially intend to stay; they earned money for their families in Italy and bought land in the United States. However, they often returned to less than enthusiastic welcomes, as the money was not felt to offset the effects on the family left behind and the "bad habits" they learned by exposure to foreign ways. Immigrants from Italy stayed in small communities and in that way have preserved much of their culture. Only a few Italians immigrate to the United States today. Italy is one of the largest producers of grapes, wine, olives, and oil in the world. The country has a private enterprise economy and is ruled by a democratic republic.

Religion

The primary religion in Italy is Roman Catholic. Divorce was legalized in 1973, followed by abortion in 1978; both stand in opposition to the tenets of the Roman Catholic Church.

Language

There are over 1,500 dialects in the Italian language. Other languages spoken include Albanian, Arabic, French, Spanish, and Sardo. The gesture for "no" is palm up with the fingers motioning inward. Dialects, subtle gestures, and double meanings make up the nuances of the Italian language. Frequent quick eye contact and touch are common.

Family Roles

The family is of great importance to the Italian. The father is said to be the head of the household, with the mother the "heart." Men are very attached to their mother (*mammismo*). Italians are physically demonstrative, gesture frequently, and stand close when talking. The elderly are beginning to live on their own, but it is not uncommon for several generations to live together. Italians protect their family and view familial obligations seriously, as those of honor. Out-of-wedlock pregnancy is viewed with disdain. Individual achievement is of secondary importance to the family, and bragging about achievements is considered rude behavior.

Health Care

Italy provides a government-run national health service. Health care funds are limited, and there are long waits and shortages of hospital bed space. Many pay out-of-pocket for private medical care. Medications are sold in drug stores, and pharmacists are qualified to treat minor injuries and illnesses. Drug stores take turns being open all night and on Sundays. People living in more rural areas, however, may have considerable difficulty obtaining services.

Traditionally, Italians view illness as a result of many factors. The people believe that illness and disability are caused by God's will. Cold drafts are felt to be responsible for colds that lead to pneumonia. Many believe that surgery will worsen their condition because the air will spread disease. Conversely, they also believe that fresh air maintains wellness. There is great concern over contamination, with the reluctance to visit or eat with someone who is ill. Some older generations believe that illness is caused by *malocchio* (evil eye) or *castiga* (curses). Many superstitions regarding pregnancy remain. Italian Americans allow their children to drink small amounts of wine.

In addition, there is a belief that illness is caused by suppression of stress and emotions. Italians are said to be more verbal in describing their symptoms than are other cultures. Prayers, tonic waters, healers, and home remedies may be tried before conventional medicine. Terminal illness is seen as God's will, and no life support measures are sought. Death is not discussed among family. Widows customarily wear black after their spouse's death, sometimes for their entire life.

The people of Italy have high rates of cardiovascular disease and stroke. G6PD enzyme deficiency and thalassemia syndromes are common. Congenital dislocation of the hip is common. Water supplies are not consistently safe. Disabled persons are mainstreamed into society with tutoring in the school system, and they receive a pension and full benefits of rehabilitation services. The mentally ill may live in special homes where they are trained to find employment, but they receive mixed acceptance in society. Physicians and therapists make house calls to the elderly. The majority of families care for the elderly in the home. Concern remains regarding long-term care of the elderly and children with severe disabilities.

Rehabilitation issues for the people of Italy include integration and the care of the mentally ill, providing respite and support for those with elderly family members, and their general avoidance of conventional medicine.

Germany

History and Economics

Germany is a culturally diverse country with large immigrant populations from Italy, Spain, and Greece. After World War II, ethnic Germans returned to what was left of Germany. The division of East and West Germany at the Berlin wall ended on October 3, 1990. Over 7 million Germans have immigrated to the United States since 1830 (Spector, 2000). Currently, 58 million Americans are of German ancestry (United States Census Bureau, 2003).

Homelessness, violence, alcoholism, and drug abuse plague Germany today. Unification brought increased taxes, budget deficits, housing shortages, and unemployment, because many left jobs in the East. The new market economy struggles. Social welfare and benefits are available.

Religion

Germany's churches are well funded by a small voluntary church tax. Churches have administrative responsibility and authority over schools, nursing homes, programs for the disabled, and hospitals. Businesses are closed on Sundays, since people are encouraged to observe a day of rest. Church attendance and influence are decreasing over time.

Former West Germans are 36% Protestant and 35% Roman Catholic. In former East Germany, 80% are Protestant, with the remaining Roman Catholic. Atheism was encouraged and taught in the former East Germany. Prior to the Holocaust, there were 530,000 people of Jewish descent living in Germany. The number today is around 105,000 (German Embassy, 2004). Continued anti-Semitism prevents many from returning to what they considered their homeland.

Language

There are dozens of dialects of the German language. People of German descent prefer to skip pleasantries and to discuss the issue at hand. They call people by title rather than name, with formal address expected until one is invited to use first names. To show respect, children often address their parents as "Sie," which is like saying Mr. or Mrs. in the United States. Germans are protective of their personal space and privacy, and touch is infrequent. The thumbs up sign may mean the number one.

Family Roles

Birth control is readily available, and in many urban areas, both spouses work and share household responsibilities. In the former Soviet East Germany, the government provided child care so that women could work. Germans are said to love order, keep a neat home, and have a strong work ethic. In rural areas of southern Germany, several generations live together. Unmarried couples are increasing; 25% of couples under age 35 years live together (German Embassy, 2004).

Health Care

Germans view health as a continuum, a state of well-being. Hard work, cleanliness, and staying warm aid in health maintenance. Stress and germs as well as drafts, unhappiness, and sedentary lifestyle are believed to cause illness. Many consult herbalists, take vitamins, or use homeopathy kits.

Many people seek only acute medical care. Socialized health care is available to all, but like consumers in the United States, Germans are not always happy with the limits on their choices of doctors and hospitals. Health promotion is gaining acceptance in this country. Alcohol use is a significant health problem and exceeds that of any other nation. Pertussis (whooping cough) is common in parts of former West Germany, as well as cardiovascular disease. The elderly are well cared for in Germany in their children's homes or in retirement communities.

The government supports family planning and sex education in the schools and media. The German Red Cross actively seeks out adolescents through mobile sex education classes. Contraception and sterilization are covered by insurance, and first trimester abortion is legal. In addition, oral contraception is free for women under age 20. Family planning clinics dispense contraception without a physician order. The adolescent birth rate was 12.5 per 1,000 compared with that of the United States at 43.7/1000 (Feijooi, 2004). Classes in prenatal care and childbirth are well attended.

Many patients do not ask questions because they perceive doing so as a challenge to the provider's authority. When dissatisfied with their care, they simply switch doctors. Germans are often stoic in response to pain.

Those with severe disabilities and the mentally ill reside in institutions where their expenses are paid by the socialized medical system. There is little adaptation such as curb cuts for those with a physical disability. Most children who are disabled are cared for in the home, and many participate in organized sports activities. Rehabilitation for those injured is purportedly excellent.

Rehabilitation challenges for the people of Germany include their hesitance to ask questions, protection of personal space and touch, and their beliefs about care of the handicapped and disabled.

Ireland

History and Economics

The desire for travel and the close proximity of Ireland to England led to the exploration of the Colonies before the American Revolution. The first-Irish to arrive were indentured servants, and others were kidnapped. It is interesting that the American Revolution gave the Irish people a chance to fight England, an opportunity that many did not pass up.

Ireland is a melting pot of Celtic people, along with English, Scottish, Welsh, French, Flemish, Norse, and German colonists. Ireland's population rapidly grew to 8.1 million people in 1841. Then the potato famine of 1845 caused a mass exodus of people to the

United States. In one tragic year, the famine and a cholera epidemic cut Ireland's population in half.

Great Britain ruled Ireland despite several unsuccessful revolts until 1922, when Northern Ireland joined England, Scotland, and Wales as the United Kingdom. The rest of Ireland became the Irish Free State, officially the Republic of Ireland, in 1949. The Republic of Ireland has a centralized, collectivist health care system based on need. Treatment for infectious disease, child health services, rehabilitation, and long-term care are free to everyone.

Irish women greatly outnumbered men immigrating to America. Much of Irish culture has not been passed on to descendants because many came without their families. Those who brought families did not settle in neighborhoods with other immigrants, because discrimination against the Irish in the United States was common in the 1800s.

Religion

Catholicism is the primary religion in Ireland. Controversy surrounds teaching contraception. Abstinence until marriage is promoted, and abortion remains illegal.

Language and Education

One-fourth of its inhabitants, mostly in the west and remote areas of Ireland, speak Irish. Almost all speak English. The Irish are well known for their articulate language and vast vocabularies. Limericks, puns, and riddles are shared and enjoyed. Schooling is free and compulsory for children age 6 to 15 years. Passing scores in three languages—English, Irish, and either French or German—is required for higher education.

Some English words have different meanings for the Irish. To describe someone as "homely" does not mean unattractive but as appreciative of hospitality. The Gaelic language has no words for "yes" and "no." Today Irish people are likely to say "it is so" for "yes." In order to avoid saying "no," one may hear "perhaps" or "we'll see." Holding up two fingers in a "V" with palm facing one's face is an obscene gesture.

Family Roles

The Irish have strong family ties and distinct roles. Traditionally, fathers rule the Irish family, whereas their wives care for household responsibilities. This tradition is evolving, with males taking on more home and child care responsibilities as women work outside the home. The traditional nuclear Irish family includes elderly parents in the home.

Modern Irish couples generally have two to three children. Older generations may have more than six children. Sexual relations are considered by some to be the woman's duty. Abstinence or the "rhythm" method is the usual form of birth control. Divorce was banned in Ireland until 1997 because of religious tenets and concern over division of land and businesses. Traditionally, property within a marriage was not viewed as shared.

Health Care

Fair complexions place the Irish at risk for skin cancer. Coal miners, who supply the country's heat, are at risk for respiratory disease and cancer. Social life revolves around pubs, where smoking is another health risk. Smoke-free businesses and smoking cessation programs are nonexistent. Drug abuse and rising crime rates are troubling problems in Ireland. Adolescent access to alcohol is gaining media attention. Coronary heart disease, phenylketonuria (PKU), neural tube defects, smoking, and alcoholism are serious threats to the Irish. Homocystinuria and PKU, congenital errors of metabolism, may cause mental retardation.

Denial is a coping mechanism used by some Irish people who delay treatment until they are no longer able to work. The Irish tend to underestimate problems, preferring denial to healthful action. Many are stoic in response to pain and feel uncomfortable revealing personal details to health care providers.

Psychiatric problems, not often discussed openly, are described in more positive, holistic terms than in the United States. Patients with depression have a "wee problem coping," and schizophrenics are "on injections" (Pyatt, 1999). Suicide is sometimes described as a "misadventure." A child with profound mental retardation is diagnosed with "severe learning disability."

Some Irish wear religious medals to ward off illness and utilize folk remedies, such as teas, cold compresses, and homeopathy before medical treatment is sought. Use of chiropractors and bathing in essential oils is used for joint pain. The Irish believe that illness is caused by stress, improper diet, lack of exercise, and obesity. Political tensions remain high, and some rural patients may fear being cared for by a provider of another religion.

Pregnancy is a special time for the Irish woman. She is careful to eat a balanced diet, believing that not doing so will cause her baby to be deformed, and receives regular prenatal care. Experiencing a tragedy during pregnancy is believed to cause congenital anomalies. As in other countries, there are long waits for government medical care.

Rehabilitation challenges for the people of Ireland include avoidance of health care until employment is affected, reluctance to share feelings and symptoms, and avoidance of confrontation. These patients will be reluctant to tell the provider that they do not agree with the plan of care.

United Kingdom

History and Economics

The United Kingdom consists of England, Scotland, Wales, and Northern Ireland. It has a rich history and plays a major role in the United Nations, maintaining peace in Europe. However, within its own borders, armed conflict continues between Ulster (Northern Ireland) and Ireland.

Public assistance with housing is available with a move toward private home ownership. Welfare and pension programs are in place. The monetary system is changing, with the United Kingdom leading the transition to the Euro as the universal form of currency in Europe.

Religion

In the United Kingdom, almost all faiths are represented. Freedom of religion is law, but fighting continues between Catholic Irish and Protestant Irish because of disparate political beliefs. The Protestant Irish took the name of Scotch Irish to indicate their loyalty. The official churches of the United Kingdom are the Church of England and the Church of Scotland, where church attendance is high.

Homosexuality and abortion are said to be less shocking to those in the United Kingdom than in the United States. Teen birth rates in England and Wales are the highest in Western Europe.

Language and Education

English is the official language spoken in the United Kingdom. In Scotland, Scottish Gaelic, a type of Celtic language, is still spoken. In Northern Ireland, Irish is spoken as a second language. In Wales, one-fourth speak Welsh. Britain has one of the highest rates of literacy in the world.

Religious education and worship are part of one's education. Schools are divided by religion, with very few children attending integrated schools. All children regardless of ability are included in the classroom setting. Education is partially funded by the parliamentary government. Students who perform well in school can get grants to advance their education.

Family Roles

Divorce, separation, and births to unmarried couples are rising. Of interest, Britain has the world's highest vasectomy rate. Women in England receive their full salary paid so that they can stay home for three months before birth and three months after birth. In addition, families receive child support that is not income-based so that all mothers can stay home with their children. Fathers are typically the heads of the household. The people tend to be less physically demonstrative than in other countries.

Health Care

The United Kingdom has a socialized medical system that is undergoing change to what resembles managed care systems. All hospitals are public, with each patient's primary physician acting as a health care gatekeeper. Medical care is quite modern and is free to all, with some charges for medications, dentures, and eyeglasses. Children, as well as elderly, unemployed, disabled, and pregnant individuals, are exempt from fees. Many patients pay out-of-pocket for their medical bills to avoid long waiting lists and the opportunity to choose their own health care provider.

Northern Ireland has the highest death rates from coronary heart disease in the United Kingdom and for men throughout the world. Health promotion activities in the United Kingdom are increasing, but most people seek only acute care. Food safety regulated by a new agricultural agency has received much attention. Cystic fibrosis and tuberculosis are significant respiratory health threats. Use of complementary medicine such as acupuncture and chiropractic care is increasingly sought for some health problems. Communication with health care professionals is often guarded, and the people are sensible about illness and pain.

The disabled are treated with dignity, are taught to be as self-sufficient as possible, and receive disability benefits. The National Health Care system provides equipment such as wheelchairs and medicines free of charge. Full rehabilitation services are available. The elderly are respected and offered free movie and bus passes in England.

Rehabilitation issues for the people of the United Kingdom include strong feelings about religion and nationality, and the tendency for guarded communication and touch with strangers.

France

History and Economics

Native-born citizens make up most of France's people. They have a mixed heritage of Celtic, German, Scandinavian, and other groups. Over 5 million immigrants live in France (World Factbook, 2004). Minorities include people from Portugal, Algeria, Morocco, Italy, and Turkey. There is hostility toward immigrants from the former French colony of Algeria and from North Africa.

France is an agricultural and industrial nation with a presidential republic government. Many French live in cities in small apartments. The affluent own second homes in quiet country villages. France is the top travel destination in the world, with an estimated 77 million tourists in 2003.

Religion

The primary religion in France is Roman Catholic, with small numbers of Islamic, Protestant, and Judaic people. Church attendance is reportedly low, and there is separation of church and state. French people are said to be very private about their beliefs. The Roman Catholic Church remains against abortion and homosexuality.

Sex education in the school systems is comprehensive. Messages about "safe sex" are broadcast on television and in locations that teenagers frequent. Oral contraception is free to all women and available without a prescription. RU-486, a drug that induces abortion, is legal in France, but parental permission is required for abortion under age 18.

Language and Education

French is the language spoken, with many dialects blending German and English. Attempts are made to protect the French language from changes. It is important to the French to appear reserved, well spoken, and cultured. Speaking with one's hands in the pockets, especially to one's superior, is socially unacceptable. Direct eye contact and frequent touching are acceptable.

Many children in France begin school as early as age 2. There is compulsory education for children up to age 16. Many go on to further their education at universities, with varying degrees of program length and internships. Government assistance with education is income dependent.

Family Roles

Having children establishes families in France, and the family is the most important social unit. Extended families are close but do not live together. The elderly often live in nursing homes, which are not paid for by socialized medicine. The French touch frequently and stand close while talking. Kissing and a handshake on greeting are common.

Health Care

Patients in France have considerable freedom when choosing physicians and hospitals, and they can go directly to a specialist. Incentives for improving and monitoring care are in place. Patient satisfaction is an increasing expectation of the public. Activist groups lobby for improvement in care, and they spur research in preventative health.

Pollution is considered the cause of much respiratory illness in this country and is the focus of eradication measures. Laws prohibit smoking in most public buildings. Preventative health programs regarding substance abuse, smoking cessation, and weight loss are increasing. Prevalence rates of fetal alcohol syndrome are 2.3/1000 (Institute for Child Health Research, Stanley, 2004). There has been considerable improvement in food safety as well, after the recent epidemic of bovine encephalopathy in the United Kingdom.

Meetings with health care providers are formal; titles are important, and behavior is polite. First names are not used, but engaging in social conversation prior to history taking is acceptable. Logical reasons for treatments increase adherence to the plan of care. The French are comfortable with touch and direct eye contact.

Older generations avoid seeing a doctor and may prefer visiting a touch healer. Other complementary medicine is infrequent. Those with evident physical disabilities are a part of society holding jobs and utilizing readily available physical therapy. Wheelchair accessibility is increasing with the design and construction of new buildings and adapted vehicles. However, as in much of Europe, people with mental illness are often institutionalized.

Rehabilitation challenges for the people of France include a reserved style of communication and a preference for the formal style with providers, limitations of insurance programs, and the stigma of mental illness.

Cross-Cultural Communication
in the United States

An estimated 8% of the people living in poverty in the United States are of European heritage (United States Census Bureau, 2003). When offering rehabilitation services, one cannot forget that poverty is a greater influence on the health behaviors of a given community than is culture alone. Even free services are costly when the patient misses a day of employment and pays for child-care expenses and transportation. The new immigrant to the United States may be living in older substandard housing exposed to high rates of crime.

Use of health care resources among many cultures is community- and family-focused. This characteristic must be taken into consideration when working with people from varying backgrounds. The collective needs of the group are often placed above individual needs. In poorer countries, funds are available only to those most likely to recover and return to society as an income-producing, tax-paying member. Conflict over decision making and use of limited funds may present real challenges for the health care provider.

Awareness of word choice and cultural diversity, individual past experience and knowledge, personality characteristics, and presence of support are essential. Because there is wide variation among ethnic groups, knowledge of place of birth, length of stay in the United States, and languages spoken and read are key pieces of information. Thus, cultural assessment is a part of a thorough needs assessment, including health maintenance practices. This information is incorporated into each individualized plan of care.

When communicating with clients in the rehabilitation setting, the health care provider is aware of the verbal and nonverbal language used during interactions. Interpreters should be utilized when appropriate (guidelines are included in the Appendix).

The provider considers the differences between client values and perception of their needs and seeks to understand the reasons for nonadherence, and renegotiates a plan of care together. Beliefs about disability and rehabilitation vary tremendously; in many European countries, the disabled and infirm are housed in institutions and are unseen by society. Disability may be viewed as punishment. Others believe that it is a blessing. The person with strong religious beliefs may feel chosen by God to care for a special child, and because the child is a "gift," there may be low expectations for self-care. This outlook may contrast with the belief that one should function at the highest level possible that is held by many Americans.

The health care provider needs to ask what the person has done for the health problem and what the person believes was the cause. Providers should address the person formally and inquire as to the correct pronunciation of the client's name. Identification of the family's decision-maker and inclusion of that person in the planning and implementation of care are essential. Finally, the provider encourages family involvement and questions, and also invites family members to sit or stand where they are comfortable, observing for cues regarding eye contact and touch.

The cultural information presented in this chapter offers a broad overview of several European countries, providing a glimpse of the adaptations required of newly arrived immigrants to the United States. As time passes, each cultural group retains certain beliefs, values, and behaviors while adapting and blending into the new culture. The clinician does well to consider this information in light of individual differences in response to illness and rehabilitation.

Summary

This chapter has discussed the European Americans as the largest cultural group in the United States. The European American immigration patterns to the United States, cultural belief systems, and their health care features and issues are described with specific references to a number of countries in the continent. The importance of cross-cultural communication with European clients in the health care system is followed by questions and case studies.

Questions

1. In a class discussion, consider what the student should do when the plan of care conflicts with the cultural beliefs and values of the client.
2. A new student from another country remarks that his professor has shortened his name because it was too difficult to pronounce. The student shrugs his shoulders and smiles. Do you feel that this situation is acceptable?
3. Draw a diagram of at least three generations of your own family, detailing their place of birth, gender, education, vocation, significant accidents and illnesses, genetic history, age at time of death, and cause of death. Circle family members sharing a home. Describe your relationship with extended family members. How are decisions made? How does the family have fun together? What is the ethnic or cultural background of the family? In what way is this background apparent in the family's way of living? What are the religious beliefs of the family? What are the dominant health beliefs of the family, and how do they affect health status? Do relatives want to be involved in health decision making?
4. Study your local newspaper. How are minorities represented? What cultural events are offered?
5. Attend a religious ceremony intended for a particular culture different from your own, and record your impressions. In class, discuss the differences you noted.
6. Cardiovascular disease is the leading cause of death for Americans and an estimated half of all deaths in European countries. Develop a health promotion plan for newly arrived immigrants, utilizing the communication principles you have learned, and offer specific information related to your field of study. Include in your plan the location for the best influence on this group's behaviors. Videotape each student teaching plan, and objectively evaluate your classmates' performance and plan.

Working with Interpreters

- Care must be taken when choosing an interpreter. Confidentiality is an issue to consider when utilizing family members and friends.

- Be alert to gender, socioeconomic, and age differences. An older interpreter of the same gender is preferred. Avoid interpreters from rival countries.
- Determine before you begin whether you want every word translated or just a summary of the conversation from the interpreter.
- Allow the interpreter time to develop rapport as well as closure at the end of an interview. Ask the interpreter for his or her assessment, since one may miss culturally significant nonverbal communication.
- Be aware that some of your conversation with the interpreter may be understood.
- Maintain appropriate eye contact with the person while asking questions.
- Hospitals and universities may have lists of available interpreters.

Suggestions for When an Interpreter Is Not Available

- Keep conversation simple; ask one question at a time and in the proper sequence.
- Use formal address, smile pleasantly, and speak slowly in a low tone. Speaking louder will not help the person understand.
- Use words that you know in the person's language. He or she will appreciate your attempts.
- Explain why you are asking the questions and how it will benefit the person.
- Verify learning by having the person repeat teaching.
- Pictures and pantomiming are useful tools in communicating.
- Determine whether the person knows another language. Many Europeans know multiple languages.
- Keep in mind that dominant language is often used during stressful situations.
- Develop patient education material in other languages.

(Andrews & Boyle, 1999)

Case Study 1

Mr. Koulomas is a 70-year-old immigrant from Greece referred for physical therapy after sustaining a hip fracture. He fell while shoveling his sidewalk. He is hard of hearing with arthritic hands. He waited several hours before calling for assistance because of embarrassment and a general mistrust of health care providers. He never married because American women "do not respect and obey their husbands here." He is concerned about leaving his 91-year-old mother unattended in his home and is inattentive to your teaching efforts. Your treatment plan includes learning to walk and dress, using adaptive equipment.

Questions

1. How would one best address the needs of Mr. Koulomas?
2. List all the reasons, other than noncompliance, that you feel contribute to his inattentiveness.
3. What additional resources would you utilize?

Case Study 2

Hanna Kaja is an 85-year-old first-generation immigrant from Wroclaw, Poland. She has come to America to join her children. She speaks no English. Her tuberculin test is positive >15 mm. She has no symptoms and received a BCG vaccine years ago.

Questions

1. What approach would most likely encourage her to comply with the treatment regimen for tuberculosis?
2. How would you collaborate with the health department in the care of Mrs. Kaja?
3. Discuss the issue of confidentiality and the use of interpreters.

Case Study 3

You are caring for a child with significant developmental delays and a seizure disorder. A large number of family members and friends are present. The mother reports through an interpreter that the child has frequent bouts with pneumonia. On examination you notice multiple round bruises on the child's back. You suspect abuse.

Questions

1. What health care practices cause unusual skin markings?
2. How would you broach the subject with the family? Use role-play to come up with a solution.

Suggested Reading

Anderson, N. (1995). European nursing: Different values. *Nursing Times 91* (42), 42–3.

Andrews, M. (1998). Transcultural perspectives in nursing administration. *The Journal of Nursing Administration 28* (11), 30–8.

Bitter, I. (2000). Mental disorders and economic change—the example of Hungary. *Bulletin of the World Health Organization 78*(4), 505.

Blunt, E. (1993). Emergency nursing in Poland. *Emergency Nursing 19*(6), 22A–30A.

Boros, M. (1998). Letters from Hungary. *Special Delivery 21*(3), 20.

Centers for Disease Control and Prevention (CDC) (2000). Prevalence of cigarette smoking among secondary school students—Budapest, Hungary, 1995 and 1999. *Journal of American Medical Association 283*(24), 3190.

Charles, J. (1992). Midwifery: Hungary for change. *Nursing Times 88*(9), 36–8.

Corduff, E. (1997). Invisible exports. *Nursing Times 93*(11), 28–31.

Davidhizar, R., Bechtel, G., & Giger, J. N. (1998). A model to enhance culturally competent care. *Hospital Topics 76*(2), 22–31.

Giger, J. N., & Davidhizer, R. E. (1999). Transcultural nursing: Assessment and intervention (3rd ed.). St. Louis: Mosby Year Book, Inc.

Giger, J. N., Davidhizar, R., & Poole, V. L. (1997). Health promotion among ethnic minorities: The importance of cultural phenomena. *Rehabilitation Nursing 22*(6), 303–7.

Grahn, G., Danielson, M., & Ulander, K. (1999). Learning to live with cancer in European countries. *Cancer Nursing 22*(1), 79–84.

Groce, N. E. (1999). Health beliefs and behavior towards individuals with disability cross-culturally. In R. Leavitt (Ed.), *Cross cultural rehabilitation: An international perspective.* London: W. B. Saunders Co.

Haradon, G. (1999). A cross-cultural immersion in post-communist Romania. In R. Leavitt (Ed.), *Cross cultural rehabilitation: An international perspective.* London: W. B. Saunders Co.

Henderson, C. W. (1998). Hungary law ends anonymity for AIDS sufferers. *AIDS Weekly Plus.* Electronic collection A20153822.

Henderson, C. W. (1998). Pediatrics Romania probes child HIV infections for first time. *AIDS Weekly Plus.* Electronic collection A53288402.

Henderson, C. W. (2000). Poland TB rate twice that of European Union. *TB & Outbreaks Week.* NewsRx.com. Electronic collection A63988492.

Kagawa-Singer, M. (1994). Cross cultural views of disability. *Rehabilitation Nursing 19* (6), 362–5.

Knutson, L. M., Leavitt, R. L., & Sarton, K. R. (1995). Race, ethnicity, and other factors influencing children's health and disability: Implications for pediatric physical therapists. *Pediatric Physical Therapy 7*(4), 175–82.

Kovac, C. (1999). Hungarians spurn private health insurance. *British Medical Journal 318* (7195), 1370.

Lack, T. (1999). Water and health in Europe: An overview. *British Medical Journal 318* (7199), 1678.

Lakey, C., Kenneally, P., Wolf, K., & Leuner, J. D. (1995). Romania: A nursing journey. *Nursing and health care: Perspectives on Community 16*(3), 144–7.

Lee, M. C., & Essoka, G. (1998). Patient's perception of pain: Comparison between Korean-American and Euro-American obstetric patients. *Journal of Cultural Diversity 5*(1), 29–37.

Leininger, M. (1995). *Transcultural nursing: Concepts, theories, research, and practice.* New York: McGraw-Hill, Inc.

Long, P. (2000). Multicultural care: Meeting the challenge. *Advance for Nurse Practitioners 8*(5), 79–80.

Luckmann, J. (1999). *Transcultural communication in nursing.* New York: Delmar Publishers.

McGinn, P. R. (1997). War weary Croatia charts a slow course to privatization, hoping to learn from others' mistakes. *American Medical News 40*(46), 9–12.

Moore, M. L. (2000). Adolescent pregnancy rates in three European countries: Lessons to be learned? *Journal of Obstetric, Gynecologic, and Neonatal Nursing 29*(4), 355–62.

National Center for the Dissemination of Disability Research (NCDDR) (1999). *Disability, diversity, and dissemination: Cultural and other considerations that can influence effectiveness within the rehabilitation system.* United States Department of Education, Washington, DC.

Papadopoulos, I. (1999). Health and illness beliefs of Greek Cypriots living in London. *Journal of Advanced Nursing 29*(5), 1097–1104.

Qureshi, B. (1994). *Transcultural medicine: Dealing with patients from different cultures* (2nd ed.). United Kingdom: Kluwer Academic Publishers, Dordrecht, Netherlands.

Simunec, D. (1995). Letter from Croatia. *Nursing Times 91*(34), 149.

Smart, J. F., & Smart, D. W. (1995). The use of translators/ interpreters in rehabilitation. *The Journal of Rehabilitation 61*(2), 14–7.

Stanley, F. (2004). Institute for Child Health Research. [On line]. Available: http://www .pediatric-neurology-paris,org, Paris, France.

United States Department of Immigration (2002). *Immigrants admitted by region and selected country of birth.* [On line]. Available: http://www.ins.usdoj.gov

United States Department of State, Bureau of European Affairs (2004). [On line]. Available: http://www.state.gov

Voelker, R. (1998). France and United Kingdom channel efforts to improve health services. *The Journal of American Medical Association 280*(8), 681–91.

Ward-Collins, D. (1998). Noncompliant: Isn't there a better way to say it? *American Journal of Nursing 98*(5), 27–31.

Welsh, J. (1994). Volunteering in Croatia. *Canadian Nurse 90*(5), 51–3.

Wilson, S. A. (1998). Irish Americans. In L. D. Purnell & B. J. Paulanka (Eds.). *Transcultural health care: A culturally competent approach.* Philadelphia: F.A. Davis Company.

World Factbook. (2004). [On line]. Available: http://www.odci.gov/cia/publications/factbook /geos

World Health Organization (1997). Health in Europe. [On line]. Available: http://www .who.dk/cpa/cpa.htm

References

Ajdukovic, M. (1998). Displaced adolescents in Croatia: Sources of stress and posttraumatic stress reaction. *Adolescence 33*(129), 209–19.

Andrews, M. M., & Boyle, J. S. (1999). *Transcultural concepts in nursing care* (3rd ed.). Philadelphia: Lippincott, Williams, & Wilkins.

Feijoo, A. (2004). Adolescent sexual health in Europe and the United States: Why the difference? [On line]. Available: http://www,advocatesforyouth.org

Galanti, G. A. (1997). *Caring for patients from different cultures* (2nd ed.). Philadelphia: University of Pennsylvania Press.

German Embassy, Washington DC (2004). [On line]. Available: http://www.germany-info.org

Gozdziak, E. M. (1996). Eastern Europeans. In D. W. Hairies (Ed.), *Refugees in America in the 1990's*. Westport, Connecticut: Greenwood Press.

Inouye, A. (2000). Unpublished interview.

Kulczycki, A., Potts, M., & Rosenfield, A. (1996). Abortion and fertility regulation. *The Lancet 347* (9016), 1663–6.

Mollica, R. F., McInnes, K., Sarajlic, N., Lavelle, J., Sarajlic, I., & Massagli, M. P. (1999, August 4). Disability associated with psychiatric comorbidity and health status in Bosnian refugees living in Croatia. *The Journal of the American Medical Association 282*(5), 433.

Pyatt, R. (1999). An internship in Ireland. *American Journal of Nursing 99*(7), 18, 20.

Roupas, F. G. (2000). Unpublished interview.

Slowikowski, C. (2000). Unpublished interview.

Spector, R. E. (2004). *Cultural diversity in health and illness* (6th ed.). New Jersey: Prentice Hall.

Tripp-Reimer, T., & Sorofman, B. (1998). Greek Americans. In L. D. Purnell, & B. J. Paulanka (Eds.), *Transcultural health care: A culturally competent approach*. Philadelphia: F. A. Davis Company.

United States Census Bureau. (2004). *International database.* [On line]. Available: http://www.census.gov

United States Census Bureau (2003). *Trends in immigration and the foreign born population.* [On line]. Available: http://www.census.gov

Wikipedia Encyclopedia (2002). [On line]. Available: http://en.wikipedia.org/

Appendix

Country	Population	Birth rate per 1,000	Infant Mortality per 1,000 Live Births	Life Expectancy from Birth	Percentage, Living Below Poverty Line
Croatia	4,496,869	9.51	6.96	74.14	*
France	60,424,213	12.34	4.31	75.8	6.5
Germany	82,424,609	8.45	4.2	78.54	*
Greece	10,647,529	10.08	5.63	78.94	*
Hungary	10,032,375	9.77	8.68	72.25	8.6
Ireland	3,969,558	14.47	5.5	77.36	10
Italy	58,057,477	9.05	6.07	79.54	*
Poland	38,626,349	10.64	8.73	74.16	18.4
Romania	22,355,551	10.69	27.24	71.12	44.5
United Kingdom	60,270,708	10.88	5.22	78.27	17
United States	293,027,571	14.13	6.63	77.43	12

*Current information is not available.

Source: U.S. Bureau of the Census and World Factbook (2004).

Note: A special thanks to the following people for their willingness to share their stories: Mary Ahearn, Frank Budzisz, Clemence Dubos, Klaus Guertler, Alice Inouye, Norbert Jausovec, Antonija Katusic, Chris Lekowski, Laura Mays, Tim Minnick, Hannah Pike, Lisi Robinson, Frank Roupas, Jack Slowikowski, Mladenka Tkalcic, Frank Williams, and Nancy Wingfield.

6

African Americans

Shirley Blanchard and Cynthia Jenkins

Key Words

African American   culture   rehabilitation
cross-cultural studies   illness beliefs

Objectives

1. Identify how cultural beliefs and practices of African Americans may influence interaction with rehabilitation providers.
2. Describe strategies for developing cutural competency in working with African Amercan clients.
3. Discuss reasons for health care disparities that may exist for African Americans.

Introduction

Effective rehabilitation with African Americans is most likely to occur when rehabilitation practitioners are willing to be respectful of and sensitive to the important differences that may exist between themselves and their clients in terms of their worldviews, historical legacies, and culturally sanctioned medical practices and beliefs. Differences between practitioner and client on any of these dimensions lend the possibility for conflict in communication and thus for potential hindrances in the healing processes. Therefore, practitioners should have at least a rudimentary understanding and familiarity with culturally sanctioned experiences, practices, and beliefs that may be of importance to African Americans. Practitioners should also be aware that just as there may be differences between themselves and their African American clients, as Americans there might be a large degree of similarity in terms of beliefs, experiences, and health practices. With added insight, the practitioner may develop an understanding of the client's needs, fears, and strengths that will aid in facilitating communication and developing appropriate treatments that support the healing process.

There are specific reasons why looking at the cultural experiences, traditional beliefs, and worldview of African Americans are important to rehabilitation. First, it is important to understand the unique challenges that African Americans have experienced during their unwilling transportation to this country and their ongoing search for respect, equality, and voice in the United States. There have been many challenges that African Americans have faced in the health care arena that run the gamut from not being able to receive adequate treatment because of race, to having difficulty accessing treatment because of poverty, and having fear of the established medical practices and practitioners (Wilson, 1999).

When working with African Americans, practitioners must acknowledge that race-related attitudes are embedded in everyone, indirectly and directly influencing how individuals are conceptualized and treated. Practitioners must define the degree to which societal norms either support or sabotage the work that they do with African American clients. They, then, must work toward ameliorating the impact on negative perceptions on the healing processes of their African American clients (West, 1993; Wilson, 1999).

At the very least, practitioners must acknowledge that historically, African Americans have been formally discriminated against and treated as second-class citizens. The residuals of slavery remain alive for African Americans, but the impact of this social experience affects all Americans. Even if only operating on a very low level of awareness for many health clinicians, societal racism influences the interaction of clinicians and clients. Health practitioners must make every effort to guard against allowing their prejudices and stereotypes to negatively taint their interactions with client (Purnell & Paulanka, 1998). In addition, clinicians should also understand and hopefully learn to appreciate the unique strengths of their African American clients and the way that these strengths can aid them in assisting the client to a higher level of health and functioning.

Because of the distrust bred through historical experiences with health care, many African Americans have continued to rely on traditional medical practices and beliefs that have been handed down through the generations. Health care practitioners wanting to deliver services and provide rehabilitation to African Americans must be aware of these traditional beliefs and practices. Smart (2001), Snow (1978), and Spector (2000) suggested that practitioners who ignore the traditional medical practices used by their clients may elicit responses such as ignoring prescribed treatment, misusing treatment, complaining about the quality of care they receive, and seeking treatment through alternative methods of healing.

Aiding in the healing processes of those from a culture that differs from our own can be made more successful if the health practitioner has at least a rudimentary understanding of potential differences in the worldview held by African American cultural members. Worldview refers to how one perceives and understands factors in life such as human nature, families, social relationships, time, space, and locus of control (Okun, Fried, & Okun, 1999). According to James-Myers (1991), because of differences in worldview, dissimilar attributions regarding a client's problems may be most likely to occur in those therapy encounters in which the practitioner and the client are of different cultural backgrounds. Therefore, successful diagnosis, treatment, and prognosis can depend on the practitioner and client, at least developing a mutual respect for the other's knowledge and beliefs about how best to accomplish the healing process.

If practitioners can elicit the patient's or family's understanding of the illness up front, they could discover reasons for mistrust or other factors that may adversely affect the healing relationship and the quality of care. Should adverse beliefs or conflicts in values occur, the practitioner ought to be prepared to acknowledge the differences and should reassure patients and caregivers that all reasonable options will be considered and that treatment plans will be client centered.

Background

How Many African Americans Are There in the United States?

Census 2000 showed that of the 281.4 million people in the United States, 36.4 million, or 12.9%, reported as black or African American. This number includes 34.7 million people, or 12.3%, who reported only black in addition to 1.8 million people, or 0.6%, who reported black as well as one or more other races (Census Brief, August 2001).

Who Are African Americans?

In the United States, the African American population consists primarily of African Americans, although sizable numbers of African and African Caribbean immigrants have become part of this group in the last 15 years. African Americans were initially brought to America from Africa as indentured servants, and they were treated in a similar fashion as European and Native American indentured servants. They first landed in Jamestown, Virginia, beginning in 1619. However, by 1661, because of the escalating demand for tobacco and cotton crops, there grew a need for consistent workers who could handle the climate and the work (Europeans and Native Americans were found to be unsuitable); therefore, Virginians legislated the "perpetual servitude" of Africans into slavery (Jones, 1997). Africans were no longer able to work off their indenture and to become freed persons. Thus began the history of slavery in the United States and the origin of the group known as African Americans.

Today, many African Americans are of mixed ancestry, including individuals with Caribbean, Native American, and European lineage. Approximately 5% of African Americans are foreign born, mainly French-speaking Haitians, Sudanese and other non-Spanish-speaking Caribbean people.

African Americans as a racial population are currently younger than the white population. Thirty-two percent of African Americans are under age 18, compared with 24 percent of whites. The median age (30 years) of the African American population in 2000 was 5 years younger than the U.S. population as a whole. African Americans are living longer than before, but still only 8% of the African American population are over the age of 65. In comparison, 14% of non-Hispanic whites were older than 65 in 2000 (Jones & Jackson, 2000).

The differences between whites and African Americans in terms of income are astounding. Black-to-white median income levels are much better for married-couple families, but significantly worse in single-parent families, which make up a greater proportion of African American than white families. Even in 1999, when the poverty rate for African Americans was the lowest ever, at 24%, this was still about three times greater than the poverty rate for non-Hispanic whites (8%).

Even when income levels by education are examined, there are still persistent differences between African Americans and whites. In 1970, college-educated African Americans made about two-thirds of what college-educated whites earned. In 2000, there are still differential earnings for college-educated African Americans and whites. The median income in 2000 for whites with a bachelor's degree or more was $41,700. For African Americans with a bachelor's degree or more, the median income was $36,600. Overall, important concerns regarding affluence and poverty status differences for African Americans and whites remain. These trends reinforce that there has been little improvement in the relative economic status of African Americans since the 1970s (Jones & Jackson, 2000).

Of this near 37.4 million people, approximately one-third, or 12.4 million, people are poor. Poverty is therefore a very pressing problem in the African American community. Individuals who are impoverished tend to suffer a series of negative social events. In the African American community, inadequate housing, unemployment, low levels of education, low access to health care, poor nutrition, and often risk-promoting lifestyle evidence this trend. According to the National Institute on Aging, it is important to recognize the affects of poverty on African American people not only for the reasons previously mentioned but also because of the long term consequences. They state, "Poor people tend to concentrate on day-to-day survival and often develop a sense of hopelessness and powerlessness. These and other factors have diminished their overall survival" (National Institute on Aging, 1999–2000, p. 3).

Where Do African Americans Reside?

When the Emancipation Proclamation was signed, less than 8% of the African American population lived in the Northeast or Midwest. However, today, according to Jones and Jackson (2000), the majority of the African American population lives in the South (54%). About 19% of African Americans live in the Northeast, as well as the Midwest (19%). Only 8% live in the West. The five states with the largest African American populations in 2000 were New York (3.2 million), Texas (2.5 million), Florida (2.3 million) Georgia (2.2 million), and California (1.5 million). Most African Americans (53%) also live inside the central cities of metropolitan areas. In 2000, 35% of African Americans lived in the suburbs (outside the central city in metropolitan areas).

What Religions Do African Americans Practice?

Spirituality and respect for elders is an integral part of African tradition. African Americans practice the three main monotheistic religions, as well as Eastern and African religions. The predominant faith is Christian; the second largest group of believers accept the ancestral religions of Africa—Vodun, Santeria, Myal—and a third group of followers practice Islam. Judaism and Buddhism are also practiced by some people within the community (Purnell & Paulanka, 1998). According to Jones (1972), some of the cultural aspects of the African religion may seem magical and mysterious, but much of it was also pragmatic, secular, and family-oriented. Overall, it enabled people to cope with their environment.

Concepts of Time and Space

Cultural variations in time and space can also have an impact on positive communications and interactions. People tend to react negatively by taking personal offense when others violate their beliefs and perceptions of these two dimensions of human interaction. It is important for practitioners to recognize their own conceptions of time and space and the way that they feel and react when others do not adhere to them. Communicating how the practitioner interprets these violations offers clients the opportunity to describe his or her experience of time and space and/or the opportunity for clients to offer reasons for their actions. It also offers both parties the opportunity to come to an agreement on how these should be handled in the future by both.

Concepts of Time

Time is often considered to be linear among Western thinkers. In other words, past, present, and future occur in this succession. Those of African descent consider time and deadlines to be a lot more flexible than those who work by the Western concept of time. African Americans tend to have what is called a "present time orientation." This does not mean that they do not recognize the past or the future, but living in the present is more important to them. Their concept of the future may also be different from the Anglo concept, and conflict is likely to occur in interactions with white middle-class people, for whom time is very specific. In a hospital setting, for instance, patients and staff members may operate on different "time clocks," causing confusion and resentment for all involved (Galanti, 1997).

African Americans often consider "CP time" (colored people time—as it's known among African Americans) when making schedules. Samovar and Porter (1995) refer to this as "hang loose" time. They know that if they schedule a gathering for 7 P.M., people will arrive by 7:30. Flexibility in scheduling is important not because African Americans don't respect time but because there are other environmental factors that may come into play that mitigate arriving on time. Also, they assume that their hosts will understand this situation or that even the hosts themselves will be late in preparing the festivities.

CP time is directly related to present time orientation because worrying about being somewhere else in the future and on time may be secondary in importance to what one is doing in the present. Nobles (1980) clarified that the African American treatment of time grows out of the African perspective on time, which is that time is a subjective phenomenon, so that the likelihood that one would feel compelled to impose his or her time perspective on others is reduced in the African system. Time for the Africans consists of experiences, and the way in which one experiences time is through his or her life. For Africans, time is not a commodity to be bought and sold or by which to be controlled. And, further, the future is contained in the present. Thus, it's not that the future isn't important; it is, but it's not more important than that life that is being lived in the present.

There is also another factor that makes lateness of appointments understandable when African Americans attend medical meetings. Many African Americans have to wait inordinate amounts of time when attending doctors' meetings, particularly in large cities. Doctors themselves often fail to see a patient at the patient's scheduled time. In many inner-city hospitals that serve low-income individuals, it is not uncommon that patients may have to wait three or four hours before seeing a physician. Therefore, being a few minutes late for an appointment may not seem to be a problem.

Concept of Space

African Americans' use of personal space has received only limited study in the past ten years. However, past research by Willis (1966) found that African Americans greeted other African Americans at greater distances than whites. Willis's research also revealed that whites greet blacks at further distances than they greet other whites. Baxter (1970) reported that among three groups, African Americans stand farther apart, followed by whites and then Mexican Americans. In 1995, Samovar and Porter reported that people from collectivistic subcultures in the United States, such as Latinos, African Americans, and Native Americans, tend to stand closer together when they are interacting with each other. However, they tend to stand farther apart when interacting with members of different cultures. For the rehabilitation professional, this information suggests that African Americans may be uncomfortable with up-close intrusions into their personal space unless a purpose for it is announced or discussed before movement toward them is made.

Language, Patterns of Interaction, and Communication

Not only does culture influence the behavior and thinking of individuals, but it also influences an individual's manner of expression and language. African Americans have characteristic linguistic and communication patterns that instead of being celebrated, have more often been stereotyped negatively by television, by the American educational system, and through other media.

Although the dominant language among African Americans is English, language used by African Americans may include the use of black dialects and pidgins, which reflect the various native African languages and languages of other cultures. Linguists define Black English as a hybrid language. It contains elements of Standard English, West African languages, and "elements manifesting the uniqueness of the African American experience in this country" (Smitherman, 1991). Black English, or Ebonics, is considered the language of the descendants of Africans who were enslaved in America. According to Boyd (1997), inner-city Black English vernacular has grammatical structures "genetically" traceable to a seventeenth-century pidgin English. Some grammatical aspects of this pidgin English—for example, its tense system and gender classes—may be "genetically" traceable to the great Niger-Congo family of languages spoken by the ancestors and distant cousins of today's African-Americans. For example, according to Smith (as cited in Boyd, 1997), certain sound configurations don't even exist in African languages. They tend to follow a very definite "C-V" pattern, or consonant/vowel pattern. In other words, when black speakers encounter European words that end in "st" or "ft" or "ld" or "nd," these are consonant clusters that are not African configurations. So, in words like "west," "test," "best," Africans will say "wes," "tes," and "bes." When they encounter "land," "hand," "band," and "sand," they will say "lan," "han," "ban," and "san." The final consonant is not being dropped, deleted, omitted, or reduced; it never existed in the first place. Therefore, what many may consider to be "bad" English for African Americans may actually be the retention of the African phonology among African Americans.

Speech may be accompanied by animated nonverbal gestures (i.e., hand movements, touching, etc.). The voice may become louder with excitement or other emotions, and gestures more animated, behavior that is sometimes mistaken for aggressiveness or anger. There is a great deal of creativity and flexibility used by African Americans in their verbal expressions (Jones, 1991), and many of these expressions have entered the common parlance of American society. Phrases such as "you go, girl" and "talk to the hand" are examples of the creativity with language.

The call and response patterns of language used in African American churches and potentially in any setting with an audience (e.g., movie theaters) should not be taken as rudeness. In the African American church, the congregation responds to the minister with enthusiastic spiritual responses and words of encouragement and agreement such as "Amen" and "preach." African Americans often respond during the course of a conversation verbally with "all right," "say it," "I hear ya," and so forth. The verbalizations are seen as the person's understanding and following closely the course of the conversation.

The significance of understanding language patterns in African Americans is underscored by a study conducted by Johnson, Saha, Arbelaez, Beach, and Cooper (2004) that found that African Americans believe that they are treated unfairly and with disrespect in the health care system on the basis of the way they speak English. They stated the following: "This lends support to the assertion that cultural differences between African Americans and their predominantly white physicians exist, regardless of language concordance. Perhaps, in subtle ways, not only Hispanics and Asians, but also African Americans, are given a message that aspects of their culture, including the way they speak English, are not looked upon favorably in the health care system" (p. 108). Therefore, it is likely that if African Americans perceive that the way they speak is either amusing to or looked down upon by the health care provider, they are less likely to attempt further or consistent communication of their needs.

Patterns of African American Families

The number of African American families is increasing. There were 8.7 million African American families in 2000. About half (48%) of all African American families today are married-couple families, a decline from 68% in 1970. Most other African American families in 2000 (44%) were maintained by women (Census Brief, August 2001).

Within the African American population, one can find various arrangements that constitute family. Thus, people may speak of family, aunts, uncles, fathers, mothers, and children without necessarily meaning that there is a genetic kinship. In general, African Americans love children and believe that those who have many children are fortunate. It is not uncommon to find families with more than four children. The head of household is frequently female. Along with cultural patterns carried over from Africa, challenges to survival due to poverty, racism, and other societal factors has necessitated reliance on networks of individuals to keep the family going. For instance young children are often raised in the households of their grandparents. The terms "sister," "bro," "cuz," "momma," and "'play' aunt" have developed as a response to solidarity and familiarity.

Among African American men age 15 and over in 2000, 45% had never been married, 39% were currently married, 3% were widowed and 10% were divorced. Among African American women, the corresponding rates were 42%, 31%, 10%, and 12% (Jones & Jackson, 2000).

Divorce is the end result for 2 out of 3 African American marriages. African American couples are three times more inclined than whites to get separated during the marriage. Divorced and separated persons are likely to experience physiological and psychological health problems. African American men, in particular, have experienced increased psychological and physiological distress in conjunction with postdivorce reactions (Lawson & Thompson, 1995). These include irrational behavior, postdivorce depression, suicide attempts, an increased use of drugs and alcohol, and a diminution of self-esteem and self-worth. Statistics reveal that the persons subject to divorce are most liable to crime, poor health, and violence (Minority Health Today, 2000).

Attitudes and Beliefs

When considering any type of interaction with an African American, the rehabilitation health professional has to be aware that African Americans, like any other marginalized group in American society, live in two worlds. They hold values, beliefs, and customs that are uniquely American, and they also hold values, beliefs, and customs that are particular to African culture. Sometimes these two worlds collide and cause conflict for an individual, but most African Americans learn to live in both worlds.

As Americans, the patient and the rehabilitation specialist will most likely share many of the same values. Hard work, sacrifice, and a decent family life are all important to African American families. In particular, education has been a primary value for African Americans over the years. Watkins, in the 1930s (as cited in Grief, Hrabowski, Freeman, & Maton, 2000) described the grandmother in the family: "In her youth, education was a symbol of great distinction and superiority and, although it is more widespread today, it still carries this connotation. She wants her grandchildren to be educated because of what it will mean to them socially and economically." However, many minority clients, although aware of the belief that "hard work equals success," "may also see the painful and stark reality of socioeconomic oppression, racism, and homophobia as significant contributors to many of their problems" (Redmond & Slaney, 2002, p. 852).

Boykin (1991) conceptualized the core cultural values of African Americans by articulating nine dimensions, which are briefly described as follows:

- *Spirituality:* Conducting one's life intuitively as though governed by supreme forces
- *Harmony:* Emphasizing versatility and wholeness
- *Movement:* Interweaving the ideas of rhythm often associated with music and dance into everyday life
- *Verve:* Preferring intense stimulation and action that are variable and colorful
- *Affect:* Placing a premium on feelings, emphasizing a special sensitivity to emotional cues, and cultivating emotional expression
- *Communalism:* Committing to the interdependence of people and to connectedness that esteems social bonds and responsibilities over individual privileges
- *Expressive individualism:* Cultivating a distinct personality and a proclivity for spontaneous, genuine personal expression
- *Orality:* Emphasizing oral and aural modes of communication
- *Social perspective of time:* Viewing time as a social phenomenon marked by human interaction and by the event shared by others

Parsons (2003) also has compiled research that suggests that African American core values may be different from the mainstream American values. Parsons describes these values as a black cultural ethos (BCE). She states the following:

> BCE esteems the intuitive whereas mainstream culture highly regards the material or the physical. Wherein the dominant culture emphasizes dichotomous thought, partitioning a whole into parts, BCE stresses harmonious thought, elevating the whole over the parts. The mainstream culture encourages the repression of emotional expression while BCE cultivates it. BCE advances the group; the dominant culture promotes the individual. The dominant culture prefers conformity whereas BCE places a premium upon distinctive personal expression. Wherein the mainstream culture emphasizes the written/visual modes of communication, BCE stresses the oral/aural modes. Lastly, in BCE time is made meaningful through social interactions whereas time derives its meaning in the mainstream culture via an association with work. (p. 27)

Rehabilitation professionals would do well to consider how incorporating some aspects of these values into their work with the African American client might enhance their work environment and strengthen communication with their clients.

Celebrations/Festivals/Ceremonies

There are very few celebrations, festivals, and ceremonies that are significantly different from the general American holidays and festivities; however, there are some that most African Americans know something about but may not necessarily attend. The health practitioner should be familiar with the significance and the dates of the major celebrations. They should consider the celebrations when scheduling appointments and incorporate where possible some of the holiday symbols into their office or practice.

Kwanzaa is a cultural holiday that is gaining in practice by African Americans. It is a holiday that pays tribute to the cultural roots of African ancestry. It is observed from December 26 through January 1st. The celebration is based on seven principles, with a special emphasis on family unity, and every day one of the candles on a seven-branched candelabrum is lighted to recognize one of the beliefs: unity, self-determination, collective work and responsibility, cooperative economics, purpose, creativity, and faith. Kwanzaa means "the first of the harvest" (Greenwood, 1997).

Juneteenth, or June 19, 1865, is considered the date when the last slaves in America were freed. Although the rumors of freedom were widespread prior to this time, actual emancipation did not come until General Gordon Granger rode into Galveston, Texas, and issued General Order No. 3, on June 19, almost two-and-a-half years after President Abraham Lincoln signed the Emancipation Proclamation. Juneteenth has therefore come to symbolize for many African Americans what the Fourth of July symbolizes for all Americans—freedom. It honors those African American ancestors who survived the inhumane institution of bondage, as well as demonstrating pride in the marvelous legacy of resistance and perseverance that they left us.

On Monday, January 20, 1986, in cities and towns across the country, people celebrated the first official Martin Luther King Day, the only federal holiday commemorating an African American. January 15 had been observed as a public holiday for many years in 27 states and Washington, D.C. Finally, in 1986, President Ronald Reagan declared the third Monday in January a federal legal holiday commemorating Dr. Martin Luther King's birthday.

Health Beliefs and Practices

Practitioners providing rehabilitation services to African Americans would be wise to consider the cultural background of the individual rather than assuming that all African Americans fit into one group. Because there is a melting pot of African Americans living in the United States, there is much diversity among African Americans in terms of health beliefs and practices. Varied health beliefs and practices among African Americans may be related to the amount of time some African Americans have lived in the United States, geographical location, their age, and income. Blacks who were born in the United States and those with other countries of origin share similar beliefs about traditional healing methods and medicine. The use of traditional healers emerged because of lack of access to health care associated with segregation. African Americans use traditional remedies to prevent, treat, and cure poor health. Some African Americans believe that folk healers have supernatural powers. Sometimes their treatments works; however, when treatment is not successful, the clients may believe that they are beyond treating.

Cause of Illness

African Americans characterize health as a continuum evolving around mind, body, and spirit (Spector, 1985). Good health is considered being in harmony with nature, whereas bad health is caused by disharmony (Jacques, 1976; Spector, 1996, 2000). Roberson (1985) found that the health beliefs of blacks living in rural communities were related to religion. Health was believed to be a blessing from God and that God's blessings offered protection against ill health, evil spirits, stress, fate, and sin. Many African Americans also believe that positive spiritual beliefs may cure illness.

Blacks may categorize illness into natural or unnatural illness. Natural illness may result from stress; cold; impurities in food, water or air; improper nutrition; or emotional weakness. Natural illness may also be a punishment for sin for the individual or other family members. Onset of natural illness may follow eating the wrong foods, drinking too much, or having bad personal relationships, and the onset may coincide with changes in the lunar and planetary cycles (Flaskerud & Rush, 1989; Spector 2000). The category of illness selected (natural or unnatural) determines which treatment method is sought by the individual and by the folk healer.

Spector (1996) described the causes of illness as being culturally based and caused by evil spirits. The following are examples of culturally based health beliefs for the cause of illness:

1. Coldness reduces resistance to illness. In winter the blood becomes thicker and protects health. Thin blood may cause illness.
2. Dirt or impurities in the body may be associated with hot conditions and may produce fever, inflammation, measles, or cancer.
3. The type of diet may cause high blood or low blood. Red foods such as beets, carrots, red wine, and red meat were considered blood builders. Colorless foods such as vinegar, lemon juice, pickled juice, and garlic reduced high blood in the body.
4. Unfriendly or hostile forces may cause unnatural illness.
5. Good health may be achieved and sustained with a good relationship with God, or with herbs and roots (Spector, 1996, pp. 191–215).

Unnatural illnesses may be caused by evil spirits. Most African Americans are fearful of unnatural illness because treatment is often not successful. Frequently voodoo is required to remove bad spirits. Guillory (1987) defines Voodoo as a blend of Christian, African, and other beliefs that combine religious and health practices. Conjurers or voodoo doctors may burn incense, light candles, or use special oils to keep away evil spirits. These special rituals may also be used to settle domestic disharmony such as keeping one's husband at home. Worry is another unnatural illness. Sustained worry prevents natural rest and may diminish appetite-depleting energy necessary for daily routines. Traditional healers believe that worry will cause "craziness."

New immigrants share beliefs more freely than those who have lived in America longer. Huff and Kline (1998) suggested that those who have lived in America longer and have achieved a middle-income range tend to believe more in the scientific medical model.

Congress and Lyons (1992) reported that socioeconomic status is also an important factor to consider when addressing cultural beliefs, health, and treatment for African Americans. African Americans in lower socioeconomic levels tend to retain the beliefs and values of their native countries. Airhihenbuwa and Harrison (1993) stated that 80% of Africans used traditional healing methods because this was the only available, reliable, and affordable system. Caribbean blacks immigrating to the United States may have limited access to health care and believe that there is a spiritual cause of disease, whereas middle-income African Americans living in America assimilate into the health values of the majority culture. According to Gregg and Curry (1994), blacks also believe that "You gotta die of something; one day you got to leave here. . . . When it's time to go, it's time to go" (p. 522). Thus, illness is a test of faith, the stronger your faith, the better the ability to overcome sickness and adversity. Lewis and Green (2000) found that African Americans who attend church three or more times per week believed that health was dependent on fate or destiny. In times of illness, black families band together for support, and they use prayer to cope with natural and unnatural illness, stress, and worry (Gibson, 1982; Spector, 2000).

Health Restoration

Prayer continues to be the most common method for treating illness. African Americans believe that they may be healed by prayer and "laying on of hands" by members of one's family or church. Often olive oil that has been consecrated is applied to the forehead during prayer; some believe that the olive oil has no magical power but is a symbol of the healing power of the Spirit. African Americans may also speak in tongues while praying. "Praying is voiced in a language that is only understandable by the person reciting the prayer" (Purnell and Paulanka, 1998, p. 61).

Various home remedies may be used to regain health. The following are some examples of home remedies that have been passed down through generations to cure illness:

1. Sugar and turpentine are combined and taken by mouth to get rid of worms and cure back pain. Nine drops of turpentine taken nine days after intercourse acts as a contraceptive.

2. Poultices (a bag filled with herbs or other medicines) are worn around the neck or attached to another body part and are used to draw out infection, fever, or cold. For example, a white potato is sliced and laid around the head to draw out a cold; when the potato turns black, it is believed that the penicillin mold destroys the infection. Fever may also be treated by placing a sliced onion on the feet and wrapping the feet in a blanket.

3. Herbs from the woods (such as sassafras) are made into a tea and used to reduce fever.

4. Salt and pork (salt pork) are used to treat cuts, wounds, and boils.

5. Hot water with lemon and honey is used to treat colds.

6. Garlic, onion, and parsley chopped and mixed is often used as an expectorant for colds.

7. Hot toddies made of lemon, peppermint, and a dash of alcohol (such as brandy, whisky, or rum) are used to treat colds and congestion.

8. Garlic may also be used to remove evil spirits or the effects of voodoo. (Spector, 2000, pp. 219–220)

Accessibility to Health Care

Barriers to accessibility for health care for African Americans were born out of necessity. During slavery, treatment for illness was inconsistent, and many blacks did not trust white physicians. Slaves relied on the use of alternative medicine such as herbs and roots.

Slaves did not seek health care outside the black community because of lack of trust, no financial resources, no knowledge of available health care, and lack of transportation, and of most importance, because the institution of slavery did not permit individual health care choices (Huff & Kline, 1999).

The type of health care provided and received depended on the whether the slave was a house slave or field slave. House servants were more likely to be literate, whereas field workers were kept ignorant of education and other resources.

Following the passage of the Emancipation Proclamation in 1893, blacks migrated to Northern states and cities. Health care gradually became available to blacks but still was inferior to services provided to whites, and it remained segregated. Incidence of some illnesses was higher for blacks living in the city than for those in rural areas because they were exposed to environmental hazards. Urban blacks generally sought health care more frequently and attempted to practice some preventive measures. In comparison, rural blacks, especially the poor, did not readily seek medical intervention, did not have transportation, and did not have the financial means to purchase health services. The result was that rural blacks experienced higher mortality rates because the disease was often in the late stages and beyond treatment (Huff & Kline, 1999). This outcome is still common today. Mistrust of the system, a history of substandard health care, and inhumane treatment in the past cause many African Americans, both urban and rural, to stay away from health care providers (Guillory, 1987).

There were several events that led to more equal accessibility to health care for blacks: (a) Civil Rights Act of 1964; (b) Medicaid-Medicare legislation of 1965; and (c) Title VI of the Civil Rights Act, which prohibited racial discrimination in any institution receiving federal funds (Thomas, 1992). In spite of these changes in legislation, black Americans continue to have higher mortality rates than whites.

Health Disparity

A critical issue that continues to plague the health care system of the United States is the disparity in the health status of African Americans and other minority Americans compared with the population as a whole (Airhihenbuwa, 1995). In particular, African Americans generally perceive that the odds are against them when it comes to health, quality of life, access to health care, and socioeconomic status. Other researchers maintain that the quality of preventive care, cultural beliefs, and racism may also contribute to the decline of the health status of African Americans (Adams, Blumenfeld, Castaneda, Hackman, Peters, and Zuniga, 2000; Airhihenbuwa, 1995; Auslander & Haire-Joshu, 1992; Fingerhut, 1992; Guerra, 1996, 1998; Johnson, 2001; Reed 1993; Smith, 1999).

There are many barriers that may be responsible for the decline of the health status and health disparities of African Americans. Important barriers include lack of financial resources to obtain insurance and to pay for services, lack of transportation and child care, lack of self-efficacy in requesting explanation of services, and inability to assimilate prescribed services into a culturally relevant routine. Language differences and the use of language may also contribute to misunderstanding and distrust. Rehabilitation practitioners may use language or terms that are not familiar to African Americans, resulting in feelings of intimidation and being "spoken down to (condescension)" (Wells & Black, 2000).

Other issues that contribute to health disparities resulting in decreased health status for African Americans include previously mentioned cultural beliefs and health practices. Specific cultural beliefs and health practices often impede utilization of modern health care services when other barriers such as income and education levels are overcome. When African Americans do utilize services, intervention is for an acute illness rather than a preventive measure. Health care utilization reports also suggest that African Americans report higher rates of dissatisfaction with health care, and they experience longer average wait times. Although low-income African Americans have the greatest barrier to care, moderate- to higher-income African Americans also face barriers (such as not being listened too, feeling invisible, and being ignored) (Adams et al., 2000; Wells & Black, 2000).

Culture of African American Eating Habits

Many aspects of eating and food choices are culturally defined. African Americans value eating well, feeding the family well, and offering meals to guests. "Food is a symbol of health and wealth for African Americans. One is expected to accept a gift of food when entering or leaving the African American home. Rehabilitation practitioners need to be sensitive regarding the gift of food. If they reject food, they are perceived to reject the giver of the food" (Purnell & Paulanka, 1998, p. 62).

Depending on the economic status, African Americans eat a diet rich in nutrients and have a preference for dark, leafy vegetables, red meat, and cheese. "African Americans believe that too much red meat causes high blood pressure and causes stroke. Foods such as milk, vegetables and meats are referred to as strength foods. Lactose intolerance occurs in about 75 percent of the African American population" (Purnell & Paulanka, 1998, p. 63).

General perceptions of African American cooking and eating habits suggest that there is a link between food and the influence of slavery. The health of a slave was affected primarily by diet. In most cases, food was adequate but nutritionally deficient because the slave master fed the slave the most economical foods possible. Slaves were given the leftover parts from animals (such as pig knuckles, tails, ears, and intestines, or chitterlings) that the slave owners considered as scraps. "The White man gave the slave food that he did not consider fit for himself" (Airhihenbuwa, Kumanyika, Agurs, Lowe, Saunders, & Morssink, 1996, p. 251).

Because there was no money for slaves to purchase other foods, the result was limited food choices and the use of available food scraps to create a meal. African Americans have come to rely on these simple but high-fat food choices as a food staple and out of necessity developed unique ways of preparing these scraps of meats and vegetables that became known as "soul food." The practice of cooking soul food has been handed down from generation to generation. In fact, being a "good" cook has been perceived as somewhat of a status symbol in the African American community (personal observation). A typical soul food meal consisted of collard greens and turnips seasoned with salted pork fat, black-eyed peas, and corn bread. Soul food was not the native food of the black community; it had its roots in slavery, not in Africa. The African diet consisted of natural, unprocessed foods such as cereals, green vegetables, peas, beans, cassava, yams, and sweet potatoes.

These simple meals and the custom of family gatherings fostered unity among the slaves (Airhihenbuwa et al., 1996). Now, instead of food being the focus of socioeconomic necessity and health, it is used for family bonding and the celebration of tradition.

In the African American culture, food is often spicy, fried, smothered in gravy, and laden with butter or other fat. Pig's feet and chitterlings have been replaced with smoked ham, barbecued ribs and pork chops, bacon, and luncheon meat. Diets now include refined white flour products and other highly processed foods that add to the increased consumption of saturated fat. Soul food must be considered as a source of obesity for both urban and rural blacks. When prepared in traditional ways, soul food may add to health risk factors for heart disease, stroke, and cancer.

The 1977 to 1978 National Food Consumption Survey results (as cited in Stolley & Fitzgibbon, 1997) reported that on average, 40% of total energy intake comes from fat. This study further suggested that cultural attitudes play a significant role in food selection and preparation for African Americans. In addition, the study showed that African Americans have a higher intake of fried foods and less dietary fiber than white Americans. The consumption of high-fat, high-cholesterol foods places African Americans at risk for increased obesity and obesity-related diseases.

Today, many African Americans attempt to preserve tradition by preparing, serving, and eating foods in the same manner as their ancestors. Research by Airhihenbuwa et al. (1996) suggested that eating practices of African Americans are strongly influenced by tradition and that many African Americans have a preference for the foods of the past. Food cost and being in a low socioeconomic bracket may also affect the way food is purchased and the way it is prepared. The literature indicates that African Americans in higher socioeconomic groups purchase cheaper cuts of meats and prepare vegetables in traditional ways even though they may be able to afford more expensive and leaner cuts of meats. For example, the New Year is celebrated by eating hog head, greens, and black-eyed peas with added pork fat such as ham hocks. Cultural beliefs suggest that this is a traditional meal that is said to bring good luck for the New Year.

In recent times, some African Americans have begun to prepare a lower-fat version of greens by substituting smoked turkey wings for ham hocks. Another positive traditional health practice is consuming the liquid in which vegetables were prepared, referred to as "pot liquor." African Americans enjoy fish (especially salmon and catfish) and poultry;

however, the health benefits may be negated by frying instead of baking or broiling and by consuming the skin. Unfortunately, foods prepared in traditional ways are increasing health-risk factors and adding to early mortality for African Americans.

For African Americans who are practicing Muslims, rehabilitation practitioners need to be aware of dietary restrictions that include a strictly kosher diet (no pork or soul food) including black-eyed peas, kidney beans, and lima beans prepared with ham or bacon, and no pork chops). Muslims believe that these foods impede digestion, that they should be used as feed for animals, and that there is no health or spiritual benefit for the body. "Muslims also believe that food affects the way a person thinks and acts, therefore food should be clean and have a positive effect on the body" (Spector, 2000, p. 224). Muslims admitted to the rehabilitation unit may refuse to eat or participate in the preparation of cooking tasks such as making pudding and jello because these products have pork derivatives and may interfere with religious beliefs. Diabetic Muslims refuse to take insulin that has a pork base or is manufactured from the pancreas of a pig (Spector, 2000).

Rehabilitation practitioners must consider cultural dietary practices when performing meal preparation in occupational therapy, when offering snacks to a diabetic patient in physical therapy, when recommending a dysphagia diet using thickeners in speech, and when having picnics in recreation therapy. Therefore, if the client is not a "ready" participant in a therapeutic activity suggested by the practitioner, the client's reluctance may be connected to cultural beliefs and practices associated with traditional food consumption and preparation.

Mental Illness

African Americans live in a world where they are expected to adapt and assimilate into the majority culture. This struggle to fit in often results in increased stress associated with rejection and isolation. Blacks present themselves as strong, unflappable, and tough even when they may be suffering emotionally. Even when African Americans are ill they have been taught to suffer in silence. Not only is suffering spiritual, but it also has historic roots in slavery. This phenomenon can be traced back to slavery when black people were expected to work and labor in the fields and to pretend to be okay (National Mental Health Association, 2000; Rouse 2001; Wesley, 2002).

Research on socioeconomic status and mental health in African Americans is well documented in the literature. Eaton and Kessler (1981) and MAASS-Robinson (2001) suggested that there is a relationship between race, socioeconomic status, and feelings of distress in African Americans in lower socioeconomic groups and in those who are upwardly mobile. In addition, Steele (1978) and MAASS-Robinson (2001) report that blacks were more likely to experience the "glass ceiling," lack of job opportunities, and each of mobility. The result is increased feelings of anger, anxiety, stress, and depression.

No ethnic group is immune to mental illness. African Americans typically do not acknowledge or seek treatment for mental illness because mental illness is not viewed as a valid health problem in the African American culture. Mental illness of any sort is considered a weakness in the African American community. When African Americans acknowledge that there is a problem, there is the burden of mistrust and the fear that the information would not be kept confidential, be misused, or be misinterpreted. Past ethical issues associated with research in African American communities and distrust of health professionals conducting research have contributed to this lack of willingness to seek treatment for mental health issues (Barbee, 1992; Smart 2001).

Because there is an insufficient number of African American counselors, clinical psychologists, and psychiatrists, African Americans may not seek mental health services from those outside their ethnic group (Leavitt, 2001; MAASS-Robinson, 2001; Smey, 2001). African Americans may delay seeking intervention because (1) of the cultural shame of having a mental health problem; (2) of the knowledge that assessment tools used to diagnose mental illness including the DSM-IV are not sensitive to the life events and experiences of African Americans; and (3) current assessments used to diagnose African Americans exclude them from the standardization process.

Other barriers to utilizing available mental health resources include having their health complaints minimized by service providers. African Americans may be told that they have hypertension and be prescribed blood pressure medication rather than being screened for a mental health issue. The result is a lack of confidence in the health system, avoidance of the issue, seeking an alternative support system, noncompliance with the recommendations made by the health care professionals, and the perception that the quality of care is poor (Jones-Warren, 1995; Rouse 2001).

African Americans may choose alternatives to conventional mental health services. Historically in the black community, African Americans rely on prayer and spiritual intervention, support form family and friends, and traditional healers rather than formal therapy as coping strategies.

Rehabilitation practitioners working in the mental health setting must realize that African Americans experience the same symptoms as others who are seeking intervention for mental illness. Their feelings of anger and hostility, stress and frustration, and anxiety and worry may be compounded by underlying life experiences of racism and discrimination. They may be irritable for no apparent reason, experience a change in eating habits or patterns, and gain or lose weight.

In order to design meaningful interactions and treatment plans for African Americans treated in the mental health setting, rehabilitation practitioners need to have a sense of their own strengths and weaknesses and to express empathy toward African Americans as well as other minorities. Henderson (1972) suggested several concepts for working with other people:

1. Every individual is a sum total of his or her experiences (objective interactions and subjective feelings), and behaves in term of those experiences.
2. Every individual has psychological drives toward health, growth, and adjustment.
3. Every individual perceives and behaves in terms of his or her needs for security, acceptance, achievement, and independence.
4. Every individual is capable of solving most of his or her problems if he or she understands the problems and learns to use his or her own resources. (Henderson, 1972, p. 58)

Other important points to remember include establishing a relationship with the client, using effective communication skills, active listening, and paying close attention to the client's verbal and nonverbal responses. African Americans are nurturing, enjoy helping others, and take pride in their personal appearance. Group activities where they are expected to share their feelings in a "mixed" ethnic group may result in limited sharing associated with distrust of majority participants. Some feelings are best expressed on a one-to-one basis with a member of the patient's family present.

Disability in the African American Culture

One in seven (14%) of working-age African Americans is disabled. African Americans who are disabled experience less employment, educational, and rehabilitation outcomes than white Americans (Belgrave, 1991). This finding may be due to the limited access to and utilization of rehabilitation services. Yet African Americans with disabilities are adjusted to their disability and cope well in the home, at the workplace, and in the community (Belgrave, 1991).

Belgrave (1991) recruited 170 African Americans from public rehabilitation agencies and facilities to participate in a study on the psychosocial aspects of disability. The age of the participants ranged from 21 to 82 with a mean age of 44.5; 47% were female and 53% male. Twenty percent were employed, and 80% were not employed; participants were receiving the following rehabilitative services: physician follow-up care, vocational rehabilitation, counseling, physical therapy, occupational therapy, and social services. Participants' disabilities were categorized into four primary rehabilitation areas: (a) speech and hearing impairments; (b) orthopedic impairments; (c) mental illness and substance abuse; and (d) other (such as sickle cell anemia, diabetes, spinal cord injury, cardiovascular disease, respiratory disease, and kidney failure).

The psychosocial variables of social support, self-esteem, health locus of control, and perception of disability were used to predict adjustment to disability. Results indicated that perception of severity of disability, self-esteem, and social support were significant predictors of adjustment to disability. Perception of severity of disability was the strongest predictor of adjustment to disability. Health locus of control and demographic variables were not significant predictors of adjustment to disability. Higher levels of self-esteem and social support were related to adjustment to disability.

The findings of the study suggest that by improving the psychosocial well-being of African Americans who are disabled may also improve rehabilitation outcomes. Because African Americans are concerned with the perception of severity of the disability, rehabilitation practitioners would be wise to assist the client to realistically recognize assets and limitations of the disability. This process would aid in facilitating a more realistic perception of the disability. Self-esteem and emotional support were significant contributors to adjustment to disability. These variables may be improved by providing positive feedback and structuring therapeutic interventions for success. Social support may be increased by remembering to include the client's family and community.

In recent years, increasing family participation in the rehabilitation process for persons with disabilities has received more consideration. Alston and McCowan (1995) suggest that family involvement can help the family member with a disability adjust to the condition. This is an important consideration when providing rehabilitation for African

Americans because traditionally they have relied on a strong extended family network when confronted with any adversity. African Americans tend to band together to support the person with a disability by providing assistance with basic and instrumental activities of daily living (such as meal preparation and grocery shopping, medication management, and transportation to scheduled appointments).

Findings by Alston and Turner (1994) reveal that African American families have unique patterns of coping with stress related to disability. Adjustment to the disability is closely related to the family's attitudes, behaviors (such as role expectations and conflict resolution), and perception of illness. In a study of psychosocial adjustment to disability among rehabilitated African Americans, Alston and McCowan (1995) and Alston and Turner (1994) found that African Americans rely on spiritual intervention, adapt family roles, and rely on extended family for assistance and emotional support.

Previously Miller (1986) demonstrated similar findings in a study of adjustment among African American patients receiving medical intervention for hypertension, diabetes, and epilepsy at a community hospital. She reported that adjustment to disability was significantly related to expressiveness, family unity, and collaboration among family members.

In spite of the positive findings reported by Miller (1986), Alston and McCowan (1995), and Alston and Turner (1994), rehabilitation research addressing cultural factors that impact African Americans' response to disability is limited in the literature.

Alston and McCowan (1995) surveyed 64 disabled male and female African Americans aged 20 to 59 using the Self-Report Family Inventory (Beavers, Hampson, & Hulgus, 1985), and the Acceptance of Disability Scale (Linkowski, 1981). The purpose of the study was to determine the influence of family on the adjustment to disability. Disabilities included sensory impairment (such as visual and hearing), substance abuse, and emotional impairment, back injury, spinal injury, epilepsy, and carpal tunnel. Family characteristics were defined as the following:

1. *Cohesion:* Contentment and happy with togetherness.
2. *Expressiveness:* Warmth and caring expressed easily among family members.
3. *Leadership:* Designated and competent family leader.
4. *Conflict:* Low level of within-family fighting and high level of problem-solving and personal accountability.
5. *Health/competence:* Described as showing love, listening, and offering positive support.

Results of the study indicated that there was a strong relationship between adjustment to disability and family cohesion and expressiveness. First, African Americans who adjust to disability come from close supportive families in which feelings are shared verbally and physically. This finding is consistent with earlier findings by Alston and Turner (1994) that African Americans share a strong kinship bond and that emotional support provided by the family prevents feelings of loneliness. Second, there was a positive relationship between level of adjustment to disability and perception of family health. A sense of family wellness and happiness was a key factor contributing to the psychosocial adjustment of African

Americans to disability and that disability does not easily disrupt the African American family unit. Third, a moderate relationship was found between adjustment and clearly defined leadership patterns. This finding reflects the tendency of African Americans to have flexibility in role adaptation in a majority society. The authors further suggest that this strength allows African Americans to readily adjust to role restructuring when a family member becomes disabled.

Finally, there was a moderate correlation found between adjustment and conflict. Family members with a few unresolved disagreements, a tendency for problem solving, and little blaming and arguing did not view this as an obstacle for dealing with the effects of disability. African American culture encourages open expression of feelings and emotions and disagreement. Thus, expression of conflict is perceived as a natural part of African American communication. This study supports the concept that African Americans learn to settle family conflict by discussing their concerns about the disability. Rehabilitation practitioners observing such an interchange among an African American patient and family in a treatment setting may conclude that there is much discord. However, in actuality this is a normal means of communication for this culture.

The strength of the African American family is important to the successful psychosocial adjustment for African Americans with disabilities. Excluding the family from the rehabilitation process may result in loss of client motivation and poor rehabilitation outcomes. Therefore, it is imperative to include the family in initial assessments, during treatment, and for any subsequent outpatient visits.

Because African Americans are verbally expressive, family members should be encouraged to discuss who will take responsibility as the primary caregiver. By presenting and discussing any general observations and potential problems in rehabilitation with the family and client present, the rehabilitation practitioner is opening the line of communication, but of most importance, is also being sensitive to the need of African Americans to operate in a family unit.

Summary

The authors have described how racial biases can adversely affect the quality of health care to the African American client. In this chapter, the authors emphasize the importance of respect, sensitivity, and understanding towards the African American experiences in the American society. After reflection on their history, the authors discuss some cultural features of the African Americans with specific focus on patterns of interaction and communication in a health care setting. Also, the health belief systems, casuse of illness, and health disparity issues are discussed in this chapter. The discussions of mental health and disability in the African American communities are followed by case studies and questions.

Questions

1. Who are the African Americans? When did they come to the United States and under what circumstances?

2. Describe some patterns of racisim and discrimination that an African American client may encounter in a rehabilitation setting.

3. Describe some important cultural factors that a rehabilitation professional must consider when working with African American clients.

4. Describe the current demographics of the African Americans in the United States.

5. Explain how the concepts of time and space influence the patterns of communication of the African Americans discussed in this chapter.

6. Discuss how disparities in health care are created for the African American population.

7. Discuss the importance of family life for this population. What are some core values inherent in their family life?

8. What is Kwanza? Describe the importance of Kwanza in the African American culture.

9. Describe nine core cultural values of African Americans discussed by the authors of this chapter.

10. Discuss some health beliefs and practices of the African American population.

Case Study

Sally Kingman is a sixty-two-year-old African American woman who sustained an aneurysm two weeks ago. Prior to the stroke, she lived independently in a small ranch style house in rural Missouri. On the morning of the event, she states that she remembers falling to the floor and passing out. She awoke briefly and was able to call a friend for help. Following emergency intervention and surgery at a regional medical center, Sally was referred to rehabilitation for evaluation. Sally has mild right upper and lower extremity weakness, and slight expressive aphasia.

Because Sally is from a rural community, she tends to be very independent and does not accept assistance in activities of daily living. She enjoys cooking soul food and enjoys visits from her three children and their families every Sunday after church.

The speech pathologist and physical therapist report that Sally is aloof and has refused the last two treatment sessions. The occupational therapist assigned to Sally's case graduated from a Jesuit University in California and has two years of work experience. During the first treatment session, Jane, the occupational therapist, addresses Sally by her first name without permission. In addition, Jane hovers over Sally's shoulder and repeatedly asks whether she understands how to put on her blouse. The following morning Sally refuses to go to therapy and states that she can get dressed on her own. Jane does not understand why Sally refuses to attend therapy. Therefore, Jane decides to discuss the matter with Sally directly. Jane begins this interaction by calling Sally "honey." Sally looks down at the floor with no response. Jane quietly leaves the room.

Questions

1. What do you think is causing Sally's silences? Is there a conflict between the therapists and Sally?

2. Which cultural factors may be impacting the communication between the client and the therapists?

3. What other factors may inhibit the relationship between patient and practitioner?

4. What are some culturally learned behaviors that Sally and the practitioners are displaying?

5. Given the situation, is space a cause for concern during their interactions?

6. How might the therapists rectify the situation with Sally? How should each subsequent rehabilitation session be structured to be more sensitive to Sally's culture?

7. Discuss some preventive health issues that may be explored with Sally and her family.

The relationship between Sally and the rehabilitation team obviously deteriorated before they could establish rapport. It is the responsibility of the practitioner to identify barriers to positive interactions with clients. A primary concern with the interaction between the therapists and Sally is lack of cultural sensitivity. If the therapists had been aware of the potential cultural differences between themselves and Sally, they would have constructed a framework for interaction with African Americans that would have put Sally at ease.

Implications for Rehabilitation

Learning Reflection   The rehabilitation therapists assigned to provide rehabilitation services to Sally Kingman must acquaint themselves with the cultural beliefs and health practices and behaviors of African Americans. How might the team learn of the culture, beliefs and practices of Sally? One of the best resources is Sally herself. Because Sally became quiet and did not answer Jane, this behavior suggests there may be a communication problem. Had Jane realized that African American elders do not like to be addressed by their first name by younger persons, she could have avoided this cultural and social faux pas. Jane could have asked Mrs. Kingman "How would you like to be addressed?" or "May I have permission to address you as Sally?" (Galanti, 1997).

Economic status may have a significant impact on Sally's ability to feel comfortable with the practitioners. Sally may perceive that the rehabilitation team represents white power figures and may react by being subservient or hostile. It is important for each team member to make eye contact with Sally to gain trust. Demeaning or condescending behavior should be avoided, including attempts to impress Sally by discussing other African American friends (Downes, 1994).

African Americans pride themselves on being strong and not needing assistance during times of adversity. Because prayer is the first line of defense and acts as a coping mechanism, the occupational therapist needs to be sensitive to the spiritual beliefs of Sally. A question such as "Will your pastor be in to pray for you today?" may open the lines of communication.

Rehabilitation practitioners must also be sensitive to the varying levels of literacy in African Americans. This is a factor when working with black elders from rural and urban communities. Typically, African Americans may become quiet or may shy away from written pen-and-pencil assessments. Avoid making the assumption that all black elders are illiterate. Most African American elders will have a relative, usually a son or daughter, read and explain any written documents. If the patient seems to require extra time, ask permission to read any consent forms, assessments, or posttreatment evaluations to the person. This approach must be sensitive and respectful so as not to embarrass the client or create an atmosphere of condescension.

Each member of the rehabilitation team may want to invite one of Sally's relatives to attend a treatment session with her. During the session, it is important for the therapist to talk directly to Sally even though the family member is present. Elder African Americans regard this directness as respect. Furthermore, this act of consideration may instill trust of the practitioner and relay the message that the practitioner is confident of hers skills and wants to have a positive outcome for Sally.

Jane's occupational therapy intervention must be based on the cultural values of Sally. After rapport is established and because Sally enjoys cooking soul food, Jane may ask Sally to define soul food and to describe how soul food is prepared. Jane could combine assessments and several treatments around cooking a traditional Sunday dinner.

Because Sally has had a stroke and may be receiving a low sodium and low fat diet, it would be important for Jane to consult and invite the dietician and a family member to a soul food cooking treatment session with Sally. This session provides the perfect opportunity to address ways to reduce fat and salt in soul food, demonstrate cooking assistive devices, and determine problem-solving and safety issues in the kitchen.

This client-centered activity puts Sally at ease because she is pursuing an activity that has meaning, that she enjoys and has prior experience with. Sally's family may want to purchase soul food items, using "new" low-fat suggestions, and share with the stroke support group or rehabilitation team. By inviting Sally's pastor to the event to pray and say grace, Sally will begin to feel that Jane is sensitive to what is meaningful and culturally relevant.

African American elders are often sensitive about dressing and undressing in front of others and especially strangers. Women in particular have been taught to undress only in front of their husbands. Male occupational and physical therapy practitioners need to ask permission to perform dressing activities, have a female practitioner present, have the client don clothing over a clean hospital gown, and always use a draping sheet to maintain privacy. Jane should explain why she wants to evaluate dressing skills and simply ask Sally "How much assistance do you need to get dressed?" Bathing and hygiene may present some of the same privacy concerns for African Americans.

Educational materials developed for the mainstream culture may not be culturally sensitive to the various educational levels, life experiences, and languages in the black community. Home programs need to be written and have picture instructions. Instructions need to include who, what, where, why, and how many. Practitioners may facilitate positive communication skills by giving and requesting information in different ways. For example, instead of asking Sally whether she understands how to get dressed, say that we need to get dressed to go for breakfast. By linking a purpose to getting dressed, Sally can see the need to perform the task in context.

Because Sally, like many other African Americans, does not trust information provided by doctors, practitioners might enlist the assistance of other African American patients on the rehabilitation unit with the same diagnosis to share their situations. By sharing their life experiences, symptoms of stroke, and spiritual and health beliefs, Sally may become more at ease and accept help. Keep in mind that consent forms signed by each participant are necessary to comply with the Health Insurance Portability and Accountability Act (HIPPA).

Rehabilitation practitioners need to be able to communicate with a diverse group of clients and patients. "In any clinical setting there are at least three sets of cultural backgrounds present—those of the clinician, those of the client, and those of the health care institution." "It is the provider's obligation to assist clients with understanding aspects of the system including cultural norms, values, and expectations that may interfere with the client's ability to make well informed decisions and manage their own health status" (Bonder, Martin, & Miracle, 2002, p. 109). Culturally sensitive practitioners need to have prior knowledge of the target group and to take the extra time to examine personal feelings, perceptions, stereotypes, and prejudices about that group. The rehabilitation practitioner must recognize the conflicts in culture and values that may occur and make every effort to take them into account when designing interventions (Campinha-Bacote, 2003). "Ask questions to gather pertinent information, be open to thinking about alternatives, and be aware of your own vantage point" (Bonder, Martin, & Miracle, 2002, p. 121). African Americans may be initially suspicious and distrustful of the majority population and may be more open to treatment if another person from the same ethnic group or family member is available during treatment. Develop the habit of including family members and being flexible in scheduling treatment sessions. Family members who work may not be able to attend treatment sessions scheduled during morning times.

Finally, be aware that the medical model may be used for serious health problems by the majority but that African Americans may elect to use traditional medicine, folk healers, and prayer instead. Since self-treatment is common, the therapist may cause less conflict by making the effort to discuss the folk-healing method into the prescribed therapeutic intervention.

References

Adams M., Blumenfeld, W. J., Castaneda, R., Hackman, H. W., Peters, M. L., & Zuniga, X. (2000). *Readings for diversity and social justice: An anthology on racism, antisemitism, sexism, heterosexism, ableism, and classism* (pp. 79–105). New York: Routledge.

Airhihenbuwa, C. O. (1995). Cross cultural health education: A pedagogical challenge. *Journal of School Health*, 58, 240–242.

Airhihenbuwa, C. O., & Harrison, I. E. (1993). Traditional medicine in Africa: Past, present and future. In P. Conrad & E. Gallagher (Eds.), *Healing and health care in developing countries*. Philadelphia: Temple University Press.

Airhihenbuwa, C. O., Kumanyika, S., Agurs, T. D., Lowe, A., Saunders, D., & Morssink, C. B (1996). Cultural aspects of African American eating patterns. *Ethnicity and Health*, 1(3), 245–260.

Alston, R. J., & McCowan, C. J. (1995). Perception of family competence and adaptation to illness among African Americans with disabilities. *Journal of Rehabilitation*, January/February/March, 27–32.

Alston, R. J., & Turner, W. L. (1994). A family strengths model of adjustment to disability for African American clients. *Journal of Counseling and Development*, 72, 378–383.

Auslander, W. F., & Haire-Joshu, D. (1992). Community organization to reduce the risk of non-insulin dependent diabetics among low income African American women. *Ethnicity and Disease*, 176–184.

Barbee, E. L. (1992). African American women and depression: A review and critique of the literature. *Archives of Psychiatric Nursing*, 6(5), 257–263.

Baxter, J. C. (1970). Interpersonal spacing in natural settings, *Sociometry*, 444–456.

Beavers, R., Hampson, R., & Hulgus, Y. (1985). Commentary: The Beavers approach to family assessment. *Family Process*, 24, 398–405

Belgrave, F. Z. (1991). Psychosocial predictors of adjustment to disability in African Americans. *Journal of Rehabilitation*, January/February/March, 37–40.

Bonder, B., Martin, L., & Miracle, A. (2002). *Culture in clinical care* (pp.109–121). Thorofare, NJ: Slack Incorporated.

Boyd, H. (Spring, 1997). Been dere, done dat! *Black Scholar*, 27(1), p. 15.

Boykin, A. (1991). The triple quandary and the schooling of Afro-American children. In U. Neisser (Ed.), *The School Achievement of Minority Children: New Perspectives* (pp. 57–92). Hillsdale, NJ: Erlbaum.

Campinha-Bacote, J. (2003). *The process of cultural competence in the delivery of healthcare services: A culturally competent model of care* (4th ed.). Cincinnati: Transcultural C.A.R.E. Associates.

Census 2000 Brief (August 2001). The Black Population: 2000, http://www.census.gov/prod/2001pubs/c2kbr01-5.pdf

Congress, E. P., & Lyons, B. P. (1992). Cultural differences in health beliefs: Implications for social work practice in health care settings. *Social Work in Health Care*, 17(3), 81–96.

Downes, J. D. (1994). *Ethnic Americans for the health professional*. Dubuque, IA: Kendall/Hunt Publishing Company.

Eaton, W. W., & Kessler, L. G. (1981). Rates of symptoms of depression in a national sample. *American Journal of Epidemiology*, 114(4), 528–538.

Fingerhut, L. A. (1992). News from NCHS. *American Journal of Public Health*, 82, 1168–1170.

Flaskerud, J. H., & Rush, C. E. (1989). AIDS and traditional health beliefs and practices of black women. *Nursing Reseacrh*, 38, 210–215.

Galanti, G. A. (1997). *Caring for patients from different cultures: Case studies from American hospitals* (2nd ed.) (pp. 11–12, 16). Philadelphia: University of Pennsylvania Press.

Gibson, R. C. (1982). Blacks at middle and late life: Resources and coping. American Academy of Political and Social Science, 464, 79–90.

Greenwood, M. (1997). Home for the holiday. *Essence*, 28(8), 105–110.

Gregg, J., & Curry, R. H. (1994). Explanatory models for cancer among African-American women at two Atlanta neighborhood health centers: The implications for a cancer screening program. *Social Science Medicine*, 39, 519–526.

Greif, G. L., Hrabowski, F. A. Freeman, Maton, K. I. (2000). African American mothers of academically successful sons: Familial influences and implications for social work. *Children & Schools*, Oct 2000, (22), 4.

Guerra, R. (1996, September). *Nebraska's racial and ethnic minorities and their health: An update.* Nebraska Department of Health, Office of Minority Health. pp. 1–39.

Guerra, R. (1998, September). *Nebraska's racial and ethnic minorities and their health: An update.* Nebraska Department of Health, Office of Minority Health. pp. 1–75.

Guillory, J. (1987). Ethnic perspectives of cancer nursing: The Black American. Oncology *Nursing Forum*, 14(3), 66–69.

Henderson, G. (1972). *To live in freedom: Human relations today and tomorrow.* Norman, OK: University of Oklahoma Press.

Huff, R. M., & Kline, M. V. (1999). *Promoting health in multicultural populations: A handbook for practitioners* (pp. 201–265). Thousand Oaks, CA: Sage Publications.

Jacques, G. (1976). Cultural health traditions: A black perspective. In M. E. Blanck & P. P. Paxton (Eds.), *Providing safe nursing care for ethnic people of color.* Norwalk, CT: Appleton-Century-Crofts.

James-Myers, L. (1991). Expanding the psychology of knowledge: The importance of world view revisited. In R. L. Jones (Ed.), *Black Psychology* (pp. 15–28). Berkeley, CA: Cobb & Henry.

Johnson, A. G. (2001). *Privilege, power, and difference.* St. Louis, MO: McGraw Hill Higher Education.

Johnson, R. L., Saha, S. S., Arbelaez, J. J., Beach, M. C., & Cooper, L. A. (February, 2004). Racial and ethnic differences in patient perceptions of bias and cultural competence in health care, *Journal of General Internal Medicine*, 19, 101–110.

Jones, J. M. (1972). Prejudice and racism, Reading, MA: Addison-Wesley.

Jones, J. M. (1997). *Prejudice and racism* (2nd Ed.). New York: McGraw-Hill Companies, Inc.

Jones, N. A., & Jackson, J. S. (2000). The demographic profile of African Americans, 1970–71 to 2000–01. *The Black Collegian.*

Jones, R. C. (1991). *Black Psychology.* Berkeley, CA: Cobb & Henry.

Jones-Warren, B. (1995). *Constructing a model for depression in middle class African-American women by exploring relationships between stressful life events, social social support, and self-esteem.* Unpublished doctoral dissertation, The Ohio State University Columbus, Ohio.

Lawson, E. J., & Thompson, A. (1995). Black men make sense of marital distress and divorce: An exploratory study. *Family Relations* (44) 2, p. 211.

Leavitt, R. L. (2001). *Cross-cultural rehabilitation: An international perspective* (pp. 70–74). Philadelphia: W. B. Saunders.

Lewis, R. K., & Green, B. L. (2000). Assessing the health attitudes, beliefs, and behavior of African Americans attending church: A comparison from two communities. *Journal of Community Health*, 25(3), 211–220.

Linkowski, D. C. (1981). *Revised acceptance disability scale.* Washington, DC: Rehabilitation Research and Training Center, George Washington University.

Maass-Robinson, S. (2001). "An open letter to my sisters: Why don't we get help for depression?" *American Journal of Health Studies Special Issue: "The Health of Women of Color,"* 17(2), 46–49.

Miller, S. (1986). Patient's perceptions of their adjustment to disability and social support in a community-based teaching hospital. In S. Walker et al. (Eds), *Equal to the challenge: Perspectives, problems, and strategies in rehabilitation of non-white disabled.* Proceedings of the national conference of the Howard University model to improve rehabilitation services to minority populations with handicapping conditions. (ERIC Document Reproduction No. ED 276 198)

Minority Health Today (July/August 2000). *Black Men and Divorce: Implications For Culturally Competent Practice)*, 1(5).

National Institute on Aging, 1999–2000. Links: Minority research and training. http://www.nia.nih.gov/news/wgma/1999/winter.pdf.

National Mental Health Association (2002). Clinical depression and African Americans. Retrieved May 13, 2002, from http://www.intelihealth.com/specials/depression/htmDepr AfrAmer.html.

Nobles, W. W. (1980). African philosophy: Foundations for Black psychology. In R. L. Jones (Ed.), *Black psychology.* New York: Harper & Row.

Okun, B. F., Fried, J., & Okun, M. L. (1999). *Understanding Diversity: A Learning-As-Practice Primer.* Pacific Grove, CA: Brooks/Cole Publishing Company.

Parsons, E. C. (2003). Culturalizing instruction: Creating a more inclusive context for learning for African American students. *High School Journal*, (86) 4, p. 23.

Purnell, L. D., & Paulanka, B. J. (1998). *Transcultural healthcare: A culturally competent approach* (pp. 60–64). Philadelphia: F. A. Davis Company.

Redmond, T., & Slaney, R. B. (2002). "The influence of information and race on counselors' attributions." *Journal of College Student Development*, 43(6).

Reed, W. (1993). *Health and medical care for African Americans.* Westport, CT: Auburn House.

Roberson, M. H. B.(1985). The influence of religious beliefs on health choices on African Americans. *Topics in Clinical Nursing*, 7, 57–63.

Rouse, D. L. (2001). Lives of women of color create risk for depression. Retrieved May 13, 2002, from http://www.womensenews.org/article.cfm/dyn/aid/666/context/archive.

Samovar, L. A., & Porter, R. E. (1995). *Communication between cultures*. Belmont, CA: Wadsworth.

Smart, J. (2001). *Disability, society, and the individual* (pp. 170–185). Gaithersburg, MD: Aspen Publication.

Smey, J. W. (2001). Understanding racial prejudice, discrimination and racism and their influence on the healthcare delivery. In R. R. Leavitt (Ed.), *Cross-cultural rehabilitation: An international perspective* (pp. 74–77). Philadelphia: W. B. Saunders.

Smith, D. (1999). *Health care divided*. Ann Arbor, MI: University of Michigan Press.

Smitherman, G. (1991). "Talkin and testifyin": "Black English and the Black experience." In R. L. Jones (Ed.), *Black Psychology* (pp. 249–267). Berkeley, CA: Cobb & Henry Publishers.

Snow, L. E. (1978). Sorcerers, saints and charlatans: Black folk healers in urban America. *Culture, Medicine and Psychiatry, 2*, 69–106.

Spector, R. (1985). *Cultural diversity in health and illness* (2nd ed.). Norwalk, CT: Appleton Century-Crofts.

Spector, R. (1996). *Cultural diversity in health and illness*. Norwalk, CT: Appleton & Lange, 191–215.

Spector, R. E. (2000). *Cultural diversity in health and illness* (5th ed.) (pp. 215–230). Upper Saddle River, NJ: Prentice Hall.

Steele, R. E. (1978). Relationship of race, sex, and social class, and social mobility to depression in normal adults. *Journal of Social Psychology, 104*, 37–47.

Stolley, M. R., & Fitzgibbon, M. L. (1997). Effects of an obesity prevention program on the eating behavior of African American mothers and daughters. *Health Education and Behavior, 24*(2), 152–156.

Thomas, S. B. (1992). Health status of the black community in the 21st century: A futuristic perspective for health education. *Journal of Health Education, 23*, 7–13.

Wells, S. A., & Black, R. M. (2000). *Cultural competency for professionals* (pp.37–40). Bethesda, MD: The American Occupational Therapy Association.

Wesley, J. (2002). Depression in African American women. Retrieved May 13, 2002, from http://www.blackwomenshealth.com/depression.htm

West, C. (1993). *Race matters*. Vintage Press. NY: Random House, Inc.

Willis, F. N. (1966). Initial speaking distance as a function of speaker's relationship. *Psychon. Psy., 5*, 221–222.

Wilson, K. B. (1999). Vocational rehabilitation acceptance: A tale of two races in a large midwestern state. *Journal of Applied Rehabilitation Counseling, 30*(2), 25–31.

7

Native Americans

Matin Royeen and Jeffrey L. Crabtree

Key Words

history

Native American

rehabilitation

collectivism

individualism

Objectives

1. Understand the history of indigenous peoples of North America.
2. Understand some of the basic characteristics of Native American health beliefs and practices.
3. Identify and appreciate the implications of Native American health beliefs for rehabilitation professionals.
4. Identify and use a strategy to maximize a culturally competent approach to delivering rehabilitation services to Native Americans.

Introduction

In this chapter we offer a brief history of indigenous peoples of North America prior to and during the time that Europeans explored, colonized, and eventually conquered these people. In addition, we briefly discuss characteristics of Native American cultures, including health beliefs and practices, and other information that will help rehabilitation professionals understand the unique Native American cultures. Finally, we offer a strategy to maximizing a culturally competent approach to delivering rehabilitation services.

From the days prior to European colonization, Native Americans likely numbered 5 million and were composed of somewhere between 1,000 and 2,000 language groups (Lynch and Hanson, 1992). As Gone (n.d.) explains, the colonization of Native Americans yields a unique political and social legacy. Native Americans, in contrast to other ethnic minority groups, are not just another race, culture, or ethnic minority. They have "an utterly unique political status afforded to citizens of tribal nations that traces its origins to the Commerce and Treaty clauses of the U.S. Constitution" (p. 3). For the purpose of simplicity, we refer to these incredibly rich and diverse people as Native Americans, recognizing that no single term precisely or accurately describes all of these peoples.

Many Native American groups and nations share certain values and experiences, and many have very different values and experiences. Consequently, we speak of Native American *cultures*, not of a single culture. It is also important to note that there are over 500 federally recognized groups of these peoples and many more that have not been recognized by the federal government. Each of these groups has its own experiences, beliefs, and values. Consequently, we acknowledge that our discussion of Native American history and health beliefs and the like is general and overly simplistic. We hope that readers will explore the beliefs and values of specific groups they serve.

Rehabilitation Assumptions and Native American Cultures

When considering rehabilitation of Native Americans, it is critical to understand that notions of disability and functional independence are unique to the dominant Western culture. According to Clay (1992), Native American cultures have no similar concept of physical disability. Rather than looking at function and dysfunction in terms of physical characteristics, Native Americans generally view function and dysfunction in terms of harmony and disharmony of spirit. Also, rather than using a term like *disabled* to describe a member of a tribe or clan, many Native Americans would assign descriptive names associated with the specific disability (Fowler, Seekins, Dwyer, Duffy, Brod, and Locust, 2000).

Furthermore, Native Americans are traditionally communitarian in nature rather than individualistic. Consequently, Native Americans do not share the same view of independence and autonomy with the mainstream culture. Native American individuals are more likely to keep group needs and goals foremost in their minds. As Gone (n.d.) stated in his assessment of the effectiveness of Western mental health interventions with Native Americans, "the dominant treatment paradigms typically . . . are suffused with concepts and categories, principles and practices that are culturally alien to most indigenous ways of being in the world" (pp. 9–10). The significant differences between basic beliefs and concepts such as dualism and individualism integral to Western rehabilitation pose a serious challenge to rehabilitation practitioners who want to provide culturally relevant services to Native Americans (Sanderson, 2000/2001, p. 3).

The First Americans: A Brief History

Despite a lack of consensus, scientists suggest that between 30,000 to 50,000 years ago, an ice bridge in the form of a glacier connecting Siberia and Alaska provided passage for the first human immigrants to the new world (Reader's Digest, 1978). Over the years, they spread to every part of the new continent from North to South America, adapting to the demands of the new environment and developing diverse cultures.

Upon arrival of the Europeans to the new world, the descendants of the early pioneers had formed a wide variety of tribes, some leading nomadic lifestyles, whereas others sustained themselves with the riches of the forests, plains, rivers, and lakes. The Europeans were fascinated and puzzled by these brown-skinned people whom they had never encountered before. Some Europeans thought that these people were refugees from the old world brought to the new world by some kind of catastrophe such as the sinking of Atlantis or the scattering of the children of Israel and the fall of Carthage (Reader's Digest, 1978). The Mormon Church and some Jewish scholars speculate that these people are the descendants of a lost tribe of Israel (Utter, 1993).

The great cultural heritage of the Native Americans dates back many centuries when their great accomplishments in arts and sciences paralleled those of Europe. Evidence of pottery, clothing ornaments, weapons, and the use of tools and metals such as copper and gold found in their burial and religious sites, reflect a well-established cultural ancestry. In 1492, after Christopher Columbus landed in the Bahamas and mistook the islands for India, he named the original inhabitants of this continent as Indians. At that time, this great heterogeneous population of 5 million Native Americans, who spoke between 1,000 to 2,000 different languages, had their own nations before their homeland was invaded by the Europeans (Lynch and Hanson, 1992). Each nation had its own form of religious, political, and social organizations. Their political, social, and economic independence was defined by the concept of sovereignty where the Native American people exercised their power free from any external pressures (Thompson, 1996).

After the European invasion of their territories, the Native Americans lost their full sovereignty. According to Thompson (1996), several factors contributed to this outcome. First, the European contacts with the Native Americans caused a tremendous reduction in the Native American population that was mainly due to disease, wars, and murders. Also, many people lost their lives as a result of forced abandonment of their homelands by the Europeans. The second factor that adversely effected the sovereignty of the Native Americans was the loss of land that was intrinsically linked to their spiritual, religious, social, and economic well-being. Also, the cultural identity of the Native Americans was destroyed when their children were sent to boarding schools away from their families, where they were not allowed to speak their own language. They were forced to wear European attire and to cut their hair. Even on reservations, some were precluded from practicing their own religion and were not allowed to participate in their cultural activities such as Ghost Dances, potlatch ceremonies, and sun dances (Thompson, 1996).

The U.S. government policies were aimed to reduce the Native American cultural base and their sovereignty, and to assimilate Native Americans into the mainstream culture. The policies of land allotment, sending children to boarding schools, and termination of the Bureau of Indian Affairs were all examples of failed assimilation attempts. Similarly, most economic developments initiated by the federal government facilitated cultural disintegration of the tribal way of life by alienating them from their cultural integrity. Despite the attempts to wipe out Native American cultures and to assimilate the people into the mainstream culture, many Native Americans held on to their cultures and maintained a strong sense of cultural identity. Smith (2000) discusses the Hopi, Hualapai, and Havasupai tribes in Arizona who exemplify how some have resisted the mainstream pathway of economic development. These tribes have chosen against tourism revenues in order to maintain the integrity of their culture. Their tribal tradition outweighed the material benefits of uranium mining in their territories. The leadership of these tribes believed that accumulation of wealth by outside interference demeans the very core values of spirituality, community living, and traditional ceremonies.

The Sacred Land of Native Americans

Initially, the new United States government wanted to deal with the Native Americans as a sovereign nation. Under the leadership of President George Washington, the Congress passed laws that no land could be secured from the Native Americans without congressional approval (Thompson, 1996). Unfortunately, this did not stop the settlers from taking advantage of the trading relationship with the Native Americans. President Thomas Jefferson thought that the Native Americans could not survive the onslaught of the European incursions and supported the idea of the Native American moving westward so that they could enjoy economic independence without any interference by the European adventures (Thompson, 1966).

The removal of the Native Americans from the East to the areas west of the Mississippi River supported the concept of separating the natives from the white Europeans who, according to Manifest Destiny, were destined by God to take control of the entire North American continent and use it for their economic benefit. The federal government relocation of the Native Americans had two goals: first, to do away with their traditional tribal way by allocating them to reservation land; and second, to make the Native Americans independent and productive members of society by means of private ownership of land (McDonnell, 1991). Both goals ultimately had the assimilation of the Native American in mind. It was expected that the Native Americans would move away from their traditional life and adopt what was considered the superior culture of the Europeans. The first comprehensive program, called the Dawes Allotment Act, was developed in 1887 to meet these goals (McDonnell, 1991). Under this act, each Native American family received 160 acres; each single person over 18 received 80 acres; and each person under 18, including the new-born, received 40 acres.

Unfortunately, the Dawes Act did not solve the Native American problem. In the twentieth century, Congress passed legislation allowing Native Americans to lease or sell their allotments during the trust period. This opened up even greater opportunities for European Americans to take advantage by developing new resources on Native American reservations. Between 1900 and 1921, the government of the United States had assigned almost 86,000 allotments, equivalent to more than 14 million acres, to Native American reservations, mostly in Oklahoma, Montana, Minnesota, Wyoming, Idaho, Washington, Oregon, northern California, and North and South Dakota (McDonnell, 1991).

The allotment policy broke down in its implementation phase, forcing many Native Americans to lease their land, making them very dependent on rental income. At this point, about 60% of the Native American people were either completely without land or did not have enough on which to make a decent living (McDonnell, 1991). The Native Americans' highly developed culture of community and living in harmony with nature contradicted the culture of white America, which valued progress characterized by efficiency, prosperity, technological advances, and exploiting the environment to meet the needs of the individual and society.

Characteristics of Native American Cultures

Given the great diversity of Native American groups and cultures, it is impossible to identify one set of beliefs and values about life, health, and wellness that influences their view and behavior related to the typical issues addressed by rehabilitation professionals. However, a number of authors (Harry, 1992; Joho & Ormsby, 2000; Robbins, 1996) have attempted to identify values and belief systems that come close to being common among Native Americans. (For one example, see Table 7.1.) In this chapter we identify four characteristics that have strong implications for rehabilitation practitioners. First, an apparently overarching belief among Native Americans is that "life is geared toward mindfully maintaining the fragile equilibrium of body, mind, spirit, and nature" (Kavasch & Barr, 1999, p. 44). A second is the belief about death and dying, perhaps best expressed by Chief Seattle who said, "There is no death, only a change of worlds" (as cited in Kavasch & Barr, 1999, p. 16). Third, in the Native American cosmology, the land is considered a place of power, a source of both practical and spiritual sustenance. The most radical view of the human relationship to the earth held by early Native Americans included the notion that one should do nothing, including planting seeds, that would wound Mother Earth (Lavender, 1992). A more moderate view of the Native Americans' relationship to Mother Earth was characterized by Old Joseph of the Nez Percé, who believed that the land could not be appropriately parceled and fenced. To him and many other Native Americans, "Land was continuous as air. It could not be alienated from the trees that grew in the high country or from the deer that browsed in the canyons" (Lavender, 1992, p. 167). The value and respect that Native Americans place on the earth is poignantly expressed by a chief of a northern Blackfoot band when he responded to a request from U.S. delegates for his signature on one of the earliest land treaties (McLuhan, 1971): "Our land is more valuable

TABLE 7.1 The Native American Shared Belief Systems Based on the Reciprocal Relationship Between Humans and Nature.

Respect for age	Children are expected to care for their elders, including extended family members such as aunts and uncles. The leadership position in the family is held by an elder, most likely the eldest female member. The elderly are consulted for their wisdom and life experiences.
Present-mindedness	Each day is lived to its fullest. The individual has little control over the future. Planning for the future is futile.
Value of extended family and clan system	The function of the family is for creation and caring. There is nothing more important than the family or clan. To be poor by American Indian standards is to be without family. In some American Indian tribes, all women who were instrumental in the development of an individual are referred to as "mother." In other tribes, first cousins are treated as brothers and sisters.
Decision making	Problem solving and decision making are group rather than individual experiences. Decisions are based on what is best for the community, not necessarily for the individual.
Cooperation	Competition is devalued and discouraged because it weakens the cohesiveness of the group. Sharing is a core value of American Indians.
Time	The completion of a task takes precedence over appointments or meetings. Time is a continuum with neither a beginning nor an end. It is not unusual for an American Indian home to be without clocks.
Status of role	Relationships are based on personal integrity, not on role, status, or the accumulation of material goods. To the American Indian, the concept of being is more important than the concept of achieving.
Natural resources and the environment	All of nature exists in harmony. Everything has a spirit. The American Indian uses only those resources needed to survive and does not change the environment to fit the needs of people but lives and accepts the environment.
Health	The basis of health and well-being is to live in harmony and balance within the world. Health is not the absence of illness or disease.

Source: Joho, K. A., & Ormsby, A. (2000). A walk in beauty: Strategies for providing culturally competent nursing care to Native Americans. In M. L. Kelley & V. M. Fitzsimons (Eds.), *Understanding cultural diversity: Culture, curriculum, and community in nursing* (p. 212). Sudbury, MA: Jones and Bartlett Publishers.

than your money. It will last forever. It will not even perish by the flames of fire. As long as the sun shines and the waters flow, this land will be here to give life to men and animals. We cannot sell the lives of men and animals; therefore we cannot sell this land. It was put here for us by the Great Spirit and we cannot sell it because it does not belong to us" (p. 53).

Finally, as stated earlier, Native Americans are traditionally communitarian in nature. Consequently, they tend to work for the good of the family, clan, or tribe. Praise of personal accomplishments may cause them embarrassment, and important decisions about health and rehabilitation are likely left to respected elders of the family or clan.

The Importance of Sport

With the great diversity of the Native American tribes—speaking different languages and following different social structures and traditions—it is difficult to generalize about certain features of their cultures, including sports. However, sports seemed to be an important part of the Native American culture and are evident in festivals, ceremonies, and other events. Games ranged from fun activities of playing with children to more significant sporting events requiring the entire community participation. According to Oxendine (1988), traditional Native American sports were significant because sports connected individuals to social, spiritual, and economic life; sports prepared the body, mind, and spirit for a healthy competition and standards of fair play for males and females; and sports provided and reinforced the notion of team membership in the community.

Culin (1975) divided the Native American games into two areas. The first category included games of dexterity that involved speed, strength, stamina, and strategy. These games required a great deal of training and preparation, and were played with a clear purpose significant to the Native American community. The second category involved games of chance played for gambling purposes. These games consisted of dice games, stick games, and the moccasin game. The outcome of the games of dexterity is generally determined by the abilities of the participants, whereas the outcome of games of chance is determined by luck. Brown (1953) states that sports in the Native American cultures began as rites and later developed into popular events. The spiritual dimension of sports was meant to bring the favor of the spirits and to rid people of evil and misfortune. The games were sometimes forms of prayers to bring rain in times of drought, to heal a sick individual, and to bring success in hunting and battle. Salter (1970) has identified mortuary practices, sickness, climatic conditions, and fertility as religio-magical connections to sports. Mortuary games were designed to honor the dead by playing his or her favorite game. The popular rain dances were performed by the Native American in order to avoid drought, too much rain, severe cold, and heat. Games for healing were used for preventive and curative purposes with the focus of stopping suffering. Some even believed that the outcome of the games was determined by supernatural powers. In some cases, the medicine men assisted by washing the feet of the runner, using warm water and herbs (Lumholtz, 1890).

Winning was important, but in the spirit of good teamwork, not of individual performance. Little emphasis was placed on individual achievements, statistics, and quantification of the games. Traditional Native American contests were not uniform, and they played their games without any set of rigid standardization. The field dimensions, uniform and equipment specifications, duration of play, number of participants, distance, and the number of points required for victory differed in various games. The more significant the event, the more the number of player participating in the game. For example, in the game of lacrosse, the number of participants varied from a dozen to several hundred. A 300-yard field was used for a small game, whereas a large game was played on a field of about one-half mile in length. Fair play and good sportsmanship were very important. The judges' integrity was never questioned. Sometimes the judges carried sticks with them during the games and used them whenever a player lost his or her temper. Trickery and deception were part of sports, and incidents of trickery among animals, humans, and supernatural creatures are recorded in Native American mythology.

The nature of games differed. Young men engaged in wrestling, tug of war, push-of-wars, and boxing. A popular gamed played among youth in different tribes was called Sitting on the Clam (Oxendine, 1988). One member of the team would bury a clam in the sand and sit on it while the rest of the player's teammates would defend the player against the opponents who were trying to break the protective circle by dragging the player off the clam. Upon successful stealing of the clam, the new team would take its turn to protect it from the opponents. Hamilton (1972) describes another popular game among the Native American youth, who would invade the nest of the wild bees. After considerable deliberation, planning, and ceremony, the young men would attack the bees' nest. The purpose was for the young men to display courage and bravery by attacking the nest, avoiding screaming or crying after repeated bee stings. After completion of this game, the young men would join another team for a search and destroy mission of another bees nest.

Inclusion of tribal artwork was used for decorating their equipment, costumes, and other implements.

The Native American Arts

Arts, crafts, and music are deeply embedded in the Native American cultural identity. Cultural and spiritual values, political statements, and religious and healing practices are often reflected in all three. Pritzker (2000) describes the prevalence of arts and crafts among the Zuni, Pomo, and Catawba tribes. The Zuni of New Mexico are well known for their weaving of blankets, pottery, and jewelry. The art of pottery is taught by a few experts, whereas the production of jewelry is based at home where parents pass on the skill to their children. In addition to the arts' serving as a big source of revenue, the Zuni government is attempting to protect its tribes by developing a certification process for the artists. The Pomo tribes of north-central California are well known for their basket weaving for many centuries. The women produce fine basketry, whereas the men make fish straps (Pritzker, 2000). Baskets with different patterns serving a variety of functions such as medicine basket, carrying basket, prayer basket, and gift basket were produced and were often buried with a corpse. The Catawba people of south Carolina were well known for the production of pottery. The artists create pottery using the traditional techniques that are passed to the younger generation within their families.

Studies of petroglyphs and pictographs on rock faces yield two types of rock art, ceremonial and biographic. The ceremonial art provides considerable cultural information about decorated shields, types of weapons, and other ceremonial regalia used by pedestrian nomads. The evidence also shows a very strong spiritual relationship between the artist and animal spirits. Turbulent changes followed in the 1700s as the scenes of warfare in the form of artwork replaced animal pictures of the earlier era. This was the transition from the ceremonial art to the biographic style (Taylor, 1994).

According to Kavasch & Baar (1999), Native Americans use a number of instruments from drums and rattles, to flutes and zithers, in sacred ceremonies, prayers, and healing rites. These instruments were meant to echo the music of nature such as thunder, rain, wind, and running water. Singing and chanting were also important aspects of everyday life from blessing a newborn child, to healing a sick person, to praying for a good harvest. The human voice was a key element in many Native Americans ceremonies such as the potlatch, powwow, and kachina rites (Kavasch & Baar, 1999).

Health, Healing, and Rehabilitation

The following discussion of health, healing, and rehabilitation is necessarily very general given that our discussion about Native Americans includes a variety of different cultures that have a profound influence on their beliefs, behavior, perceptions, and the like (National Center for the Dissemination of Disability Research, 1999). According to Rhoades & Rhoades (2000),

> A generally accepted Indian concept of health is that it is a tangible reality, not simply the state of being free of disease. This health, or wellness, is often described as the ability to exist in a harmonious relationship with all other living things, but also with a number of spirits, including a great and all-powerful spirit. The emphasis on the spirit world, supernatural forces, and religion stand in sharp contrast to the secular emphasis on disturbed physiology and purely physical explanations of Western medicine. (p. 404)

More specifically, in this generalized Native American view, an individual's psychological, emotional, spiritual, and physical well-being are all connected. According to this holistic view, good health results from the presence of harmony with family, friends, nature, and the universe (Huttlinger and Tanner, 1994). Some believe that harming Mother Earth causes self-harm that results in illness. Generally speaking, the primary causes of illness include witchcraft, violation of taboos, the loss of soul, spirit possession, and annoying the elements (Rhoades & Rhoades, 2000; Sobralske, 1985). These etiologies, in many Native American cultures, account for most of the specific diseases identified by the mainstream medical culture. For example, in a study of Muscogee (Creek) Indians, Wing and Thompson (1995) found that participants did not differentiate the causes of alcoholism from those of other illnesses. In order to maintain good health, people should pay special attention to relationships, kinship obligations, and giving generously to others (Basso, 1989).

Traditional Native American Healing

Traditional Native American medicine is a complex system that operates at multiple levels: "personal care of most common maladies not requiring special expertise, 'folk' healing by 'lay' individuals with special skills, and an elaborate system of practitioners who dedicate a substantial portion of their lives to the 'healing arts'" (Rhoades & Rhoades, 2000, p. 402). Traditional Native American medicine is inexorably connected to religion and the spirit world. Traditional practitioners, sometimes called shamans and singers in the Navajo tradition, acquire special powers to communicate with the spirits, heal the sick, and foretell the future. They can acquire these powers through something as "simple" as a dream, through what is called a vision quest or through mind-altering drugs. Although the traditional healer exercises great powers, this power is not considered a personal attribute of the healer but is seen as a higher power invoked by the healer (Davies, 2001; Rhoades & Rhoades, 2000).

Conditions caused by these traditional Native American etiologies are generally treated by religious practitioners such as the shaman, who can invoke supernatural powers to cure the conditions. The symptoms of disease (pain, rash, cough, loss of function) are treated by more naturalistic methods such as the use of herbs, heat, cupping, and the like (Kavasch & Barr, 1999; Rhoades & Rhoades, 2000)

Reflecting on Native American healing, Null (1996) describes a Lakota [Sioux] story. During a famine, a woman wearing a white buffalo skin and carrying a sacred pipe appeared. She showed the people the pipe ceremony that consisted of offerings made to the four directions and singing songs while playing the drums. She taught people that thanking Wakan Tanka, or the Great Spirit, with the pipe would provide blessings on earth. She taught the people about the unity of the earth, sky, and all life. The woman turned into a buffalo, changing colors several times. At the end, she changed into a white buffalo calf and disappeared into the distance. Before disappearing, she told people that she would return at the proper time. According to Null (1996), her promise of return was fulfilled with the birth of a white buffalo in Jamesville, Wisconsin. In its birth in the summer of 1994, this buffalo has changed its colors from white to black, then to red to yellow and back to white. North represents white, south represents red, west represents black, and east represents yellow in many Native American cultures. This buffalo has a significant symbolic meaning to the Native Americans, who interpret the birth of this white buffalo calf to mean that all the four energies come together in peace as one human race.

The Native American symbols such as the shield often play a role in healing, wellness, and spiritual protection. Shields used for spiritual protection were circular designs that contained symbols of an animal or an insect to which the individual felt close. Another powerful instrument used to symbolize peace and harmony and promote healing was the medicine wheel. The medicine wheel is frequently a large design, often made of available stones, laid out in a circle divided by lines of stones that radiate outward to the enclosing circle. According to Kavasch and Baar (1999), medicine wheels constructed since European colonization generally have four main spokes. North represents purity and renewal, South signifies rapid growth and trust, East signifies illumination and wisdom, and West reflects strength and introspection. Each direction covers three separate months, with each month having specific characteristics. The medicine wheel shows individuals the proper path of life directed toward accomplishing goals that require the following steps of sacrifice, prayer, transformation, and thanksgiving.

Ceremonies and Rituals

Native Americans use ceremonies and rituals for all manner of health and wellness purposes from healing to living in peace and harmony with nature. In the following sections, we describe some of the ceremonies that deal directly with health and healing to help provide the reader some insights into the purpose and meaning of sacred practices. Not all of the ceremonies and rituals discussed here are used by all Native Americans, and there are many variations of these ceremonies and rituals throughout Native American cultures.

Ghost Dance

This ceremony is performed for regeneration and restoration of the Earth. According to Null (1996), this dance acquired additional meanings and spread very rapidly to other American Indian nations. The performance of the ghost dance provided healing for those who had lost their loved ones. Others believed that wearing certain designs on their clothing would provide protection for them in battle. The magical and spiritual power of this dance served as a unifying force for the Native American people. Native Americans will never forget the sad memory of the Wounded Knee massacre of 1890 in which U.S. government troops killed many dancers during a peaceful Ghost Dance ceremony.

Pipe Ceremony

In essence, the pipe ceremony marks a very strong bond between the earth and the spiritual energies of the universe. Null (1996) cites an Ogalala Sioux author (Eagle Man) who begins the ceremony by seeking powers of energy from the four directions. The West provides rains, a source of life for all organisms. The North is the source of strength, endurance, and truthfulness in life. The East brings the power of the sun that gives knowledge and spirituality without which mankind could be harmed. Finally, the South brings medicine, growth, and bounty for all. In order to acknowledge the spirit of Mother Earth, the Eagle Man touches the pipe to the ground, promising to protect Mother Earth, and then the pipe is held up toward the sky, since the sun provides life for the earth. Finally, the Eagle Man thanks the six powers of the universe The smoking of the pipe ceremony carried the people's word to the Creator, and in return, the Creator would send blessings to the individual smoking the pipe. After smoking the pipe, the Native American would always keep their word. The government took advantage of this feature of the Native culture where the signing of the treaties was accompanied by pipe ceremonies.

Purification Ceremony

This ceremony, also known as the sweat lodge ceremony, integrates the spiritual and the physical world through the process of purification. The traditional healer serves as the leader of the ceremony and assists the participants to become aware of the healing process within themselves. After the initial period of contemplation and prayer, the traditional healer sends four sacred herbs in four different directions. Sage gets rid of the negative energies, whereas sweetgrass brings powerful individuals from the other side to heal. Cedar, a sweet purifier, is very attractive to the energies of the invisible world. The last herb is tobacco, which is used to bless the earth. The participants crawl around a pit full of grandfather hot rocks, which are brought in one at a time. The first four rocks are placed in four directions and are sprinkled with different herbs and other things that the traditional healer may bring. After the water hits the rocks, the steam fills the air and unifies everyone. Sitting in a circle, each participant offers prayers to the Almighty, the sky, the earth, and the great spirits. More thanks are given, people sing songs for bringing in spirits, and healing begins when the physical world interacts with the nonphysical world. The traditional healer calls in the spirits, and each participant verbalizes his or her request and asks for healing. The purification ceremony serves as another healing vehicle for those people suffering from disease (Null, 1996). Lyons (1998) provides a comprehensive description of the healing practices of the Native Americans in the past 350 years.

Smudging Ceremony

According to Kavasch & Baar (1999), most Native American cultures have smudges, or smudging ceremonies, during which the participants burn herbs for prayers and purification. The herbs are not intended to burst into flames but rather are to smoke slowly. The participants burn sage as a purifier to banish trouble and bad spirits, and sweetgrass to welcome good spirits and good energies. Smudging is often done during healing prayers and ceremonies to connect participants with spirit helpers. In addition, these herbs are often burned during funerals and death feasts because it is believed that their smoke carries prayers and sadness upward to the ancestor's spirits.

Many of the ceremonies and traditional healing practices discussed here may seem odd to the Western rehabilitation practitioner. However, these practices are embedded in Native American cultures (Rhoades & Rhoades, 2000). An appreciation of the meanings of these practices provides a foundation for providing culturally competent rehabilitation services to especially traditional Native Americans.

An Integrative Approach to Practice

Although the following integrative approach to practice (James & Prilleltensky, 2002) was developed for ethnically and culturally diverse mental health practices, it provides rehabilitation practitioners with a framework for addressing diverse cultural issues imbedded in services provided not only to Native Americans but also to virtually all ethnically and culturally diverse populations. The authors describe the integrative approach as "a cycle of activity that includes philosophical, contextual, experiential, and pragmatic considerations" (p. 5 of 30). Addressing these four considerations helps practitioners integrate into their practices cultural elements that often go ignored or, if addressed, are considered in isolation.

The following is an overview of the integrative approach with a summary example of the practical application of this approach in providing services to Native Americans. With each overlapping condition, the practitioner seeks information from the rehabilitation client, caregiver, family members, and others who have information that will help maximize the effectiveness of culturally competent interventions. (See Table 7.2 for a summary of the integrative approach.)

TABLE 7.2 Integrative Approach: Considerations, Questions, Resources, and Outcomes.

Considerations	Key Questions	Resources	Outcomes
Philosophical	What is the client's and the caregiver's vision of the good person, the good society? What are each person's dominant values?	Client's and caregiver's moral, religious, and social guide and the family.	Understanding of the client's and the caregiver's meaning of a good person, the good life, and the good society.
Contextual	What are the client's and the caregiver's social, cultural, religious, and moral norms? How do these affect their concept of life, mental health, and physical function?	Client's and caregiver's moral, religious, and social guide and the family.	Identification of the client's and the caregiver's prevailing norms and the social conditions affecting beliefs about life, mental health, and physical function.
Experiential	What is missing from the client's and the caregiver's social context needed to improve the mental health and physical function of the client, caregiver, family, and community?	Client's and caregiver's moral, religious, and social guide and the family.	Identification of the client's and the caregiver's needs related to mental health and physical function as expressed by the client and other stakeholders.
Pragmatic	What can be done to improve the mental health and function of the client, caregiver, and family?	Rehabilitation practitioners in consort with the client, caregiver, and family.	Personal change in response to rehabilitation practitioners' culturally competent assessments and interventions.

Source: James, S. & Prilleltensky, I. (2002). Cultural diversity and mental health: Towards integrative practice. *Clinical Psychology Review, 22*(8), 1133–1154.

Philosophical Considerations

Philosophical considerations have to do with the client's beliefs about the good life: what it means to be a good person living in a good society and what social values people have that shape their beliefs about physical function and mental health. The practitioner should ask, for instance, whether the client believes in the liberal notions of individualism or in more traditional notions of collectivism. Native Americans are likely to believe in collectivist notions of the individual's role in the family and tribe. A Native American will likely say that the good life is one of cooperation and of working for the good of the family, clan, or tribe. Good people are respectful of their elders and do not seek riches or reward for themselves, only for their clan or tribe. The good society is one that is committed to the welfare of the collective group and one that is a good shepherd of the land and its bounty. These expressions of people's philosophical beliefs give the reflective rehabilitation practitioner an understanding of the social values of their clients and provide a backdrop for understanding specific behaviors and attitudes of their clients.

Contextual Considerations

Contextual considerations are basically the "actual state of affairs in which people live" (James & Prilleltensky, 2002, p. 1140). Native Americans generally live as though their spiritual and physical life are inseparable. Health, in that view, is dependent upon what "sort of life one is leading, whether one is at peace with everyone else, and whether one's own life is in balance" (Robbins, 1996, p. 149) Significant contextual considerations include Native Americans' family unit, their experiences with Western health care services, the Western medicine beliefs of the etiology of various diseases, and Native Americans' beliefs about traditional medicine. For example, because the Native American family traditionally includes the clan and tribe as well as the immediate kin (Robbins, 1996), young Native Americans will likely defer important decisions to older members of their family and tribe, and will look to traditional healers to cure illnesses.

After years of dealing with the mainstream American culture, Native Americans may be suspicious of Western rehabilitation practitioners. This inclination, added to the tendency of many Native Americans to maintain a family hierarchy, the reluctance to talk openly about their problems in front of a stranger, the avoidance of direct eye contact, and the tendency to be silent unless spoken to, can lead the rehabilitation practitioner to believe that Native Americans are subassertive and uninterested in therapy.

Western medicine medicalizes social ills such as alcoholism, diabetes, and other "lifestyle" illnesses and considers them as a problem of individuals instead of family or social problems (James & Prilleltensky, 2002). Consequently, the rehabilitation practitioner will need to address social context problems that need intervention at the family and community levels.

To paraphrase Joho and Ormsby (2000), it would be preposterous to assume that Native Americans disregard the benefits of typical Western rehabilitation interventions. However, providing services to help the person who has recently had a stroke to ambulate, communicate, and perform daily tasks as safely and independently as possible is only a piece of the total healing process. Native Americans might also expect to use a traditional healer to help determine, from the traditional Native American perspective, the cause of the stroke, and through various ceremonies, to regain their spiritual balance (Hodge & Fredericks, 1999; Joho & Ormsby, 2000).

Experiential Considerations

While the philosophical and contextual considerations prompt questions about clients' worldview and their cultural, social, religious, and moral norms, the experiential consideration assumes that the lived experience serves to identify the specific and broad needs of the clients. This consideration encourages us to cast a broad assessment net to gather information about our clients' disabling, subjective experience. When we ask open-ended questions like *What is missing in your life?* and *What is a desirable state of affairs for you?* rather than just focused questions like Why can't you transfer or safely live alone? we come to appreciate the social and spiritual context of the client, and we are more likely to offer culturally relevant services.

Gathering information about clients' disabling experience includes giving clients the opportunity to perform, during therapy, in ways that express their cultural values and beliefs. Specifically, by having Native American clients engage in the normal routines and perform in culturally acceptable ways, rehabilitation practitioners come to understand how those clients express their intentions, to gain insight into clients' meanings, and to come to understand how their clients respond to the intrinsic and extrinsic limits and constraints placed on their performing. (Crabtree, 2003).

Pragmatic Considerations

According to James & Prilleltensky (2002), "The main question answered by this set of considerations is what can be done. This question is meant to bridge the gap between the actual state of affairs on one hand, and desirable and ideal visions on the other" (p. 17 of 30). It is important to note here that the authors of the integrative approach assert that one should not limit intervention only to the individual and to "therapy." They suggest that because the individual is never removed from his or her context, social action and community interventions are often needed and useful. The ideal outcome of examining this consideration includes personal and social interventions "that respond to the local context and that are sensitive to the needs of the individuals and communities" (p. 18 of 30).

Case Study

Tom, a 30-year patient, was brought to OT and PT services by members of his family. He was involved in a car accident that caused a broken right hand and broken left knee. Tom had difficulty with movements of both hand and knee following surgery. He is a brick layer, and both his hands and his feet are important for financial survival. The OT and PT both discuss the extent of Tom's problems with him and members of his family during the initial visit. During the interview, Tom is not very talkative and answers questions only with his eyes down. Additionally, older members of the family answer questions for Tom, who appears to be passive and disinterested. Both the OT and the

PT feel that Tom is not taking any initiative for his own recovery. Furthermore, Tom is not very sure how the OT and the PT intervention can help him.

Questions

1. Why do you think that Tom is accompanied by members of his family? Isn't he old enough to be able to deal with the OT and the PT?
2. Discuss and explain Tom's patterns of communication with the rehabilitation professionals.
3. Provide some reasons for Tom's uncertainty about the PT and the OT intervention.
4. Describe some expectations of the rehabilitation professionals in the area of communication with Tom.
5. Provide five specific culturally based recommendations for the rehabilitation professionals.

Summary

Providing effective and relevant services to virtually any rehabilitation client can be a challenge. Providing services to members of specific ethnic and cultural groups compounds that challenge. In this chapter, we offered a brief history of indigenous peoples of North America prior to and during the European exploration and colonization. In addition, we briefly discussed characteristics of Native American cultures, including health beliefs and practices, that will hopefully help rehabilitation professionals understand the unique Native American cultures. Finally, we offered a strategy to maximize a culturally competent approach to delivering rehabilitation services.

Questions

1. Describe the way that Native Americans lived before the arrival of the Europeans to the New World.
2. How did the newly arrived European treat the Native Americans?
3. Describe how some of the federal government programs affect the cultural identity of the Native Americans.
4. What are some important cultural characteristics of the Native Americans?
5. As a practitioner, how would you utilize these characteristics as an effective tool with the Native American client?
6. On the basis of the traditional Native American belief system, what are the underlying causes of illness?
7. Describe some ceremonies and rituals of the Native Americans.

8. Should some of these rituals be included during interventions? If yes, describe how.
9. Describe some important considerations in the treatment of the Native Americans mentioned in this chapter.
10. How would you utilize these points toward effective intervention with the Native American client?

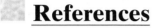 # References

American Indian Disability Technical Assistance Center (no date). How has the U.S. Government addressed disability issues? Retrieved from http://ruralinstitute.umt.edu/Indian/Factsheets/USDisLeg.htm.

American Indian Disability Technical Assistance Center. (no date). How have American Indian Tribes addressed disability issues? Retrieved from http://ruralinstitute.umt.edu/Indian/Factsheets/AmITribes.htm.

Basso, H. (1989). Southwest Apache. In D. E. Walker (Ed), *Witchcraft and sorcery* (pp. 167–190). Moscow, Id.: University of Idaho Press.

Beauvais, F. (1992). An integrated model for prevention and treatment of drug abuse among American Indian youth. *Journal of Addiction Disease. 11*(3), 63–80.

Brown, J. (1953). *The sacred pipe: Black Elk's account of the seven rites of the Oglala Sioux*. Norman, OK: University of Oklahoma Press.

Carmichael, D. L., Hubert, J., Reeves, B. & Schanche, A. (1994). *Sacred sites, sacred places.* New York: Routledge.

Cassidy L. (1988). Occupational therapy intervention in the treatment of alcoholics. In D. Gibson (Ed.), *Treatment of Substance Abuse: Psychosocial Occupational Therapy Approaches.* New York: Haworth Press, pp. 17–26. (ADAI bk) Call No: RC 564 T74 1988.

Clay, J. (1992). Native American independent living. *Rural Special Education Quarterly, 11*(1), 41–50.

Collins, L. (1994). Sociocultural aspects of alcohol use and abuse: Ethnicity and gender. *Drugs and Society, 8*(1), 89–116.

Crabtree, J. L. (2003). On performance. *Occupational Therapy in Health Care, (17)*2, 1–18.

Culin, S. (1975). *Games of North American Indians.* NY: Dover.

Davies, W. (2001). *Healing ways: Navajo health care in the twentieth century.* Albuquerque: University of New Mexico Press.

Eckardt, M. & Martin, P. (1986). Clinical assessment of cognition in alcoholism. *Alcoholism: Clinical and Experimental Research, 10*, 123–127.

Fowler, L., Seekins, T., Dwyer, K., Duffy, S., Brod, R., & Locust, C. (2000). American Indian disability legislation and programs: Findings of the first national survey of tribal governments. *Journal of Disability Policy Studies, 10*(2), 166–185.

French, L. (1990). Substance abuse treatment among American Indian children. *Alcoholism Treatment Quarterly, 7*(3), 63–76.

Gangle, M. (1987). The effectiveness of an occupational therapy program for chemically dependent adolescents. *Occupational Therapy in Mental Health, 7*, 67–88.

Gone, J. P. (no date). *American Indian mental health service delivery: Persistent challenges and future prospects.* Retrieved from htttp://www.lsa.umich.edu/psych/clinical/jgone/AIMHExt.doc. Scheduled to appear in J. S. Mio & G. Y. Iwamasa (Eds.), *Culturally diverse mental health: The challenges and resistance.* New York: Brunner-Routledge.

Hamilton, T. (1972). Native American Bows: Philadelphia, George Shunway Publishing.

Harry, B. (1992). *Cultural diversity, families, and the special education system.* New York: Teachers College Press.

Hennecke, L. & Gitlow, S. (1983). Alcohol use and alcoholism in adolescence. *New York State Journal of Medicine, 83*, 936–940.

Hodge, F. S. & Fredericks, L. (1999). In R. M. Huff & M. V. Kline (Eds.), *Promoting health in multicultural populations: A handbook for practitioners* (pp. 269–289). Thousand Oaks, California: Sage Publications.

Huttlinger, K., Krefting, L., Drevdahl, D., Tree, P., Baca, E. & Benally, A. (1992). "Doing battle": A metaphorical analysis of Diabetes Mellitus among Navajo People. *American Journal of Occupational Therapy, 46*(8), 706–712.

Huttlinger, W. & Tanner, D. (1994). The peyote way: Implication for culture care theory. *Journal of Trans-Cultural Nursing, 5*(2), 5–11.

Indian Health Service (1996). *Trends in Indian Health.* Washington, DC: U.S. Department of Health and Human Services, Public Health Service.

James, S. & Prilleltensky, I. (2002). Cultural diversity and mental health: Towards integrative practice. *Clinical Psychology Review, 22*(8), 1133–1154.

Joho, K. A. & Ormsby, A. (2000). A walk in beauty: Strategies for providing culturally competent nursing care to Native Americans. In M. L. Kelley & V. M. Fitzsimons (Eds.), *Understanding cultural diversity: Culture, curriculum, and community in nursing* (p. 212). Sudbury, MA: Jones and Bartlett Publishers.

Kaufman, J. (1986). Indian alcoholism: A national plague. *NIHB Health Reporter, 4*, 55–8.

Kavasch, E. B. & Barr, K. (1999). *American Indian healing arts.* New York: Bantam Books.

Kimball, H., Goldberg, I. & Oberle, W. (1996). The prevalence of selected risk factors for chronic disease among American Indians in Washington State. *Public Health Reports, 111*(3), 264–271.

LaFrombois, T. (1988). American Indian mental health policy. *American Psychologist, 43*, 388–397.

Lang, K. (1988). Ethnographic interview: An occupational needs assessment tool for American Indians and Alaska Native alcoholics. *Occupational Therapy in Mental Health, 8*(2), 61–80.

Lavender, D. (1992) *Let me be free: The Nez Perce tragedy.* New York: Harper Collins Publishers.

Lindsay, W. (1983). The role of the occupational therapist in treatment of alcoholism. *American Journal of Occupational Therapy, 37*, 36–43.

Lumholtz, C. (1890). Tarahumari life and customs. *Scriber's Magazine, 16*, 296–311.

Lynch, E. & Hanson M. (1992). *Developing cross-cultural competence: A guide working with young children and their families.* Baltimore: Brooks Publishing.

Lyons, W. (1998). *Encyclopedia of Native American healing.* New York: W. W. Norton and Company, Inc.

Mail, P. (1985). Closing the circle. A prevention model for Indian community with alcohol problems. *HIS Primary Care Provider, 1*, 2–5.

McDonnell, J. (1991). *The dispossession of the American Indian 1887–1934.* Bloomington, IN: Indiana University Press.

McLuhan, T. C. (1971). *Touch the earth: A self-portrait of Indian existence.* New York: Promontory Press.

Mooney, J. (1890). The Cherokee ball play. *The American Anthropologist, 3*, 105–132.

Mooney, J. (1893/1991). *The ghost-dance religion and wounded knee.* New York: Dover Publications.

Moyers, P. & Barrett, C. (1992). Neurocognition and alcoholism: Implication for occupational therapy. *Occupational Therapy in Health Care, 8*(2–3), 87–115.

National Center for the Dissemination of Disability Research (1999). *Disability, diversity, and dissemination: A review of the literature on topics related to increasing the utilization of rehabilitation research outcomes among diverse consumer groups. Part 1—Theoretical framework.* Retrieved from http://www.ncddr.org/du/researchexchange/v40n01/

Nelson, E., Moon, W., Holtzman, D., Smith. P. & Siegel, P. (1997). Patterns of health risk behaviors for chronic disease: A comparison between adolescent and adult American Indians. *Journal of Adolescent Health, 21*(1), 25–32.

Nobokov, P. (1981). *Indian running.* Santa Barbara, CA: Capra Press.

Null, G., (1996). Native American healing. Retrieved from www.garynull.com/Documents/nativeamerican.htm.

Oxendine, J. (1988). *American Indian sports heritage.* Champaign, IL: Human Kinetics Books.

Pritzker, B. M. (2000). A Native American encyclopedia: History, culture, and peoples. Oxford: Oxford Digest University Press.

Reader's Digest (1978). *America's fascinating Indian heritage.* Pleasantville, NY: Reader's Digest University Press.

Rhoades, E. R. & Rhoades, D. A. (2000). Traditional Indian and modern western medicine. In E. R. Rhoades (Ed.), *American Indian health: Innovations in health care, promotion, and policy* (pp. 401–417). Baltimore: The Johns Hopkins University Press.

Robbins, M. J. (1996). In M. C. Julia, G. B. Winbush, G. H. Waltman, K. V. Harper, A. D. Kulwicki, E. L. Chung, H. Burgos-Ocasio, M. J. Robbins & S. S. Ratliff, *Multicultural awareness in the health care professions* (pp. 146–163). Boston: Allyn & Bacon.

Salter, M. (1970). *Games in Ritual: A study of selected North American Indian Tribes.* Unpublished doctoral dissertation, University of Alberta, Canada.

Sanderson, P. L. (Winter 2000/Winter 2001). American Indian rehabilitation's national agenda: Building and refining efforts. *American Indian Rehabilitation Newsletter.* Retrieved from http://www.nau.edu/~ihd/AIRRTC.doc.

Sobralske, C. (1985). Perceptions of health: Navajo Indians. *Topics in Clinical Nursing, 7*(3), 32–39.

Smith, H. (2000). *Modern tribal development: Paths to self-sufficiency and cultural integrity in Indian country.* Walnut Creek, CA: Altamira Press.

Stensrud, M. & Lushbough, R. (1988). The implementation of an occupational therapy program in an alcohol and drug dependency treatment center. *Occupational Therapy in Mental Health, 8*(2), pp. 1–15.

Sugarman, J., Warren, C., Oge, L & Helgerson, S. (1992). Using the behavioral risk factors surveillance system to monitor year 2000 objectives among American Indians. *Public Health REP, 107,* 449–456.

Taylor, C. (1994). *The plains Indians. A cultural and historical view of the North American plains tribes of the pre-reservation period.* New York: Crescent Books.

Terrell, D. (1993). Ethnocultural factors and substance abuse: Toward culturally sensitive treatment models. *Psychology of Addictive Behaviors, 7*(3), 162–167.

Thompson, W. (1996). Native American Issues: A reference book. ABC-CLIO/contemporary World Issues Series. Santa Barbara, CA.

USA Today (September 18, 2002). Interior Secretary in contempt of court over Indian royalties.

Utter, J. (1993). *American Indians: Answers to today's questions.* Lake Ann, MI: National Woodlands Puplications.

Van Deusen, J. (1989). Alcohol abuse and perceptual motor dysfunction: The occupational therapist' role. *American Journal of Occupational Therapy, 43*(6): 384–390.

Waters, F. (1963). *Book of the Hopi.* New York: Ballantine Books.

Weatherford, J. (1991). *Native roots: How the Indians enriched America.* New York: Fawcett.

Wing, D. & Thompson, T. (1995). Causes of alcoholism: A qualitative study of traditional Muscogee (Creek) Indians. *Public Health Nursing, 12*(6), 417–423.

8

Asian Americans

Asha Asher

Key Words

Asian Americans
Japanese Americans

Chinese Americans
cross-cultural studies

health-related beliefs

Objectives

1. Discuss important cultural values that influence health behaviors in this population.
2. Describe how communication strategies used by this population may lead to misunderstandings with health care providers.
3. Discuss attitudes toward mental health issues for this population.

Introduction

Persons of Asian American descent make up about 4.2% of the U.S. population (U.S. Census Bureau, 2000). Although the 2000 census lists 25 separate Asian ethnicities, most of the data related to them are limited to the Chinese, Japanese, Filipinos, and in some cases, Vietnamese. Because of this restriction, significant gaps remain in understanding the diverse health and social services needs of Asian American children and families.

Leung (1996) offers a possible explanation for this lack of data. Initially, Asians experienced significant discrimination in this country and were frequent targets of violence. Consequently, the community learned to rely on support systems developed within their own ethnic groups. This arrangement resulted in the belief that there was no need for services by external providers; consequently, few data are available on rehabilitation needs of this population. However, people from underrepresented cultures can and do benefit from rehabilitation services, as long as the services provided are culturally appropriate and meaningful (Jenkins, Ayers, & Hunt, 1996). Leung and Sakata (1988) stressed that rehabilitation workers need to look beyond the model minority theory that all Asian Americans are high academic achievers and high wage earners and that they are ethnically and racially homogenous. The ethnic and cultural differences between the groups are complex. Not only are there vast geographical distances between the Asian countries, but languages, as well as ancient cultural heritages with unique customs, also separate the people (Leung & Sakata, 1988).

An important variable to consider when working with individuals or families from Asia is the generational status, or the time spent in this country. With time and exposure to the mainstream culture, new cultural values are absorbed and integrated with those from the culture of origin to create a unique blend of cultural values. Apart from the historical experience of discrimination that Asian Americans have faced in the past, the third and fourth generations of Asian Americans today continue to face subtle discrimination. For example, they still carry labels such as Chinese American, which are not applied to persons of European descent. They continue to be asked, "Where are you from?" (Parmar, 2003, p. 5). Parmar clarifies that the question may arise because of many reasons, including geographic or anthropological inquisitiveness or because of issues of color. However, this question causes pain, because it implies that the person questioned is seen as an outsider, or "The Other" (Parmar, 2003, p. 5).

Although several studies address the health-risk factors relevant to Asian groups, few studies have data comparing the health factors of the different ethnic groups (e.g., Chinese versus Koreans). Dietary practices, social-cultural values regarding health care, use of alternative medicines, and societal attitudes toward mental health issues are some of the many factors that impact the success of health care interventions.

Several cross-cultural studies have yielded information that is important for health maintenance of Asian-American groups. Enas (1996) found that in Asian countries, cerebrovascular disease (CVD) or stroke is more common which may be related to high salt intake. As immigrants from Asian countries transitioned to an American diet, with high cholesterol or animal fat, Enas found that the Asian Americans experienced increased rate of coronary artery disease (CAD), which is more common in Western societies. To lower

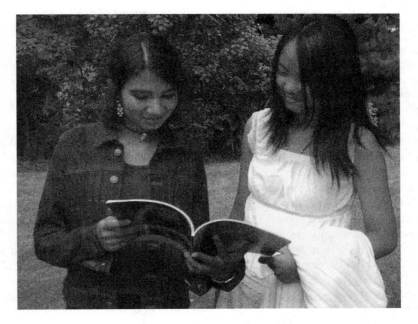

FIGURE 8.1 Teenagers Ruchi and Alice construct their identity in the mid-west, combining the cultural values of their families, of their current environment, and of the countries India, Taiwan, and Canada that they grew up in.

the health risks associated with acculturation, Louie (1999) recommends education regarding the disease process, and the use of traditional or alternative ethnic foods substitutes to ensure follow through.

A study by Koh, Sun, and Zhang (1996) found that cancer is a major concern for Asian Americans. Cervical cancer was a problem special to Asian American women, whereas stomach and liver cancers were of special concern to men from this population. Rates of other cancers were comparable to those found in the general population in California. Liver cancer was found more often in immigrants arriving from areas where chronic hepatitis B infection is endemic. On the basis of the high numbers of Asian males that smoke, Chen and Hawks (1995) project that in the future, higher rates of death due to lung cancer and cardiovascular disease are likely. The authors believe that asthma and elevated blood pressure are other hazards that the Asian American community is likely to face. Comparing the prevalence of type 2 diabetes in Asian Americans with that in other racial/ethnic groups, McNeely and Boyko (2004) found that after adjusting for Body Mass Index (BMI), prevalence of diabetes in Asian Americans was about 60% higher than in non-Hispanic whites. This study indicates that for any given BMI, Asian Americans are more likely to develop diabetes than non-Hispanic whites.

Health education programs are often limited by social attitudes and stigma, thereby preventing the Asian American from accessing resources. The following studies point out several factors that health education programs must consider to be useful to the target population.

Discussing the risk behaviors with respect to AIDS, Hofstede (1984) explains that the trait of collectivism, which is common in the Asian culture, plays a role in perpetuating a lack of information. Collectivism emphasizes group goals and concerns, and draws a distinction between in-groups and out-groups. Because of the low reporting rate of homosexuality, AIDS is often perceived as an out-group disease, resulting in lack of concern regarding individual risk status. The Asian expectation is that the male (especially the first-born) will marry and carry on the family name, and if this does not happen, it may alienate the individual from society. Homosexuality brings family dishonor and possible ostracism by the family and community (Choi et al., 1995), and this attitude leads to a lower rate of direct communication and self-disclosure about sexual behavior. The reduction of interpersonal communication affects exchange of information about AIDS in the Asian communities, leading to increased isolation, and reduces the effectiveness of educational and health promotion programs.

Choi (1996) found that Asian Americans have a high rate of tuberculosis (TB). Choi suggested that myths surrounding TB, language and communication issues, and access to care were some factors limiting the treatment of the disease. Shame, denial, and anger presented additional barriers to treatment. Health care programs must discreetly disseminate information and ensure privacy, especially regarding diseases that are socially unacceptable such as tuberculosis or AIDS.

Stigma and shame are associated with mental illness in the Asian American community (Meadows, 1997). Clients or families may describe somatic complaints rather than admitting to affective symptoms such as depression. Mental health workers should tactfully explore the possibility of underlying mental health issues when a client presents with persistent physical symptoms, realizing that admitting to mental health problems may be seen as a betrayal of family honor. Treatments suggested may have to overtly address the physical symptoms, which would allow the client and family to follow through with treatments while preserving the dignity of the family.

Mental health tools used in Western medicine, including the group process, assume a strongly individualized sense of self (Roland, 1988). These tools work well with the Western sense of self, which has an "I-ness" characterized by a self-contained set of ego boundaries with sharp distinctions between self and others. Roland, a psychiatrist, found that his South Asian patients often had a collective identity, which enabled people to live in harmony with each other. Although this familial identity or, "We-self," enabled them to function within extended families, it prevented his South Asian patients from responding to the Western therapies. Therefore, mental health workers need to review the appropriateness of Western tools when working with the Asian American population.

In a similar vein, Perez-Arce, Carr, and Sorenson (1993) questioned the appropriateness of behavioral treatment applications in working with Asian American populations. When delivering a cocaine treatment program to a predominantly minority population, the authors found that most Asian patients did not complete the program. Perez-Arce, Carr, and Sorenson (1993) felt that the expectations placed by the program were in conflict with the cultural values shared by persons from Asian backgrounds. Asian American values guiding a person's behavior include the need to preserve family loyalty and harmony, and avoidance of direct confrontation or criticism especially with persons considered higher in the social hierarchy. A treatment approach that expects all clients to treat each other as peers regardless of their age, occupation, or experience, which promotes same-sex bonding as a support mechanism, and additionally utilizes a direct confrontation and feedback approach as its basis, is in direct contrast to the principles valued by Asian American clients (Perez-Arce, Carr, & Sorenson, 1993). These behavioral treatments may not be appropriate for many Asian-American clients, and their utility needs to be reviewed before use.

Asian Americans often straddle mainstream American culture while maintaining many of their traditional cultural patterns. This tendency carries over to the use of health care services. Often traditional herbal medicines and other therapies prescribed by alternative medical professionals or by family elders are taken together with modern medicines prescribed by Western doctors. Because some herbal medicines contain potent drugs, their interaction with the Western medicine may produce tragic results (Coward & Ratanakul, 1999). Developing an atmosphere of trust when working with clients from minority populations allows clients to share their use of alternative medical therapies without fear of censure.

Heath care workers commonly face problems when getting informed consent from clients from a different culture. Barnes, Davis, Portillo, and Koenig (1998) highlighted some of the issues faced. Health care personnel often have little time, and the client may be given minimal information before being asked to sign papers. The client may not perceive that there is truly a choice available with regard to the intervention. Alternatively, the client may appear to agree to the prescribed regimen to avoid disrespect to the health care worker, who is seen in a position of authority. The agreement may be offered to allow the health care worker to "save face," without the intention of following through by the client. Additionally, clients may have difficulty in understanding the implications of the information shared by medical staff because of limited language proficiency. Even clients with good verbal skills may not understand the metaphors used locally (such as, "you are treading water"). When under stress, clients may be more comfortable conversing in their original language.

Use of interpreters to gain consent, when available, may be limited by many factors. Even if the language is the same, the interpreter may speak a different dialect. The interpreter may be from the general geographic area where the client originates, however he/she may not be fluent in the exact regional language. For example, the interpreter may speak Hindi, which is spoken mainly in the north of India, and not Tamil, which is spoken in the south. If the interpreter is of the opposite gender, the client may not be comfortable discussing personal or gender-related information with the stranger. Additionally the client may not wish to share intimate information with interpreters, for fear that it would be spread within their community and become a source of humiliation. Therefore, although they may help communication, the utility of interpreters is often less than desired.

Barnes, Davis, Portillo, and Koening (1998) advocate that after adequate information is given in a format that is understood by the client, the medical personnel must accept the choice of the client and/or the family and understand that there may be divergent priorities for desired treatment outcomes. The client or the family may choose quality of life over longevity. The client may also make decisions based on family needs, including the financial and physical hardship faced by the family. The medical decision may not be based on medical needs alone, and it must be respected.

Chinese

Chinese immigrants first came to the United States in large numbers during the 1850s to work in the California gold fields and to help build the transcontinental railroad (Wong & Lopez, 1995). Many people of Chinese origin have migrated to the United States from places outside China, notably Indochina after the fall of Saigon. Most of the Chinese-Vietnamese were typically Cantonese speaking and often were literate in Chinese as well. Others include the Chinese-Khmer and the Chinese-Lao who were able to escape political instability. A number of Chinese also entered the United States from Central and South America, adding to the heterogeneity (both social and economic) of the Chinese American population.

A strong sense of cultural identity can create a bond among the Chinese from different backgrounds. However, because of the diversity of their origins (Mainland China, Taiwan, Vietnam, Central America, or other), cultural beliefs and values vary greatly. Currently, a little less than two-and-half million persons of Chinese origin live in the United States (U.S. Census Bureau, 2000).

Several languages and several different dialects are used by the Chinese Americans, depending on their origins. These include Putonghoua or Mandarin, Cantonese, Min, Haka, Toishanese, and Fukinese (Chan, 1998). Health care workers should consider the exact language spoken when trying to locate an interpreter for translation.

Rice, potatoes, noodles, cornmeal, tofu, and other grains are used as staple foods. Many cultural traditions also reflect genetic make-up. Few dairy products are used in Chinese cuisine, a practice that may be a result of the lactose intolerance commonly seen (Kittler & Sucher, 2001). Fruits and vegetables are eaten when seasonally available. *Man tou* (steamed bread) is a staple in the northern provinces, duck is a specialty of Beijing, and spicy foods are found in the Sichuan province. Food is eaten with chopsticks, and a porcelain spoon is used for soup. Zhou and Britten (1994) found in a survey of students from China and other Asian countries that most of the Chinese frequently cooked in steel woks, which increased the iron content of food.

China was influenced by three major religions, Confucianism, Taoism, and Buddhism. The "three teachings" (the three established religions) are further complemented by ancestor worship, which is characterized by three basic assumptions:

1. All living persons owe their fortunes or misfortunes to their ancestors.
2. All departed ancestors have needs that are the same as those of the living.
3. Departed ancestors continue, as in life, to assist their relatives in this world just as their descendants can assist them.

Belief in the mutual dependence and interaction between the living and the dead thus reinforces efforts, which include a variety of traditional rituals, to maintain a positive and close relationship with one's departed ancestors as well as with living kinsfolk. The basic Chinese philosophical/religious orientation has remained rooted in the secular world and has been relatively consistent throughout the past 2,000 years. Adherence to the "three teachings" reflects a polytheistic orientation that stresses complementarity rather than conflict among Confucianism, Taoism, and Buddhism. It reflects a collectivistic society, in which human relationships are inclusive, rather than exclusive (Chan, 1998).

In accordance with Confucian principles, the family is the basic unit or backbone of society. While guiding and protecting the individual, the family serves as a tie between the individual and the society. The value of family engenders primary loyalty, obligation, cooperation, interdependence, and reciprocity. Each individual is viewed as an integral part of the family, and the members engage in sustained efforts to promote the welfare, harmony, and reputation of the family. Family values include reverence for elders, ancestors, and the past (Chan, 1998).

Children are viewed as an extension of their parents, bringing meaning to their lives. Many traditions and customs are observed to protect the child's vulnerability, for example, the use of charms to protect them from evil spirits. Initially, children are viewed as helpless and not responsible for their actions. Throughout infancy and childhood, the child is provided with a very nurturing, indulgent, secure, and predictable environment, including demand feeding and sleeping with a family member. Toilet training is started early, with the mother predicting the child's schedule. Strict demands are not placed on the child (Chan, 1998).

Freedman (1974) compared Chinese infants with European American infants. He found in comparison with the activity displayed by the European American infants, infants of Chinese descent displayed very little spontaneous motor activity. In addition, Chinese American newborns tended to be less changeable and less perturbable, tended to habituate more readily, and tended to calm themselves or to be consoled more readily.

There is a transition in the expectations placed on the child through the preschool years, with the child assuming greater responsibility for his or her actions. The school-aged child is increasingly included in adult activities such as weddings, funerals, and other social functions. Children are reminded of their obligations to uphold the family honor. The individual's behavior reflects on the whole family. Highly valued achievements such as academic excellence are a source of shared pride among family members. Discipline is often administered through the use of guilt and shame. Behaviors that are punished include disobedience, aggression (particularly sibling directed), and failure to fulfill one's responsibilities. The child can absolve himself or herself of this "loss of face" by actively displaying changes in behavior, and not just with verbal apologies.

As the child acquires younger siblings, the child is routinely delegated the task of caring for them and for modeling acceptable behaviors. The sibling roles are formalized by kinship titles that may specify ordinal positions among them. A classical parental response to sibling rivalry would be to scold the older child for not setting a good example and the younger child for not respecting the older sibling. Observance of these roles and codes of conduct results in a persistent awareness of the effects of one's behavior on others. The children are socialized to think and act in proper relation to others and must learn to transcend their physical concerns. Although Asian parents tend to promote family interdependence, they may, however, simultaneously encourage the development of individual independence outside the family (Chan, 1998).

Socially, aging is described in relation to how people take, make, and play their roles in a given society and how a given society or environment impacts on individuals as they advance in age (Zhan, 1999). From traditional Chinese perspectives, old age itself has been considered as an "accumulation of wisdom" and the "fulfillment of happiness." *Xi Young Hong*, a Chinese saying, refers to the time of the sunset (an analogy to aging), which brings with it a bright red color to symbolize happiness. Health is the foremost indicator of happiness in one's later life. To bring *Xi Young Hong*, many Chinese elderly people pay attention to their body and mind. Zhan (1999) investigated health practice among Chinese elderly women living in the United States. The women in the study identified five unique measures of health promotion: exercise (including walking and tai chi, a traditional Chinese exercise involving a series of slow movements that require body and mind concentration), regular check-ups (did not include comprehensive services such as dental services and mammograms), education (regarding health maintenance), involvement (in church, family, and community activities), and the balance of yin and yang (particularly regarding diet). Facilitating factors that promoted health included medical insurance, social support, and spirituality. Social supports that the Chinese elderly depended on included family (mostly daughters) and friends.

Zhan found that in the traditional philosophy of Confucianism, which promotes strong social and family bonds, the Chinese elderly are revered and respected. However, the custom of extended families has dissipated in the United States with increasing numbers of young people living alone, thus adding to the loneliness of the elderly. Spirituality was noted as an important way to promote mental well-being.

Chinese philosophy does not view a human in fragments as body, soul, and spirit (Hui, 1999). Since human beings are considered products of nature, humanity and its natural environment are inseparably and interdependently related. The Chinese understanding of nature and the cosmos is expressed in three important philosophical concepts: *chi* (material or vital force), *yin and yang*, and *wu-hsing* (five elements). Health implies that the *chi* between the organs of the person are flowing normally as detected by the pulses of the body. Yin and yang operate in opposition to each other to reach a state of dynamic equilibrium. All bodily functions are the result of the harmony of yin and yang. Additionally, the five phases, or elements—wood, metal, water, fire, and earth—are believed to be fundamental categories of all matter in the universe.

Hui (1999) explains that traditional Chinese medicine involves the various interactions between the organs of the body, as well as the influence of environmental factors on the human body and emotions. A person enjoys perfect health when he or she has a strong and an unobstructed flow of *chi*, is under the influence of well-balanced yin-yang forces, and is accompanied by a harmony with the five phases, or elements, of the environment. In that state of "*zheng chi*" (literally, vital energy) "pathogenic factors" will not be able to interfere with the health of the person, and health is maintained. When the yin-yang forces are out of balance and the operation of the five phases or elements has been disrupted by the seasons or the weather conditions, then the *chi* of the human body is said to have been weakened, allowing the "pathogenic factors" to cause the diseased state. In other words, the state of health is a state of equilibrium between the "*zheng chi*" of the body and "pathogenic factors." Chinese traditional medicine focuses primarily on the maintenance and promotion of the "*zheng chi*" (building up body resistance) and only secondarily on the pathogenic factors. Therapeutic intervention to dispel pathogenic factors is reserved only for acute conditions, and even then, health-maintenance procedures are usually simultaneously administered.

Health maintenance involves the following:

1. Maintenance of inner harmony and balance between yin and yang forces.
2. Employment of exercise (tai chi, qigong), massage (to maintain the flow of chi in the body), and therapeutic diet (including herbs and metals), and lifestyle arrangements and practices (including location of one's home and dietary adjustments to the changes of the seasons).

Asian Indians

The term *Asian Indian* was first used to identify people from the country of India and those who claimed Indian descent but were not born in India (Manian, 1997). This distinct identity reflects immigrants and their descendents who came from the Indian diaspora in South and Southeast Asia, Africa, South America, and the islands of the Caribbean and the South Pacific. They may claim a non-Indian nationality (such as South African, Malaysian, Guyanian, Fijian, Sri Lankan, or Nepalese) but remain culturally Indian, practicing the customs and traditions of Asian Indians. They follow religions prevalent in India, including Hinduism, Buddhism, Christianity, Islam, Sikhism, and Jainism. They socialize with Indians, eat Indian food, and wear Indian clothes. Also, they involve themselves in Indian community organizations and associations, and they read Indian newspapers, journals, and magazines.

Although most Asian Indians are at ease adopting the Western culture outside the home, within the home Indian customs, habits, religion, and tradition are maintained. Indian Americans may speak more than one of the 19 different languages recognized in India (for example, Hindi, Marathi, Telegu, Malyalam). Many of these scripts are written left to right but may be written just below the line (as opposed to the Roman script, which is placed on the line). Urdu is written in a right to left direction. Although there is tremendous diversity in regional cultures, networks and alliances are often formed with others of Indian origin, because of the small numbers in a given place. Families join together for social and religious functions, and they often compromise on the customs observed. For example, if a significant number of guests follow a vegetarian diet, nonvegetarian items may not be served.

Kollipara and Britten (1996) confirmed previous findings that most Indians living in the United States continue to retain their native food practices. They found that use of the traditional iron *Karhai*, which is shaped like a shallow bowl used for cooking vegetables, and a *tava*, which is a flat skillet generally used to roast *rotis*, results in increased iron content of the food. More acidic, moister foods, and foods cooked longer in iron *karhais* and on the *tava* added more iron. Many shades of vegetarianism are seen in Indians; some restrict themselves only to food of plant origin, others use eggs and fish, and either mutton, beef, or pork as dictated by religion. Milk and milk products provide both protein and calcium.

Food is an important part of any social or business interaction in the Indian home. A guest is greeted with some sweets and a glass of water before any small talk is initiated. Health care providers may be offered food during home visits. Traditionally, an important task of the woman of the house is ensuring that the dietary needs of her family, especially those of the children, are met. In large households, at least one of the women assumes the job of serving the meal in several portions, coaxing the family until she is satisfied that everyone has consumed the right balance of nutrition. On special occasions, the man of the house together with his wife will personally check that the visitors eat well. At social gatherings in the United States, generally the children are served the meal first, followed by the men. Once they ensure that their family is well fed, the women apply the same diligence to their own meal. At this time, the men or older siblings entertain the younger children, allowing the women to eat without interruptions.

Generally, women are responsible for household chores such as cooking and other household tasks, whereas men attend to other chores such as car maintenance or house repairs. Shoes are not worn inside the house, particularly not in the kitchen. Many Indian households in the United States follow traditional behavior patterns in terms of food preparation. This tradition includes wearing "home" clothes during cooking, that is, clothes that are worn outside the home and may have been exposed to pollutants are not worn during cooking. Cooking is generally started with thorough hand washing. In a non-vegetarian household, implements such as pots and knives used for cooking the meats may be kept separate or thoroughly washed before being used for other foods. Traditional Indian food is not easily manipulated by Western silverware. Since it is eaten with the fingers, before eating and after the meal hand-washing is a must. The food is generally eaten only with the fingers of the right hand, and decorum requires that no more than the last phalange of the fingers is soiled. Small pieces of the *Roti* (bread) are broken off and used to sandwich a piece of the cooked vegetable or meat. Ideally, rice and curry (which indicates sauce) are also eaten with the same decorum, but nowadays a concession may be made in the use of a spoon to handle the curries. In daily transactions, the right hand is used preferentially for giving and receiving anything and for eating. The left hand is used for cleaning after body functions. Transfer of hand dominance to the left because of loss of function may therefore pose additional emotional issues that need to be resolved. Water is considered an appropriate cleansing material. In India, one takes a bath by pouring water from a bucket onto the body, soaping the skin, and then using more water to rinse off. Bathing requires that the dirt is removed from the body and flows away. Consequently, many people of Indian origin may find it more acceptable to take a shower than to use the bathtub in the United States. The elderly who have been brought up outside the United States may find it hard to get accustomed to the use of toilet paper or to use cream cleansers with babies. As one lady tersely corrected a young mother finishing a diaper change with her baby, "You just spread the dirt all around!"

A few communities from the Hindu tradition continue to follow the custom that during the three or four days of the menstrual cycle, a woman does not participate in household or religious duties. Although this custom appears to discriminate against women because of their biological functions, the women often welcomed the monthly break during which they were absolved from household responsibilities. They could devote time to reading or indulge in their hobbies such as sewing or embroidery, while the children and the men in nuclear families, or other women if it was a large household, carried out the chores. The men and children learned that the housewife was not always available to cater to their needs and became more self-reliant. The custom also helped young girls to understand that menstrual function was a normal part of every woman's life. On reaching maturity, one young girl shared excitedly with her sister, "I get to sit aside!" If it were absolutely essential for a menstruating woman to continue her chores (such as when she was hosting a large gathering), simple rituals would reinstate her back into the workforce.

The Indian equivalent for "thank-you," *dhanyavad* or *shukriya*, is used only under extremely formal circumstances. When one receives help from another, it cannot be repaid with mere lip service. Gratitude may be expressed by acknowledging the assistance received. Convention requires that the receiver remain in debt to the giver and should remember the favor. As occasion arises, the receiver helps out the benefactor without being asked to.

Indians also respect the ancient custom of *atithi satkar*, or hospitality, dictated by the legendary Manu, "the law-giver." Any visitor to the home is received with warmth and honor. Food and shelter are offered, and if needed, the family gives up its comfort (bed, privacy) to accommodate the visitor. According to the laws of Manu, this hospitality was to be offered for up to three days. In return, the guest was expected to share the stories of his or her travels with the family and neighborhood, disseminating information (in the days before technology) about distant lands. Although Manu originates from the Hindu tradition, the warm hospitality is typical of any Indian household.

India is home to several major religions. Hindus comprise 82% of India's population, Muslims 11%, Christians 2.3%, Sikhs 1.99%, Buddhists 0.77%, and Jains 0.4% (Singh, 1988). Besides these, other religions form 0.43% of the country's population, including Zoroastrianism, Judaism, and Bahai. The two major religions (Hinduism and Islam) share as much as 97% of cultural values between them. Some of the norms shared include succession by an elder son and ritual use of oil and color. Common traits shared include food habits, material culture, and folklore. Buddhist, Jain, and Hindu literature contain a cluster of story collections known as "Katha literature." These include the "Jataka" tales, the "Panchatantra" tales, and the "Kathasarita sagara." Although the stories have been collected in several written versions, oral versions continue to circulate. The stories often have religious and moral instruction intertwined within its structure. These stories are in addition to the sacred texts of the religions, which also use the structure of oral teachings such as illustrations and parables. The use of storytelling as a medium for religious instruction extends far back into Indian history (Narayan, 1989).

Family Structure

The family is the basic social unit and takes precedence over the individual. Several generations may live under one roof. Although some communities follow a matriarchal lineage, family lineage is generally patriarchal. Marriage is a joining of two families rather than of two individuals. The woman joins her husband's family, and the family celebrates the arrival of a new daughter (in-law), sister (in-law), or aunt. In every family, kinship titles are used to address persons older to the individual such as "Dada" or "Taiee," used in Western India to address an older brother or sister. The title entitles the elder to respect and control, but the privilege includes responsibility for the youngster who uses the title. The kinship titles differentiate between relations. For example, a "mama" is a mother's brother, versus a "kaka," who is the father's brother.

In many parts of the country, the individual name or given name is written first, and the family name is written last. Males use their father's name as the middle name. An unmarried woman uses her father's name as her middle name and that of the husband on marriage. Some communities use an individual's given name as the first name and that of the husband or father as the last name. Among followers of the Sikh religion, Singh is a respectful title for a male, and Kaur for a female, and they may be used as a middle name. A new immigrant may find it confusing to translate this into the Western system of first and last names when filling in official forms.

Through infancy and into toddlerhood, the child's every need is attended to, and he or she is not allowed to cry. If a child is upset, the mother is immediately held responsible for finding out what is bothering the child and for distracting the child. Food is often used as a distracter. Because feeding the family is an important maternal task, Indian children may not be held responsible for feeding themselves until they are older. Even when children are able to physically eat independently, an adult will hover around, turning every meal into a social occasion. Generally people are cautious about praising or openly appreciating anything, especially their children, for fear of invoking the "evil eye" or "Nazar." A small black spot applied to a child's face, serves to ward off the "evil" eye.

Discipline is often administered in a circumstantial way. Children are expected to behave because doing so will make their family look good; infringement of the behavioral code reflects poorly on the family and would make the caregiver appear ineffective as a disciplinarian. Children follow expectations because there is a strong bond with their caregiver, whom they wish to please. Thus from an early age, the child is inducted into the social code of the family.

The ages at which children are given responsibilities vary by community. Often, once a younger sibling arrives on the scene and the child gets a kinship title of seniority, small responsibilities are placed on the child. It may involve something as simple as watching to check when the baby awakens. Girls are often given increasing responsibilities at home including greeting visitors and helping the mother in the home. Boys are directed to work outside the house. Any effort by the children is applauded, thus enhancing their self-esteem. Gradually, age-appropriate responsibilities are placed on the child.

In the United States, there may be little variation between the responsibilities placed on girls and boys of Indian origin. Children are taken along for any social gatherings, whereas babysitters are generally restricted to work-related parental absences. Thus, there is flexibility of sleep routines, and children often get to bed very late on the weekends. The children of the host family are responsible for entertaining the visiting children regardless of their ages.

Issues of Aging

As the younger members of the household are ready to assume responsibilities, the elders are advocated to step aside, offering guidance as needed. In most communities, the son and his wife look after the physical needs of his parents. The parents in turn may assist with the social and religious education of the children, that is, by sharing the rich folklore of the community and by entertaining the young children of the family. Children spend a lot of time with the grandparents, giving young parents much-needed privacy. Even when aging grandparents have little physical energy, they are entrusted with special tasks; for example, they may complete special prayer routines that ask for particular favors such as success in an examination for a grandchild. This role gives the elders a sense of involvement in the routine life of their family. The close ties between the generations are seen in most Indian households regardless of their religious backgrounds.

In the United States, aging parents face many problems. Parents are brought over to the United States because of filial duties. Often their children and grandchildren are busy with their daily routine, and the elders have little to do. Because of the diversity of the population from India, it is difficult to find a support group with a common language and similar social customs; therefore, it is difficult to adjust to life in the United States. Traditionally the daughter-in-law would look after the elders' physical needs. Within dual-income families, however, she is often overworked and cannot handle the extra workload, resulting in strife.

Health Beliefs

A body free from disease is essential to an individual to complete his or her life tasks, including spiritual responsibilities. Wellness is seen as a balance between the physical, psychological, social, and spiritual realms of an individual. Illness is viewed as a state of imbalance between these, caused by many factors including disruptions in sleep or diet. Diagnosis of a disease condition includes examination of symptoms and manifestations of the disease, and also examination of the physical constitution and psychological disposition of the patient. The major task of those who desire a healthful state is maintaining a balance of substances in the body and establishing a harmony between the body and its environment. Alternative medical disciplines common in India, including homeopathy, ayurveda, unani, acupressure, acupuncture, and faith healing, are often used in addition to Western medicine.

Japanese

The first Japanese immigrants to the United States arrived between 1890 and 1924 (Kitano, 1976). Currently in the United States are the *Sansei* (third-generation immigrants) and the *Yonsei* (fourth-generation immigrants), who are well educated and affluent as a group. In general, they have moved away from the traditional Japanese communities. Immigrants arriving after 1965 are referred to as the *shin-issei* generation (Kitano and Kikumera, 1988).

The Japanese use several different scripts for writing—Kanji, Hiragana, Katakana, and Romaji. The script is traditionally written vertically from right to left, and top to bottom. It may also be written horizontally from left to right. The Japanese place great worth on nonverbal language or communication. One is expected to sense a person's feelings on a subject without verbal communication. Japanese society is group-oriented, and loyalty to the group and to one's superiors takes precedence over individual needs. Politeness is extremely important. A "yes" given quickly may be out of politeness and may indicate only that a person is listening. Negation may not be stated directly, but a "I will think about it" may indicate "no."

A bow is a traditional greeting between the Japanese; the manner of a bow can indicate respect and humility. Formality is observed, and titles are important in introductions. For example, the suffix -san is used with the family name. First names are used only within the family and with friends. Name cards (offered and accepted with both hands) generally accompany introductions. Second- and third-generation Japanese-Americans may be comfortable when addressed informally; however, new immigrants should not be addressed by their first names.

One characteristic highly valued by the Japanese is *Gaman*, or self-control. Downes (1994) explains that this restraint of emotions and self-sufficiency may lead patients to avoid complaining even in the presence of severe pain. Hashizume and Takano (1983) clarify that Japanese also avoid verbal confrontation. Because they are habituated to interact with humility and politeness, they may be misunderstood or inadvertently overlooked.

The Japanese diet consists of rice, fresh vegetables, seafood, fruit, and small portions of meat. The high sodium content is due to the extensive use of soy sauces, monosodium glutamate, and pickled foods (Downes 1994). Food is eaten with chopsticks, with the right hand. Generally the food is prepared into bite-sized portions and is picked from the bowl held in the left hand. Soup may be consumed directly from the bowl.

Conformity in appearance is a general characteristic of the Japanese. By tradition, the Japanese will conform to the dress of the group, that is, will remain in harmony with the group. The traditional kimono may be worn only for formal occasions. Conformity is also seen in the interpersonal relations, in which the group is more important than the individual. This concept affirms an individual's place and role, and also gives the individual a sense of identity within the group. This collective sense of identity may make it difficult for some to make individual decisions in a client-centered approach used in rehabilitation settings (Iwama, 1999).

Time is a highly valued commodity with the Japanese. They are generally very punctual and expect appointments to end at predetermined times. Education is highly valued in Japan. Children attend *jukku*, or evening school, to gain a competitive edge at the college entrance examinations. Admissions at a prestigious university would ensure a secure job and eventually a good position in society.

The common religions of Japan are Buddhism and Shinto. Traditionally, most Japanese practice a combination of Buddhism and Shinto; for example many may observe Shinto rituals at birth or marriage but may observe a Buddhist funeral. The Japanese also celebrate the different seasons.

The family is the foundation of Japanese society and is bound together by a strong sense of reputation, obligation, and responsibility. A person's actions reflect on the family. Affection, time together, and spousal compatibility are less important than in other cultures. The father is the head of the home, whereas the mother is responsible for managing household affairs and raising children. The practice of filial piety places the responsibilities of children on their parents. In return, the parents can expect to be respected and cared for in their old age.

Issues of Aging

Children take on the responsibility of caring for aging parents. Placement in long-term-care facilities may be resorted to if the situation is unmanageable; however, this decision may be accompanied by feelings of guilt. The Japanese recognize the sixtieth birthday with an elaborate celebration. Elders symbolically pass family care-taking to the next generation, absolving themselves of adult responsibilities and returning to the joys of childhood and personal pursuits. They also have the assurance that they now will be cared for with respect and with appreciation for sacrifices made on behalf of their families (Doi, 1991).

Heath Beliefs

Religions influence some of the health beliefs of the Japanese. Shinto religion believes that disease is caused by bodily contact with substances such as blood, corpses, or skin diseases. Purification rites are part of the Shinto religion, which is reflected as a Japanese characteristic. This includes the bathing rituals and use of herbal cathartics and laxatives. Additionally, harmony with nature, family, and society is valued. Generally, Western medicine is used as well as traditional medicines depending on the situation.

Health-Risk Factors and Considerations for Health Care Decision-Making

Common health problems experienced by Japanese Americans include hypertension and stress-related diseases such as ulcers, colitis, and depression (Hashizume & Takano, 1983). Diabetes risk in Asians appears to increase with prolonged exposure to Western lifestyle. Thus diabetes risk may be higher in predominantly U.S. born groups, such as Japanese Americans, than in Asian American groups with a higher proportion of recent immigrants (McNeely & Boyko, 2004).

Diego, Yamamato, Nguyen, and Hifumi (1994) noted increased suicide among elderly Chinese and Japanese. They suggest that the higher rate of suicide is due to acculturation of their children and subsequent cultural conflicts. The traditional Japanese view suicide as acceptable because of their emphasis on feeling useful. For example, the elderly who are isolated, suffering from chronic health problems, or disabled may feel worthless or believe that they are a burden and thus may consider suicide.

Lock (1983) suggested that some Japanese might inwardly resist the tradition of conforming to the group, leading to psychological suppression. This in turn may be responsible for somatization observed in some Japanese; that is, the person may project physical symptoms rather than admit to psychological problems.

Meadows (1997) believes that Japanese families would be concerned if they were seen accessing mental health services and therefore avoid doing so. People in the community would "know" of the family's shortcomings, adding to their shame. Meadows advocated the use of culturally appropriate adaptations such as scheduling with breaks between two consecutive patients, minimizing the chances of incidental contact.

Filipinos

The country of the Philippines is a chain of islands in the Western Pacific ocean off the southeast coast of mainland China. It stretches for 1,000 miles between Taiwan in the north and Indonesia in the south. The region has seen many foreigners who were attracted to the area because of commerce, colonial conquest, religious fervor, or war. Jacinto and Syquia (1995) trace the history of the islands and the immigration of their inhabitants into the United States. The original inhabitants were called the Aetas. They were forced to flee to the hills by the Malays, who intermingled with the Indonesians to evolve into the people now considered Filipino. The other settlers include Chinese merchants; Indonesians, who brought Hinduism and Buddhism into the country; Indians who brought in a Sanskrit-based written language; and Arabs, who brought in Islam. The arrival of Europeans in the fifteenth century marked the beginning of a long and an oppressive occupation. The Portuguese attempted to subdue the region in 1521 but were defeated. The Spaniards conquered the region in the sixteenth century and ruled for nearly 300 years. The accompanying Franciscan and Dominican clergy introduced Roman Catholicism. By the late nineteenth century, the sporadic attempts at liberation by the Filipino people coalesced into a struggle for independence. Just as this struggle was bearing fruit, the United States defeated Spain in the Spanish-American war of 1898 and thereby took over the Philippines. The United States subdued all Filipino resistance, and the Philippines became America's first colony. The United States implanted an American-type education, which replaced the influence of the Spanish rulers. The Americans, in turn, lost to Japanese invaders in April 1942. Filipino guerrillas successfully ended Japanese occupation three years later, with the assistance of additional United States troops. The islands were finally granted independence from the United States in 1946.

The Filipinos were one of the earliest Asian groups to cross the Pacific and enter North America. Filipino crews manned the Spanish galleons that traded with Mexico. Some of the crew jumped ship along the Louisiana Gulf Coast and established themselves in the area. They intermarried with the native population, built villages on stilts, and fished for their livelihood.

The first wave of recent immigrants came between the years 1920 and 1940. They were referred to as *pinoys* and mostly found jobs as agricultural workers. They often faced harsh working conditions and were targets of racist attacks. In spite of the oppression, the *Manongs*, which is a respectful term to address elders, managed to band together and contributed substantially to the American workforce. Additionally, a group of students arrived in the United States to study. Known as *pensionados*, they were groomed to assume leadership roles in the colonial government. This first group has been referred to as bachelor workers (Jacinto and Syquia, 1995).

The second wave of immigrants arrived between 1945 and 1965. These were generally educated and skilled workers who came with their families. Many in this group had been promised U.S. citizenship if they served in the U.S. armed forces during World War II. However, this promise was not fulfilled until the end of 1992 (Downes, 1994).

After the 1965 federal immigration act, which abolished the quota system based on national origins, the number of Filipino immigrants to the United States increased substantially. These immigrants came mainly from the cities and were generally well-educated professionals.

The Spanish named the islands *Philippines* in honor of King Phillip. Because there is no "f" sound in their language, the natives referred to themselves as "Pilipino." In the United States, their name is generally spelled as Filipino. Pilipino is the official language of the Philippines, but in the United States, the language is commonly called Tagalog, the name of an ethnic group from the northern Philippines. Pilipino is spoken by about 80% of the population, with Cebuano and Ilocano being the two other languages widely spoken in the country. The country has 40 other languages and 87 dialects, which have evolved because the geography of the area isolated people. A student in the Philippines may be conversant with at least three languages: the local dialect that is spoken at home, Pilipino in a social situation, and English at school.

Filipinos value smooth social relationships, and their communication patterns are shaped by this outlook. Direct disagreement or conflict is avoided (Downes, 1994). Mediators may be used to resolve conflicts, thus allowing the involved parties to maintain their dignity during conflict resolution.

Filipino food has a blend of Malaysian, Polynesian, Spanish, and Chinese influences (Kittler & Sucher, 2001). They have three main meals, in addition to two minimeals or snacks. Food is generally eaten with a spoon, and a fork may be used to push food onto it.

Religion plays an important role in the Philippines, which is the only Asian nation that is predominantly Christian. The majority of Filipinos are Catholic; however, other evangelical missionaries have also established communities on the islands. Five percent of the population is Muslim. A small percentage of the population is Buddhist, whereas in remote areas, traditional folk beliefs that originated from before the Spanish rule continue to be practiced.

Various authors have reported differing interpretations of the Filipino family system. Agbayani-Siewert and Revila (1995) stated that the Filipino family is structured differently from other Asian families. Age entitles the elderly to respect; however, it does not automatically ascribe them with authority. The authors explain that the ties with the kin group are very important, and the family will rally around if a kin member is in trouble. Andres and Ilada-Andres (1987) state that family hierarchy is not patriarchal but is more egalitarian, whereby husband and wife share almost equally in family and financial decisions. However, other authors (Ceria and Shimamoto, 1996) state that traditional Filipino families are very authoritarian. Within a family, authority is hierarchical, flowing from oldest to the youngest. Ceria and Shimamoto explain that the four primary rules in traditional Filipino culture are (a) authority of male members, (b) seniority of age, (c) obedience of youth, and (d) collective responsibility.

The Filipinos keep in close contact with the extended family, which is enlarged by the presence of the *compadre*, or the godparent system. The godparents participate in the religious education and may assist financially at other times.

Jacinto and Syquia (1995) describe the basic principles with which the Filipino children are raised. *Amor proprio* is a sense of self-esteem or a sense of self-worth. It results in the Filipinos' being defensive toward any negative remarks, and accounting for their extreme sensitivity. Therefore, the Filipinos are also respectful and ensure that they preserve the self-esteem of the people they deal with. *Hiya* is a form of self-depreciation and shame. It is related to the concept of "face" and a concern with how one appears in the eyes of the others. *Pakikisama*, or getting along with others, was a means of enforcing smooth interpersonal relationships even if it involved conceding to others' wishes. Mediators are often used to complete transactions with the least amount of confrontation and to minimize the possibility of shaming someone or having him or her lose face. *Utang na loob* means a debt of gratitude or reciprocity for a favor. It involves reciprocal obligations that weave participants into a fabric of social alliances. It requires give-and-take and provides a sense of social security. *Bahala na* means leaving things to fate or God. It is a fatalism or resignation that helps a person cope with outside forces, which are beyond his or her control. It enables the Filipino to face disaster or tragedy with equanimity. *Kapwa tao* is a core value of shared identity. It is the sense of belonging to a group and of being no different from the group. Thus, in the Filipino culture, children are socialized into the family group, are very respectful of an individual's feelings, and are conscious of being a part of the group.

Children are highly valued in the Filipino culture and are considered a gift from God. Babies may not be taken out of the house until 3 or 4 weeks of age. Various folk practices are used to protect the child, such as keeping garlic and salt near a baby as a protection from evil spirits, wrapping a coin on the infant's umbilical cord to help heal it faster, and pinning religious medals onto the baby's clothing to keep the baby safe (Chan, 1998).

During infancy the child receives constant attention and is rarely allowed to cry. This practice is facilitated by the presence of extended family members within the home. The child is fed on demand and sleeps initially with the parents and later with siblings. Through early childhood, conforming to family expectations of respect for authority and obedience to caregivers are customary. Typically the mother is the chief disciplinarian. Sibling-directed aggression and hostility toward kinship group members is condemned.

Issues of Aging

As explained before, age entitles the senior Filipino to respect. Moneda and Gibson (1996) discuss the situation of elderly Filipino parents who joined their children living in the United States during the 1970s and 1980s. These immigrants came to live with their children who had acquired economic stability and housing. Many of the elderly experienced shock and loneliness, finding themselves isolated from people familiar with customs of their country. While their children worked, they often were left home alone. Many were given household and babysitting tasks that were emotionally unfulfilling and often unfamiliar. Members of this elderly group often had chronic health problems that needed attention, and many felt displaced and confused.

Health Beliefs

Ceria and Shimamoto (1996) found that although magic and superstition remain an important part of Filipino thinking, the average-age Filipino willingly accepts medical care when offered. This modern medical care may be supplemented by *hilots*, who cure by massage, or other alternative medical practices may be used. Certain Chinese oils or ointments and other folk remedies, which include the use of hot/cold classification of illnesses, and the concept of wind illnesses (based on the system of Chinese medicine) are also used. For example, *Yentosa* is used for treating joint pains, which are believed to be caused by the presence of "bad air." A coin is wrapped in cotton, the tip of the cotton is wet with alcohol, lit with a match, and placed on the aching joint, and covered with a glass. The flame gets extinguished almost immediately, creating a vacuum inside the glass, which is believed to suck the bad air out of the joint. Other types of healers, who use prayer or "laying of hands" to transmit positive energy to the patient, are also used. These folk healers may complement modern health practitioners by providing psychological, emotional, and spiritual support. The average Filipino may interpret illness as occurring only when one is in acute pain, extremely ill, or unable to walk (Ceria and Shimamoto, 1996). Consequently, they may not access preventative medical care.

Vietnamese

Vietnam is at the crossroads of two major cultures: the Chinese culture in the north and the Indian culture in the west (Chuongh, 1994). There are several ethnic minorities in Vietnam including the Chinese, mountain tribesmen, and cambodians. Smaller ethnic groups include the Malays, Indians, Pakistanis, and French. Vietnam has a long history of foreign aggression. The foreign powers that ruled earlier include China, France, and Japan. During a twenty-year period ending in 1975, the civil war between North Vietnam (which was aided by China and the Soviet Union) and South Vietnam (which was aided by the United States) took a heavy toll on human life in the region.

Immigration History

Vietnamese people began migrating to the United States in 1975, after the fall of the Republic of South Vietnam and the neighboring pro-American governments in Laos and Cambodia (Chuongh, 1994). In 1973, after more than a decade of military involvement in southeast Asia, the United States signed the Paris Peace Agreement, halting all military activities in Vietnam and leaving the governments of South Vietnam, Laos, and Cambodia to fight their own wars. The communists took over the entire region, and the first wave of refugees rushed to friendly embassies to secure passage out of their countries. More than 130,000 southeast Asian refugees, mostly of Vietnamese origin, arrived in the United States. Many of the refugees were from middle-class backgrounds with extensive exposure to Western education. They also migrated together as families and the familial support helped mitigate the difficulty of migration. In a two-year period, the number of refugees jumped to 400,000. It included the people who chose perilous escape routes via the sea and refugee groups from Laos and Cambodia.

In 1982, the governments of Vietnam and the United States set up the Orderly Departure Program, which offered the possibility of a legal exit from Vietnam. It allowed families to reunite officially and decreased the number of Vietnamese attempting hazardous escape in small, open boats. The profile of these immigrants varied and included merchants of Chinese ethnicity. In 1987, the U.S. Congress passed the Amerasian Homecoming Act to allow children fathered by U.S. soldiers to immigrate to the United States. Under this legislation, more than 30,000 Amerasians and their close Vietnamese family members were admitted to this country. Many of these newcomers arrived in their teens and have found adjustment to U.S. life extremely painful.

Vietnamese is the national language of more than 56 million speakers in Vietnam and of over 1 million Vietnamese immigrants overseas. The language is diversified into three regional dialects—northern, central, and southern—which differ slightly in pronunciation and vocabulary, but not in grammar. The script for this is based on the Roman alphabet.

Nonverbal communication is important between Vietnamese people (Huynh, 1987). Respect is conveyed by use of titles, waiting quietly, for example, until the teacher has spoken, and avoiding eye contact. The smile is another symbol of conveying respect; it may be used as an expression of an apology for a minor offense or as an expression of embarrassment for a blunder. For casual and informal circumstances, feelings of thankfulness or apology are not expressed by verbal expressions such as "Thank you" or "I am sorry" but by nonverbal behavior such as silence or a smile. Children are not thanked for small services but are acknowledged with a smile. Compliments are accepted with a smile or denied, saying that one does not deserve the compliment.

The Vietnamese usually have three names, for example, Nguyen Hy Vinh. The first name is usually the family name, whereas the last name is the given name. The Vietnamese use the given name for identification. Terms such as *first name* and *last name* may confuse a Vietnamese who is new to the American culture. A Vietnamese is called by his or her given name and referred to by the full name. A man whose name is Nguyen Van Tam will be called Tam by his friends but Mr. Tam by others. After marriage, a Vietnamese woman keeps her maiden name. In informal circumstances, she will be referred to by her given name or that of her husband, but in formal circumstances, she will be referred to by her maiden name in full preceded by the title "Mrs."

Usually a Vietnamese person has two ages, one related to the chronological age and the other to "Tet," or the Lunar New Year. A person who is born prior to the Lunar New Year will be a year old on Tet regardless of whether he or she was born a few days prior to Tet or a whole year prior. When required to write the name and birth date on a form, the person new to this country has to sort through which name to put first, which age to give (the one calculated by the Tet or the chronological), and how to write the date (date-month-year or month-date-year). Few people appreciate the intricacies involved in this simple task!

The Vietnamese generally eat three meals per day. The Vietnamese use chopsticks, forks, or fingers to eat. Milk-based calcium intake is low, perhaps because of lactose intolerance. However, the calcium may be provided from other sources such as fish (Kittler and Sucher, 2001).

The predominant religion in Vietnam is Buddhism. Christianity, Taoism, and Confucianism (which is more a religious and social philosophy) are the other religions practiced in the country. One important feature of the religious attitude of the Vietnamese is its great tolerance. There never has been religious fanaticism or religious warfare in Vietnam. The religious belief of the common Vietnamese is a synthesis of the three traditional religions (Buddhism, Confucianism, and Taoism) that have coexisted peacefully in Vietnam for centuries.

The average Vietnamese is not an individualist; the individual's interests and destiny are rarely conceived outside the framework of the immediate and extended families. The Vietnamese immediate family generally includes husband, wife, children, and also the husband's parents and the wives and children of the sons. The extended family consists of the immediate family and close relatives sharing the same family name and ancestors who usually live in the same community. The Vietnamese father, who is the head of the family, shares collective and bilateral responsibility with his wife and children in legal, moral, and spiritual matters. In Vietnam, the youngest son inherits the family home and cares for the elderly parents.

Bringing up children is an important responsibility. Parents share the honor and fame of their virtuous children, but also the disgrace if the children are dishonorable. Children are taught the rules of respectful behavior at home. They are expected to love, respect, and obey their parents when they are young and to support their parents when they are old. Filial piety extends beyond the death of one's parents, in the form of ancestor worship and the maintenance of ancestral tombs. Younger siblings are required to respect and obey older siblings. The oldest brother will substitute for the parents in case of emergency. The family ties extend to the extended family.

Health Beliefs

The Vietnamese may believe that everything in the cosmos influences an individual and that spirits and deities control the universe. Illness may be the result of destiny or disharmony caused by wandering spirits of the dead. Traditionally, many of the health beliefs rely on the concepts of Chinese medicine involving the balance of hot and cold in the body. Western medicines are believed to be "hot." Minor health problems may be taken to a traditional healer and more severe problems to a Western doctor. Cultural healers play an important role. Their methods include the use of magic, prayers, talismans, bloodletting, pinching the skin, roots and herbs, coin rubbing, cupping, herbal steam inhalation, and the use of balms.

Health-Risk Factors and Considerations for Health Care Decision Making

Refugees from Vietnam experienced several health problems linked to the immigration experience, which often involved risky journeys with exposure to the elements and unhygienic conditions. Problems that developed included intestinal parasites, tuberculosis, hepatitis, trichinosis, and other infectious diseases. Several mental health concerns such as depression also affected this population. The Vietnamese believe that evil spirits cause mental illness as a punishment. Because of the stigma attached, mental health problems may be expressed as physical, and treatment will be more acceptable if a physical component is included.

Koreans

The first group of Korean immigrants to the United States arrived in the early 1900s. They were recruited as laborers to work on sugar plantations in Hawaii. The workers had to endure harsh working conditions and low wages, but generally they survived with the hope of eventually returning to the home country. This hope was lost when Japan occupied Korea and the workers had to create their own support communities within the United States (Kim & Kim, 1997).

The second wave of immigration, which arrived after the Korean War, consisted of Korean wives of U.S. military personnel, war orphans, and college students. Although some Korean wives had successful marriages, others suffered physical and mental abuse at the hands of their husbands. They had limited abilities to be self-sufficient. Americans adopted around 45,000 Korean orphans between the years 1962 to 1975. According to Kim and Kim (1997), the recent immigrants came for better educational and economic opportunities, as well as reunion with family members.

The Korean language has many words derived from Chinese and many grammatical features in common with Japanese. It is written from left to right.

Koreans commonly use chopsticks and spoons during meals. The Korean diet is limited in milk or milk products but is rich in soups made from fish, vegetables, and meat (Kittler & Sucher, 2001).

Several different religions are prevalent in Korea. Kim and Kim (1997) describe the influence of different religions on Korea. The original and continuing core of Korean religious experiences, especially in the rural area, is Shamanism. The term *shaman* has been widely adopted by anthropologists to refer to specific groups of spiritual healers in diverse cultures. The Korean shaman, usually a woman, is called a *mudang*. A *mudang* can enter altered states of consciousness (i.e., trances) that are often brought about by chanting and dancing to the accompaniment of a drum. While in a trance, the *mudang* can acquire knowledge and power to heal the patient and to help the family and community (Kister, 1997). Shamanism focuses on practices and experiences rather than beliefs and dogma.

Confucianism has shaped the way Koreans live and is an idealistic ethical-moral system intended to govern all the relationships within the family and the state in harmonious unity. It emphasizes filial piety, reverence for ancestors, loyalty to friends, work ethics, self-cultivation, and scholarship. Confucianism reached into the farthest corners of Korean society. In contemporary Korean society, Confucian values, manners, and family and social relationships are deeply ingrained, even though many Koreans are unaware that these are Confucian values.

Around 300 A.D., Buddhism, which entered Korea from India and China, was embraced as a state religion, although governmental systems were already run along Confucian lines. Buddhism teaches that pain and suffering are part of living and that human suffering is brought on because humans are trapped in a cycle of desire that can be ended only by casting off all things that make up the self. Even today, Buddhism remains a powerful influence in Korea.

Christian missionaries entered Korea as early as the seventeenth century. Factors influencing the growth of Christianity included a strong desire of Koreans for Westernization and modernization; teachings that opened the way to learning and understanding modern thought, including political ideas of democracy; and missionaries who opened up education to everyone including women, in contrast to the earlier practice that allowed education only to privileged upper-class boys (Kim & Kim, 1997).

The family is the foundation of Korean society. Korean life is influenced by Confucian values such as filial piety and ancestor worship (Kim & Kim, 1997). The father is the head of the family and is given the most respect, followed by the oldest son. The women may be given less respect; however, they retain their maiden name on marriage. A Korean name consists of a one-syllable family name followed by a one- or two-syllable given name. Kim and Park (Pak) are the most common family names. Extended families often live together, with the oldest members being given the most respect. Family genealogies document a person's birth, relations, achievements, and place of burial, and a family's status is enhanced with the extent of its records. As with many other Asian cultural groups, family conflicts and, at times, breakdowns occur associated with the changing role of women resulting from acculturation into the American society (Min, 1995). As women work outside the home to contribute to the economic survival of the family, they are less likely to accept the traditional male superiority, thus leading to stress (Min, 1995).

Most Korean couples would prefer to have a male child. Koreans believe that before birth, a baby can already hear the mother's voice and develops feelings. During pregnancy the mother-to-be follows advice shared for over 500 years and completes activities that are related to the baby's intellectual stimulation and emotional growth. After birth, the mother and baby are confined to the home for at least a month. Only the close relatives who are free from any visible signs of illness are allowed to visit them, and a baby is usually segregated for about three months. Big celebrations mark the child's completion of the first 100 days and the first birthday (Hyang Sook, personal communication, 2001). Education is greatly valued by Koreans, and children are generally encouraged to get a college education. There are fewer opportunities for physical activities in Korean schools, since the main focus is on academics.

Issues of Aging

It is customary for the Korean elderly to live together with their children and grandchildren. Elderly family members are honored and respected. A study conducted by Wallace et al. (1996) of elderly Koreans living in the Los Angeles county found that they practiced a higher number of healthy behaviors as compared with the white population. These behaviors included annual physical and dental examinations, physical activity, eating breakfast, and not snacking between meals, a low rate of alcohol consumption and smoking, and getting seven to eight hours of sleep at night. The Korean elderly reported a similar prevalence of most chronic diseases as the white population except for lower numbers of osteoarthritis, stroke, and cancer. Higher numbers of Koreans reported kidney problems. The authors felt that increasing physical activity levels, increasing use of preventative medical and dental care, and reducing smoking among men could optimize preventative health care. The authors stressed that physical activity should be encouraged by offering traditional Korean exercises, walking, or other culturally appropriate modes of physical activity.

Koreans may utilize a combination of medical approaches, using treatments from traditional shamans, herbalists, Confucian beliefs, Chinese medicine, and Western medicine. According to Downes (1994), traditional Korean health clinics (*hanbang*) and health practitioners (*hanui*) are found in the United States. Treatments such as steam baths, ginseng, and deer horn are used in addition to the traditional Chinese medical treatments such as acupuncture. Pang (1989) states that the advantages of the traditional clinics include low cost, convenience of hours and drop-in feature, and client input into the treatment procedures.

Health-Risk Factors and Considerations for Health Care Decision Making

Shin (1999) states that women show a high ratio of musculoskeletal and coronary circulatory diseases as compared with the Korean men. A higher rate of mental disorders is also noted because of the social pressures to conform to a conventional role, resulting in internalizing of psychological troubles. Whereas a small increase was found in the use of alcohol and drug use among Korean women, a decrease in the rate of smoking was found. In the United States, a study by the California office of AIDS study found a low incidence of AIDS among people of Korean origin (2.7 per 100,000).

Koreans believe that mental illness may occur as a result of the patient's being haunted by evil spirits. The family may attempt exorcism before medical treatment is sought (Meadows, 1997).

Summary

Several factors involving self-care should be kept in mind when rehabilitation needs of Asian-Americans are evaluated. The client may be habituated to different foods and differing methods of eating them, such as chopsticks or fingers, and may have difficulty using Western eating utensils. Awkwardness in using silverware in the American tradition may indicate a lack of experience with the implements in the premorbid condition, rather than a disturbed praxis. Similarly, visual scanning may previously be done in different ways (right to left, left to right, top to bottom) depending on the language script the client is used to in the premorbid condition. Retraining of visual scanning should take this factor into account. If there is a loss of use of one limb, the issue of hand dominance may need to be clarified. The left hand may be culturally less acceptable, and the client may need to work through that emotional issue before making a successful change.

Researchers have presented evidence of biological variations in normal development and health risk-factors. Many cultural practices (such as vegetarianism in Indians or the use of soy products by the Japanese) may have evolved as an adaptation to the genetic differences (higher levels of lipoproteins in Indians or lactose intolerance in the Japanese) and should be respected. However, service providers need to understand the observed practices and to ensure that they are acceptable under the circumstances in question. For example, massaging babies is an ancient Indian practice that may not be appropriate for a child with spasticity.

Communication practices may be different when dealing with Asian Americans. They use subtle nuances in communication, emphasizing nonverbal communication. Face saving is important, and clients often defer to perceived authority so as not to embarrass the authority figure. Additionally, English as a second language may add to the difficulties experienced in communicating. Clients may need help to understand that they truly have a choice in making health care decisions. This understanding may allow greater compliance with suggested health care remedies.

A sense of trust and partnership needs to be established between clients and service providers. Clients would then feel comfortable sharing information regarding the use of alternative therapies, thus allowing service providers to watch for hazardous combinations of Western and Eastern therapies. Knowledge of these alternative therapies may additionally allow service providers to associate two treatments together, for example, using Western psychiatric medicine together with the traditional regimes of balanced diet and exercise.

Asians often have a collective identity of self, which involves the reciprocal responsibility required to live in harmony within the hierarchical structure of family and society (Coward & Ratanakul, 1999). Therefore, health care providers will have to pay more attention to the extended family and the environmental context in which the person lives. The concept of family may need to be redefined to include the extended family and individuals who the patient feels are most significant in their lives (Kagawa-Singer 1994). The health care workers need to be aware that clients may need support from their extended family to make critical health care decisions.

Keeping in mind issues of informed consent and patient rights, the service providers must skillfully orchestrate an accord between patient, family, physician, nursing staff, and other staff, to decide how to share information regarding the patient and to honor the patient's wishes. In many cultures the elderly relinquish their responsibilities of decision making to significant members of the family. These elderly feel that it is a privilege not to have to make decisions. Rules and policies must be flexible enough to accommodate these needs. Standards of care established should include cross-cultural information.

Advocating for culturally relevant epistemology in occupational therapy, Iwama (2003) expounds the difference between Eastern and Western belief systems. Western ideology promotes individualism, independence, self-determinism, and actualization. In contrast, East Asian cultures value interdependence, social belonging, and harmony with their circumstances (Iwama, 2003). Asian Americans today construct their own distinctive blend of cultural values, depending on the degree of acculturation to the West. Providers of rehabilitation services must consider the individual needs shaped by these values to make health care intervention meaningful to both the service provider and the receiver of the service.

Case Study

Alka was quite upset with her mother-in-law, who had recently migrated to the United States. Alka was concerned with Ma's insistence on living exactly as she did in her home country, India. Alka was particularly vexed with Ma's early morning rituals. Ma woke up early, swept and cleaned her own room, had a bath, and then performed her *puja*, or prayer ritual. She would insist on going outside to face the sun while she recited the ancient Sanskrit words that women had recited through the ages. The prayers would bring good luck to her husband and children, in this life and further on.

"This is New York, the temperature outside is below freezing, her hair is still wet, she will not wear shoes because her entire life she has used only open chappals, she does not wear a coat, because it is too heavy, and the only time she used a sweater was when she was ill. Do I have to wait till she gets pneumonia before she will listen to reason?" Alka vented a long list of frustrations.

Alka and her husband lived like a typical yuppie family, adopting local customs and clothing suitable to the climate. However, Ma had a harder time accepting the change. The winter clothing, never needed, in a warm tropical climate, was heavy. The stiff shoes interfered with the gait pattern she had used for more than seventy years, and she was afraid that she would fall when she wore them. The traditional occupations of a women in India restricted her indoors. However, the ancient sun-worship ritual obliged her to stand directly in the sunlight, whose importance in averting seasonal affective disorder is now acknowledged by science.

Questions

1. What solutions can you think of to help the mother meet her needs for morning sunlight and to protect her from the weather?
2. What are some practical reasons that the heavy clothing would be a problem?

Questions

1. Discuss how the valued Japanese characteristic of self-control could cause communication problems and hinder progress in rehabilitation with a client.
2. What type of role conflicts might occur for a middle-aged Japanese female client who needs rehabilitation services?
3. On the basis of your understanding of the way mental illnesses are viewed in the Asian American community, discuss approaches to treatment for this problem.
4. In what ways might the beliefs about family in the Asian American cultures interfere with the type of teaching done for rehabilitation clients in the United States?

5. Discuss how cultural differences in the use of nonverbal communication between provider and patient could lead to misunderstandings.

6. Explain how knowledge of dietary practices within the Asian cultures can be used to provide competent care.

7. Discuss barriers to health education within the Asian cultures.

8. Compare and contrast health beliefs of the Chinese culture with a more Westernized model.

9. Discuss how activities performed in rehabilitation, such as feeding oneself or reading, may have to be modified on the basis of the client's cultural background.

10. Compare and contrast your own health-related beliefs with those of one of the Asian cutures.

References

Agbayani-Siewert, P. & Revilla, L. (1995). Filipino Americans. In Pyong Gap Min (Ed), *Asian Americans, contemporary trends and issues*. Thousand Oaks, CA: Sage Publications.

Andres, T., & Ilada-Andres, P. (1987). *Understanding the Filipino*. Quezon City, Philippines: New Day Publishers.

Barnes, D. M., Davis, A. J., Portillo, C. J., & Koenig, B. A. (1998). Informed consent in a multicultural cancer population: Implications for nursing practice. *Nursing Ethics, 5*(5), 412–423.

Ceria, C. D., & Shimamoto, Y. (1996). Healthcare problems among Filipinos in Hawaii with a focus on the Filipino Elderly. In L. Zhan (Ed), *Asian voices, Asian and Asian-American health educators speak out* (pp. 68–81). Sudbury, MA: Jones and Bartlett.

Chan, S. (1998). Families with Asian Roots. In E. Lynch and M. Hanson (Eds.), *Developing cross-cultural competence, a guide for working with young children and their families*. Baltimore: Paul Brookes Publishing.

Chen, M. S., & Hawks, B. L. (1995). A debunking of the myth of healthy Asian Americans and Pacific Islanders. *American Journal of Health Promotion, 9*(4), 261–268.

Choi, K., Salzaar, N., Lew, S., & Coates, T. (1995). AIDS risk, dual identity, and community response among gay Asian and Pacific Islander men in the United States. In G. M. Herelk and Green (Eds.), *AIDS, identity, and community: The HIV epidemic and lesbians and gay men* (p.115–134). Thousand Oaks, CA: Sage Publications.

Choi, P. S. (1996). Tuberculosis concerns for Asian Americans and Pacific Islanders. *Asian American and Pacific Islander Journal of Health, 4*(1/3), 127.

Chough, C. H. (1994). *Vietnamese students: Changing patterns changing needs*. San Francisco: Many Cultures Publishing.

Coward, H., & Ratanakul, P. (1999). *A cross cultural dialogue on health care ethics* (p–6). Waterloo, Ontario, Canada: Wilfrid Laurier University Press.

Diego, A. T., Yamamoto, J., Nguyen, L. H., & Hifumi, S. S. (1994). Suicide in the elderly: Profile of Asians and Whites. *Asian American and Pacific Islander Journal of Health, 2*(1), 50–57.

Doi, M. L. (1991). A transformation of ritual: The Nisei 60th birthday. *Journal of Cross-cultural Gerontology, 6*, 153–163.

Downes, N. (1994). *Ethnic Americans for the health professional.* Dubuque, IA: Kendall/Hall.

Enas, E. A. (1996). Cardio-vascular diseases in Asian Americans and Pacific Islanders. *Asian American and Pacific Islander Journal of Health, 4*(1/3), 119–120.

Fisher, H. W. (1959). The diseases of the Filipino men. *Hawaii Medical Journal, 18*(3), 252–254.

Freedman, D. G. (1974). *Human infancy: An evolutionary perspective* (p. 173). New Jersey: Lawrence Erlbaum Associates.

Hashizume, S., & Takano, J. (1983). Nursing care of Japanese American patients. In M. Orque, B. Bloch, and L. Monroy (Eds), *Ethnic nursing care: A multicultural approach.* St. Louis: C. V. Mosby.

Healey, L. A., Skeith, M. D., Decker, J. L., & Bayani-Sioson, P. S. (1967). Hyperuricemia in Filipinos: Interaction of heredity and environment. *American Journal of Human Genetics, 19*(2), 81–85.

Hofstede, G. (1984). Hofstede's culture dimensions: An independent validation using Rokeach's value survey. *Journal of Cross-cultural Psychology, 15*, 417–433.

Hui, E. (1999). Concept of health and disease in traditional Chinese medicine. In H. Coward & P. Ratanakul. (Eds.) *A cross cultural dialogue on health care ethics* (pp. 34–46). Waterloo, Ontario, Canada: Wilfrid Laurier University.

Huynh Dinh Te (1987). *Introduction to Vietnamese Culture.* Multifunctional Resource Center, San Diego State University, California.

Iwama, M. (1999). Cross-cultural perspectives on client-centred occupational therapy practice: A view from Japan. *OT Now. Nov./Dec.,* 4–6.

Iwama, M. (2003). Toward culturally relevant epistemologies in occupational therapy. *American Journal of Occupational Therapy, 57*, 582–588.

Jacinto, J. A., & Syquia, L. M. (1995). *Lakbay, journey of the people of the Philippines.* San Francisco: Many Cultures Publishing.

Jenkins, A. E., Ayers, G. E., and Hunt, B. (1996). Cultural diversity and rehabilitation: The road traveled. *Rehabilitation Education, 10*(2), 83–103.

Kagawa-Singer, M. (1994). Diverse cultural beliefs and practices about death and dying in the elderly. In D. Wieland, D. Benton, B. Kramer, & G. D. Dawson (Eds.), *Cultural diversity and geriatric care: Challenges to the health professions* (pp. 101–115). New York: Hawthorn.

Kim, L. I., & Kim, G. S. (1997). *Korean American immigrants and their children.* San Francisco: Many Cultures Publishing.

Kister, D. A. (1997). *Korean shamanistic ritual, symbols and drama of transformation.* Budapest: Akademiai Kiado.

Kitano, H. L. (1976). *Japanese Americans.* London: Prentice-Hall.

Kitano, H. L., & Kikumera, A. (1988).The Japanese-American family. In C. H. Mindel & R. W. Habenstein (Eds.), *Ethnic families in America, patterns and variations* (pp. 41–61). New York: Elsevier.

Kittler, P. G., & Sucher, K. P. (2001). *Food and Culture.* Belmont, CA: Wadsworth Thomson Learning.

Koh, H. K., Sun, T., & Zhang, Y. Q. (1996). Cancer in Asian American and Pacific Islander populations. *Asian American and Pacific Islander Journal of Health, 4*(1/3), 121–124.

Kollipara, U. K., & Britten, H. C. (1996). Increased iron content of some Indian foods due to cookware. *Journal of American Dietetic Association, 96*(5), 508–510.

Leung, P. (1996). Asian Pacific Americans and Section 21 of the Rehabilitation Act amendments of 1992. *American Rehabilitation, 22*(1), pp. 2–6.

Leung, P., & Sakata, R. (1988). Asian Americans and rehabilitation: Some important variables. *Journal of Applied Rehabilitation Counseling, 19*(4), 16–20.

Lock, M. (1983). Japanese responses to social change—making the strange familiar. *The Western Journal of Medicine, 139*(6), 829–834.

Louie, K. (1999). Health promotion interventions for Asian American Pacific Islanders. In L. Zhan (Ed.), *Asian Voices, Asian and Asian-American health educators speak out.* Boston: Jones and Bartlett.

Manian, P. (1997). *Asian Indian children, straddling two cultures,* San Francisco: Many Cultures Publishing.

McNeely, M. J., & Boyko, E. J. (2004). *Type 2 Diabetes Prevalence in Asian Americans. Diabetes Care, 27*(1), 66. Retrieved January 27, 2005 from http://proquest.umi.com/pqdweb?

Meadows, M. (1997). Mental health and medicine: Cultural considerations in treating Asians. *Minority Nurse Newsletter, 4*(4), 1–2.

Min, P. G. (1995). *Asian Americans: Contemporary trends and issues.* Thousand Oaks CA: Sage Publications.

Moneda, A. G. V., & Gibson, S. E. (1996). The golden health promotion program for the golden dreamers. In L. Zhan (Ed.), *Asian voices* (pp. 16–25). Sudbury, MA: Jones and Bartlett.

Narayan, K. (1989). *Storytellers, saints, and scoundrels, folk narrative in Hindu religious teaching* (p. 43). Philadelphia: University of Pennsylvania.

Pang, K. Y. (1989). The practice of traditional Korean medicine in Washington DC. *Social Science Medicine, 28*(8), 875–884.

Parmar, P. (2003). Introductions. In P. Parmar and N. Somaiya-Carten (Eds.), *When your voice tastes like home.* Toronto: Second Story Press.

Perez-Arce, P., Carr, K. D., & Sorenson, J. L. (1993). Cultural issues in an outpatient program for stimulant abusers. *Journal of Psychoactive Drugs, 25*(1), 35–44.

Roland, A. (1988). *In search of self in India and Japan, toward a cross-cultural psychology*. Princeton, NJ: Princeton University Press.

Shin, K. R. (1999). Korean women and health. In L. Zhan (Ed), *Asian Voices, Asian and Asian-American health educators speak out* (pp. 43–57). Sudbury, MA: Jones and Bartlett.

Singh, S. K. (Ed.) (1988). *The People of India*. Excerpts published as *Rediscovery of India*. India Abroad Publications, Chicago, January 2, 1998.

U.S. Census Bureau. (2000) *Census 2000*. Retrieved June 29, 2004, from http://www .census.gov/prod/2002pubs/c2kbr01-16.pdf.

Wallace, S. P., Villa, V., Moon, A., & Lubben, J. E. (1996). Health practices of Korean elderly people: National health promotion priorities and minority community needs. *Family community health, 19*(2), 29–42.

Wong, S. C., & Lopez, M. (1995). *California's Chinese immigrant students in the 1990s*. San Francisco: Many Cultures Publishing.

Zhan, L. (1999). Xi Young Hong: Health practice in Chinese older women. In L. Zhan (Ed.), *Asian voices: Asian and Asian American health educators speak out*. Sudbury, MA: Jones and Bartlett.

Zhou, Y., & Britten, H. C. (1994). Increased iron content of some Chinese foods due to cooking in steel woks. *Journal of the American Dietetic Association, 94*(10), 1153–1156.

Sincere thanks to Dr. Nina Asher, Ed.D., Assistant Professor of Education and Women's and Gender Studies, Louisiana State University, LA, for a constructive critique of the initial compilation of this chapter.

9

Arab Americans

S. Omar Ahmad, Naser Z. Alsharif, and Matin Royeen

Key Words

Arab	Islam	Middle East
Arab American	Mohammed	North Africa
Muslim		

Objectives

1. Provide an overview of the region known as the Middle East.
2. Discuss some diverse cultural features of the people originating from this part of the world.
3. Provide general information about some countries in the region.
4. Offer specific rehabilitation cases dealing with Arab American patients.
5. Present specific recommendations for the rehabilitation practitioner working with Arab American patients.

Introduction

This chapter is divided into two sections. The first section provides an overview of Arab Americans related to immigration, demographics and rehabilitation care of the Arab American patient in the United States. The second section briefly discusses a number of countries including Kuwait, Iraq, Lebanon, Saudi Arabia, and Afghanistan a non-Arab country in the region. The authors hope that readers can appreciate the great contributions of the different civilizations that have existed in this important part of the world throughout history.

The term *Arab Americans* refer to those U.S. citizens and permanent residents whose ancestry and roots go back to the Arabic-speaking nations of southwestern Asia and northern Africa, a region also known as the Middle East. However, it is important to note that some authors include the non-Arab countries of Afghanistan, Iran, and Turkey as part of the Middle East. The main focus of this chapter is those Arab-Americans residing in all states with greatest concentration in California, Michigan, New York, Illinois, Maryland, Massachusetts, New Jersey, Ohio, Texas, and Virginia (Abraham & Shryock 2000; Ameri, 2000; Barakat, 1993; El-Badry, 1994; Hoogland, 1987; Suleiman, 1999; Zogby, 1991). The Arabic language serves as one of the most significant unifying force among Arab Americans despite the fact that these people speak different Arabic dialects. The 28-character Arabic letters written from right to left are held in high regard for their artistic form in the Arabic culture. Although bonded with a great common cultural heritage, Arab Americans practice different religions, which include Christianity, Islam, Druze, Judaism, and others. Some Arab American families have been living in the United States for many generations and may not be able to speak Arabic.

Rehabilitative Care of Arab-American Patients

The rehabilitative care of any ethnic American group begins with a basic understanding of the demographics, history, immigration patterns, and values and beliefs of that ethnic group. Similar to other ethnic groups in the United States, the Arab Americans are subject to stereotyping by the media with a tremendous influence on public opinion (Shaheen, 1984, 2001). Therefore, a balanced understanding of the background of Arab Americans should serve as an effective tool for those health professionals involved in the rehabilitative process of this population. For Arab Americans, history dates from the late 1800s to the present and incorporates several distinct waves of immigration and ideology. The majority share the same aspirations as other groups of immigrants to be successful as American citizens. However, many aspects of demographics, sociopolitical history, and religious beliefs may complicate the understanding of this group of patients. This chapter will attempt to provide a background for understanding the factors that may influence the rehabilitative process for Arab American patients.

Background

Demographics

It is difficult to define who an Arab is. When attempting to define the group, we face many preconceived notions about who they are and where they exist (Zahir & Pollara, 1998). The homelands that Arab Americans come from are located from the southwest of Asia to the north of Africa. Though some debate exists, the countries that are generally accepted as the Arab homelands are Algeria, Bahrain, Egypt, Iraq, Jordan, Kuwait, Lebanon, Libya, Mauritania, Morocco, Oman, Palestine, Q'atar, Saudi Arabia, Somalia, Sudan, Syria, Tunisia, United Arab Emirates, and Yemen. Arab populations, however, have maintained a strong feeling of unity as a people (Wesfield, 1990) that is established on a common history, language, and culture.

Arab countries comprise a large geographical area (approximately 14 million square kilometers) but range in populations from the densely packed streets of cosmopolitan Cairo to the Bedouin tribes of Saudi Arabia. The Bedouin people constitute less than 1% of the total Arab population of 250 million. There are an estimated 3 to 4 million Arabs in the United States, and they are almost divided equally between Muslims and Christians (Lipson & Meleis, 1983). They share a common Semitic heritage and speak Arabic. In the Arab world, 90 percent of Arabs share Islam as their religion, but it is important to note that there are Arabs that practice Judaism as well as Christianity. In fact, the Arab Christian communities in Palestine, Lebanon, Syria, Egypt, and Iraq are the oldest Christian communities and trace their history to the time of Jesus and the apostles. Islam, however, dominates the area culturally, socially, and in some countries, politically. Many of the old Arab-Christian communities share many of the practices and beliefs of their Muslim neighbors. Many of those practices are influenced by the Arabic culture and religion.

In the beginning of the seventh century A.D., the entire Mediterranean world, a majority of Persia, Egypt, the Byzantine Empire, and Palestine were Christian. Additionally, a Christian and a Jewish minority were living in the Arabian subcontinent. During the life of the prophet Muhammad, the Arabian subcontinent had been incorporated into the fledgling Islamic empire. Within a few decades of the prophet's death in 632 A.D., the Persian and Byzantine Empires, Egypt, as far west as Spain and Sicily, and as far east as China, had been incorporated into the Islamic empire. This incorporation ushered in a period of relative stability in the Islamic world, as inhabitants of the new territories were allowed to practice in peace their respective religions of Christianity and Judaism, which Muslims believe is contrary to Western literature, stating that Islam spread by the sword. In fact, it has been documented that it took two to three centuries for the bulk of the populations in the new territories to accept Islam (Lewis, 1982).

In the year 1098 A.D., groups of Franks began military actions against Palestine and western Syria that came to be known in western Europe as the Crusades. For two centuries, Palestine was contested and finally reverted to the Islamic Empire. Following the Crusades, a close trading relationship was established with western Europe that persisted for centuries. The Islamic Empire encouraged trade and contact with these European merchants and saw it as a benefit for the region. During the ensuing two centuries, the Islamic

World was itself invaded by the Mongol hordes from the East, which were consequently converted to Islam and effectively increased the size of Islamic holdings in Asia.

In 1492 A.D., Muslims and Jews were forcibly removed from Spain during a period called the "Expulsion," thus ending Islamic control in western Europe. During the Ottoman Empire that continued until the eighteenth century, there was a period of relative geographic stability in the Islamic world. During the reign of Queen Elizabeth I of England, the Ottoman Empire signed treaties with England and other European empires, resulting in structured alliances. During this same period, most of the African holdings of Islam fell to the rush of western European colonial powers through superior technology and partitioning of larger parts of the Islamic world. This trend continued until the twentieth century and still continues to affect foreign policy in these regions.

When treating Arab and Arab American patients, it is important to understand how historical events can affect trust and the establishment of supportive and caring relationships; such historical events can influence a therapeutic relationship. Historically, western Europe has devised many ways to partition and separate indigenous populations for the purpose of control and maintenance of political domination. Prior to the influx of European control, the Arab world was less structured by geographic division, with feudal governments dividing resources by mutual agreement and not including firm territorial division. Many "countries" in the Islamic empire did not have formal names, with territorial designations held over from antiquity, such as Byzantium and Palestine (Lewis, 1982). Christianity and Judaism were well understood in the Arab world, both having maintained large populations throughout the history of the empire; however, the Arab world was poorly understood by the colonial powers. In fact, there was little or no perceived need to understand it by the colonial Europeans, thereby resulting in significant distress by the Muslim populace and the roots of colonial discontent and jingoism which can be felt today. Current events have appeared to reinforce a feeling of alienation by the Arab and Arab American populace that may need to be addressed in a therapeutic context. Respect for traditions and beliefs must be given, as well as a willingness to interview and seek out information that will assist in treating the patient as a valuable individual. Additional care must be taken to establish trust with Arab American patients. Failure to do so may result in a social power imbalance that may impair full participation in the therapeutic relationship and may produce poorer treatment outcomes.

Immigration Patterns

Arab Americans live everywhere in the United States. However, there are many cities with large population such as the Detroit-Dearborn area and New York City with an estimated 300,000, each, and California with almost half a million. It has been documented that there were three waves of immigration. The first wave of Arab immigrants (Syrians) occurred between 1880 and 1930. In search of better economic opportunities, some became farmers and factory workers, whereas others engaged in successful business endeavors such as jewelry, carpets, and dry goods (Elkholy, 1988; Naff, 1980; Thernstrom, Orlov, and Handlin, 1980). The second wave of Arab immigrants started after World War II and continues today. These immigrants are highly educated people, some of whom came to the United States after being expelled by the newly formed state of Israel in 1948. Military revolutions in

Egypt and other countries in the region brought other educated people and intellectuals as immigrants to the United States.

In recent times, thousands of Muslim students have come to the United States in pursuit of technical training and college education, so that the skills learned abroad could be used in their home countries (Meleis, 1982). As a result, many have chosen to seek citizenship or employment in the United States. It is important that the rehabilitative practitioner recognize that the cultural and health practices of Arab Americans may vary according to whether they are first, second, or in some cases, third generation Americans. Therefore, it is no surprise to have Arab Americans in the clinic who are as much Americans as white Americans. More and more new immigrants are very familiar with American culture because of their fascination with the American culture. Further, typical behavior identified later in the chapter does not apply to all and the religious adherence of each individual family will affect many of the "expected" typical behaviors.

It is essential for any health care professional to have some basic understanding of Arab American patients. Unfortunately, Arab Americans are one of the most misrepresented and misunderstood groups in the United States. Arab stereotyping in the American popular culture is very common. Often Arabs are depicted as greedy billionaires, bombers, belly dancers, oil sheiks, slave traders, and terrorists. Whether in print or on screen, it is rare that a humanistic and realistic picture is presented. Between 1985 and 1995, Professor Jack Shaheen tracked features that were telecast in St. Louis, Missouri, on both cable and network. He documented 15 to 20 movies per week that mocked or denigrated Arab Muslims and 150 movies that have regularly inserted unsightly Arab Muslims and prejudicial dialogue. Although there has been some sensitization to the portrayal of Arabs in the media, much work is still needed to present accurate and balanced information regarding them. Arab Americans are dismayed by continuous bigotry and stereotyping and are disturbed to experience the consistent masking of the human side of Arabs and Muslims and to see it replaced with abstract emotion and misrepresentation. As with any other ethnic group, including adults and children, they are longing to read, hear, and see positive images of grandparents, uncles, aunts, and friends living in the old countries. The majority of these people are as friendly and familiar as the Waltons or the Huxtables. They are also most concerned about the effect of this negative stereotyping on their children, since the scars of bigotry can last forever. Following the bombing of the Murrah Federal Building in Oklahoma City, the American-Arab Anti-Discrimination Committee compiled a total of 119 hate crimes against people of Arab decent and Islamic property that were documented in the *Washington Post, Dallas Morning News, Tulsa World, Syracuse Herald-Journal* and many other newspapers. Beyond the general stereotyping, there are a number of facts that are important to be familiar with to dispel many of the misconceptions about Arabs in general and Arab Americans in particular. Islam and Arabs have a great respect for women. In fact, it was Islam that assigned women equality with men and afforded them the same rights to possess property, keep their name after marriage, retain guardianship over their minor children, undertake professions, and sue in court. In addition, polygamy is illegal in most Arab countries and represents a very insignificant percentage of all marriages. Furthermore, presently the education of women is given a high priority in all Arab countries, and many women hold key positions in teaching and administration, as writers, doctors, pharmacists, lawyers, engineers, computer scientists, and so on.

The great diversity of the Arabs defies a homogenous explanation of immigration. In the United States, immigration patterns differ greatly as one analyzes the different groups that have made the United States their home. There are vast differences in education, socioeconomic status, and race. There are Arab Americans who have descended from Armenians, Chaldeans, and Assyrians who have maintained their own distinct cultural markers and health beliefs (Kurdahi-Zahir Hattar-Pollara, 1998). Though their own health care beliefs may differ, the reactions that these groups may have to Western medicine are similar.

Case Study 1

Yousef S. is a 53-year-old male being seen by Paula, an occupational therapist in an outpatient clinic after hip replacement. In her review of the medical records, she notices that Yousef S. is an Arab American. Paula knows little about Arab American culture, so she decides to ask some probing questions about the patient's background and health beliefs.

The patient comes to the clinic with his 20-year-old daughter, Samira. The patient appears anxious, uncertain, and hesitant when the therapist calls the patient into the treatment area. The patient insists on having his daughter with him during the session. Paula sets up the treatment environment to provide adequate personal space and adequate privacy. Then, Paula begins the interview by introducing herself. She asks some questions about his family and living situation. She makes sure to speak in a friendly and inquisitive manner, and not trying to get "right down to business." When the patient begins speaking to her, she notices that he has a heavy accent, which she realizes causes her some discomfort. Yousef lives with his daughter and her family. Initially, Paula keeps turning to the daughter to assist in understanding Yousef, but then she simply repeats the question and apologies for her difficulty in understanding. In this manner, she shows respect for Yousef and helps him to feel comfortable in communicating with her. During her initial interview, Paula discovers that he has been in the United States for six years. Through respectful, open-ended questions she is able to determine that he is a 53-year-old man who is a supervisor at a shipping company and has a very physically demanding job.

Yousef has appeared a half-hour late for the past three sessions to the outpatient clinic. Paula is very concerned, since the late arrival has been impacting her clinic schedule. Yousef's daughter has been accompanying him to the clinic regularly, and Paula decides to use the time in the clinic to discuss what may be causing him to miss his appointment. Initially, she approaches Yousef and Samira and asks, "This is the third time you are late for your appointment. Is there some sort of problem?" At this point, Yousef and his daughter appear very embarrassed, and they promise to be on time for the next session.

Questions

1. In order to provide most effective intervention, what specific steps would you take as a therapist to learn more about Yousef's cultural background?

2. Discuss some effective ways of communication styles with your Arab American clients. Do you think Paula's direct confrontation to being 30 minutes late was the most effective way?

Paula was able to do several things right in the previous scenario. She was able to identify that she had preconceived notions about Arab American culture and was able to gather some information prior to the session. She was mistrustful of the patient because of the association of Arab Americans to recent terrorism in the news, but she was able to increase the comfort of the patient by having some friendly small talk prior to initiating treatment and asking open-ended questions that allowed the patient to answer as his comfort level improved. Initially, she looked to the daughter to help with translation but corrected her behavior to respond to the patient, showing respect for his communication and recognizing possible cultural issues. We will follow Yousef throughout the chapter.

It is essential to understand the importance of time to a culture. In the West, a premium is placed upon time. We use palm pilots, personal electronic assistants, and computers that beep and hurry us on to appointments at a rigid and insistent rate. Meetings are frequently punctuated by frequent glances to watches and the clock on the wall. We tend to parcel out events in terms of time: one hour for this meeting, fifteen minutes for that, and so on. This is the hallmark of an industrialized society that focuses on the value of individualism, or a cultural focus on the self and the nuclear family versus less industrialized cultures that are considered more collectivist, or concerned with a larger collective community (Levine, 1997). Middle Eastern and subcontinental cultures tend to operate on "event time," or the day is punctuated by specific events, not parceled out by clock time. For instance, it may be considered rude to abruptly end a conversation because an appointment is scheduled; rather, the appointment will have to wait until the conversation is finished. Many of the Arab patients you meet may have grown up in a society where the trains may not have run on time and an appointment for 10:00 A.M. may have really meant, show up at noon.

Research has demonstrated that trying to make people radically change their perception of time can cause great stress (Levine, 1997). For instance, having recently traveled to Saudi Arabia, an Arab country that conforms principally to event time, I stood in a line for over two hours to receive a stamp for my passport. As I stood in the line, I felt more and more anxious and agitated. The locals around me, however, were talking, were laughing, and generally were much more healthy than I. I had a mismatch of my perception of the importance of time from that of the other travelers in the line. I was forced to comply with a different time paradigm. Your patients may well feel that their sense of time and time value are violated if you do not make an attempt to respect their idea of socio-temporality. Conversely, it is important to remember that individuals who have immigrated to the West may not share the values of the cultures that they have left or that they may have adapted to the pace of life in the West and share a common view of time.

In the previous scenario, Yousef and his daughter were confronted for tardiness to the session. As may be expected, the abrupt admonishment may have caused irreparable harm to the therapeutic relationship. Let's alter the scenario: Paula is concerned by the lateness of the patient to his treatment times. Paula realizes that there may be some issues with the patient that may transcend his desire to arrive on time. Paula asks the patient, "How is everything going with you, Yousef?" The patient responds that he is doing well. Paula then addresses the tardiness, "I'm a bit concerned that you have been a little late for your appointments. Is there anything that I can do?" Yousef responds, "I have been having trouble getting here because the busses run late and inconsistently to my neighborhood." Paula treats the patient in a respectful manner and seeks to gather information through positive information-gathering. In fact, the assumption of socio-temporal incompatibility was wrong in this case! It was good that Paula stayed away from making culturally biased assumptions.

Values and Beliefs of Traditional Arab Culture

Family Structure

Arab culture is considered highly stable from an anthropological perspective, and there are many common cultural factors which can be typified that can be considered when treating Arab American patients (Wesfield, 1990). Arab culture typically shares strong and well-established family roles that affect the sense of identity of the individuals seeking health care. In Arab culture, the family is the strongest social unit from which the societal values derive (Kurdahi-Zahir & Hattar-Pollara, 1998). The extended family can exert social control when issues of health care are being discussed, and often a decision cannot be made until other family members are consulted. However, doing this may not be possible, since the extended family may not be present in the United States. The father and grandfather typically exert the most control and wield the greatest social power when a decision regarding health care is to be made (Moracco, 1983). This tendency is positively exhibited by the typically high degree of social and community support of individuals and families of Arab Americans, which can be accessed in the treatment of the Arab American patient (Khalaf, 1971). Collectivism creates a stark contrast to the typical American fierce individualism that is supported by the Constitution and laws stressing individuality. The Arab American patient may be placed in a situation of great stress if forced to make a decision for himself or herself without the consultation of the family. The rehabilitative practitioner should consider this when treatment planning with patients and their families.

Arab family life is typically patriarchal, and the family roles are determined by both age and gender. The father is considered the head of the household and is the person primarily responsible for health care decisions for his social unit. Children are expected to put the family's need ahead of their own and are expected to look to the parents to make health care decisions (Barakat, 1993). The mother's role is to attend to the home, to care for the children, and to meet the social needs of the family. The mother is responsible for seeing the children through different developmental milestones (Barakat, 1993). In addition to the defined roles of the family, age is an important determinant of social power in the Arab family. It is typical in the Arab family to consult older adults before making health care decisions, and their words may carry more power than technical expertise or education. Older men typically carry the most social power, and older women carry more power than does a younger male (Sadawi, 1983). In the case of a sick child, the mother may be the first to decide that the child will go to the doctor. Next, she may discuss the treatment options with the father of the child. The father may then seek counsel with the extended family, including the grandparents of the child, as well as other members of the family who may want their opinions to be heard. The mother will then relay the father's decision to the doctor. Again, depending on the background of each family and the time when they immigrated, the process may not involve what has just been discussed, and the parents together will be making all the decisions. However, as discussed, these family roles may now be the exception rather than the rule, especially for women who lived in or emigrated from countries such as Egypt, Jordan, Lebanon, and Palestine, since many are well educated and have joined the workforce in their native countries and are continuing to do so in the United States. Additionally, the roles in the family have become less stable as the immigrants choose to modify their roles and are affected by the individualistic American culture.

Traditional Arab culture values personal relationships with the health care provider as well as with individuals encountered in the health care area. Sheets and El-Azhari (1998) report that this tendency is often in conflict with traditional task-oriented Western values. The traditional Arab will require a period of friendly, personal discourse about a neutral topic before a trusting relationship can begin to develop. It is essential to develop this "context" before entering a therapeutic relationship (Hall, 1977). For example, if a health care professional enters the room, hurries through a medical history, and initiates treatment, the Arab patient may be very uncomfortable and may fail to divulge important information. In fact, this haste may be considered extremely rude and constitutes a loss of credibility for the clinician. This can be expressed by the patient with poor follow-up, decreased compliance, or a cessation of treatment. To assist in the therapeutic relationship, a pretreatment meeting may be arranged, or the initial treatment visit may be used to perform an extensive interview with the patient and his or her family to increase the comfort level of the patient and family. Courtesy and personal value are highly respected in Arab culture, so small talk with the patient prior to the initiation of personal questions—or ones that may be perceived as personally intrusive—is recommended (Lipson & Maleis, 1983).

Islamic Law Regulating Patterns of Life

Traditional Arab Muslim culture follows strict proscriptive guidelines set down by Islamic law in what is called *Al-Halal Wal Haram Fil Islam* (what is lawful and prohibited in Islam) as are written in its holy book, the *Qur'an*, and the *Sunnah*, or words of his messenger, Muhammad (peace be upon him). These writings describe a set of guidelines that indicate which vocational and recreational activities members of different age groups and genders may be engaged in, and they have been incorporated into the *Shari-ah*, or Islamic Law. Not all Arabs are Muslim, nor do all Muslim Arabs comply strictly or exclusively to these rules. Even Middle Eastern countries rely less on these guidelines in modern times, but some very traditional Arab Muslims may adhere to them. They may, however, provide some guidance when evaluating occupational patterns and structuring interviews with Arab and Arab Muslim patients.

Art

Arab culture has an extensive and a complex history in the fine arts. This may provide a therapeutic medium or a context for therapy that the rehabilitation professional may use to both establish rapport and provide a treatment context. The history of fine arts in the Arab world can be traced prior to the time of the pharaohs, recorded by the Assyrians, Abyssinians, Hiitites, Persians, Greeks, and with current Islamic influence. The Egyptian art dating back 3,000 years served as a medium of communication whereby gods and pharaohs expressed their might and accomplishments to an illiterate and agricultural community through images and symbols carved on temple walls (Malek, 1993). By the late sixth century, Islamic civilization spread across the Arab world, and previous notions of beauty and art no longer held true. Islamic art had its beginning in the mosques under public tutelage and began to extol the virtues of Islam. The social culture adopted the approval and disapproval of different art forms, and every piece of artwork received intense public scrutiny (Arnold & Guillaume, 1931). The Arabic script that is found in the Qur'an evolved into a unique and distinctive art form that penetrated many arts from calligraphy to sculpture, pottery, architecture, poetry, painting, masonry, woodwork, and metallurgy (Arnold & Guillaume, 1931).

Islam keeps strict guidelines upon what type of artistic pursuits that an individual may engage in. For example, an individual may participate in a sculpture class only as long as the subject matter that he or she seeks to replicate adheres to Islamic law (Al-Qaradawi, 1980). The individual is prohibited from creating artistic objects that attempt to revere the human form, demonstrate vanity, replicate an image of the prophet, or demonstrate that which is *Haram*, or unlawful to Islam. These rules include photography, paintings, and other artistic pursuits (Al-Qaradawi, 1980). There is a history of debate and discussion as it relates to art in the Arab culture. Even so, many Arabs will choose not to engage in these types of artistic occupations because of strict control of the subject matter; however, there is a strong history of woodworking, weaving, painting, calligraphy, poetry, and song in Arab culture that provides a wealth of treatment opportunity. Choosing an artistic pursuit in which the product is useful (not merely artistic) may assist in the assimilation of the Arab patient into art groups. Opportunities also exist for allowing the individual to share the contributions of Arab culture in these areas, and typically, debate is welcomed. These pursuits can provide the rehabilitation professional with opportunities for fine and gross motor tasks, graded cognitive tasks, sensory-motor experiences, and limitless other treatment opportunities, using a culturally relevant and meaningful task.

Exercise

Exercise is a common avenue that rehabilitation professionals access with patients of many diagnoses. It is easy to identify the role and importance of sports in the Arab world. Either sport or exercise may be used by the rehabilitation professional during treatment. The *Sunnah* describes several athletic pursuits that are *Halal*, or permitted, by Muslim culture. They are recommended as a source of enjoyment and recreation, but they must, at the same time, prepare the individual for worship and other obligations. In these pursuits, all athletic and training situations are permissible for either pleasure, for rehabilitation, or as an organizing personal influence as long *as the activities do not violate the cultural and religious values* (Al-Qaradawi, 1980). Specific sports that receive wide appeal in the Arab world are soccer, track and field, various equine events, wrestling, and martial arts. Recently, sports such as basketball and handball have increased in popularity. Additionally, any of the athletic activities that typical American children may engage in are possible in American Muslim culture.

Rehabilitative efforts may be assisted by pointing out that various prescribed physical activities may assist with religious obligations. For instance, if an Arab man has had a knee replacement, exercises will help the patient assume positions necessary to complete his daily prayers. It is important to note that in less culturally assimilated households, after young childhood, athletic events are performed only with members of the same gender (Sarwar, 1989).

Vocational Engagement

Arab Americans are involved in almost every facet of the American economy. Immigration has brought Arabs of various training and experience to North America. There is a strong Arab history of trading in both ideas and goods that is carried on in their new surroundings. There are Arab professors, computer programmers, doctors, lawyers, cab drivers, businesspeople, and a wide range of other professions that represent the complete socioeconomic strata. It is important to remember that up to half of the Arabs in the United States are Christian and are not held to the same religious obligations as Muslim Arabs; the degree of cultural assimilation will affect choices in occupation and activities.

There are a few vocational occupations that may be considered *Haram*, or disallowed, in traditional Arab Muslim culture. There are several limitations for Muslim businesspeople that should be recognized when occupational engagement is considered. The first is in trading or selling traditionally prohibited materials including pork, wine, liquor, and any other intoxicants. In addition, the sale of idols (including religious statuary) and crosses is traditionally prohibited. Many Arab Muslims will not seek a vocation in areas that involve speculation for profit, which includes professions such as futures and commodity sales, speculation on stud horses, gambling, and land speculation. Jobs in businesses that collect interest or lend money for a fee are also prohibited (Al-Qaradawi, 1980). In the United States, engagement in professions that are traditionally seen as *Haram* can cause great psychological distress in the patients involved in them, because it may be seen as very offensive to the individual's family and socioreligious group. Conversely, those individuals who have assimilated into the culture may not share those values and may have been causative factors in leaving their countries of origin.

Fasting

Sawm, or fasting, is a closely held tenet of Islam. During the Islamic month of *Ramadan*, the Arab Muslim will abstain from eating, drinking, smoking, and conjugal relations during daylight hours. The Islamic calendar is lunar, meaning that it is based on the phases of the moon rather than on the sun, as is the Western calendar. This difference may cause some confusion among Westerners, as it appears that the month of fasting follows no predictable pattern. For that reason it is very important to clarify with the patient whether he or she has been fasting and to adjust treatment accordingly (Sheets & El-Azhari, 1998).

A common complaint among health care professionals is that during *Ramadan*, patients will forgo or delay taking medication from dawn to dusk or cease its use entirely (Pirotta, 1994). This problem can be lethal for patients with diabetes, cardiac concerns, and pulmonary dysfunction, so it is important for the therapist to consider these factors in the care of Arab patients. There has been increasing debate within Islam about what actions constitute breaking the fast. Intentionally allowing any substance to enter the body through the nose or the mouth, intentional eating or drinking, or conjugal relations are prohibited and will break the fast. There is controversy regarding injections, inhalers, eye drops, or other medication in the Muslim community, so it is important to know what the individual's intentions are during *Ramadan* before recommending treatment (Sheets & El-Azhari, 1998). Another consideration is the recommendation of physical occupations such as lawn care, vocational activities, or intense exercises, because the individual may be dehydrated and may not have the opportunity to rehydrate for several hours.

Case Study 2

Usma is a 23-year-old first-generation American whose father was born in the United Arab Emirates. Usma has a history of insulin dependent diabetes mellitus and is under Thomas's care. It happens to be in the Islamic month of *Ramadan,* and Usma has come to the hospital through the emergency room with many of the signs and symptoms of hyperglycemia. The patient was stabilized, and upon questioning the patient, Thomas expresses outrage when Usma says that she is not taking her insulin throughout the day and refuses to take her regular blood tests while fasting. He says, "Keep on acting foolishly, and you may die! You have a deadly but controllable disease, so you must manage it effectively!" Usma listens to Thomas quietly, is discharged, and returns within a week with the diagnosis of diabetic coma.

Questions

1. Why is Usma being accompanied by her father?
2. What is *Ramadan?* Discuss the reasons for Usma's refusal to take insulin during the day.
3. How do you describe Thomas's attitude after Usma's refusal to take insulin?
4. As a rehabilitation practitioner, how would you deal with Usma in this situation?
5. What recommendations do you have for Thomas?

This is, unfortunately, a likely scenario. It is important that the health care professional work very closely with the patient, the family, and a Muslim sheik or the head of the Islamic Center or mosque in the community, so that both the religious needs and the medical needs of the patient are met without compromising the patient's health. Patients have to be well educated about the importance of taking medications and following a diet in the overall control of their disease. The family and the religious leaders, moreover, have to provide support so that these needs are met. Potential solutions to meet the medical and the religious needs of the patient have to be clearly identified.

Now let's look at a revision of the previous scenario.

Thomas engages Usma in some small talk and asks why she has not been taking her insulin and regulating her blood sugar. Usma responds that to bleed or to take medicine will break her fast, so that during the month of *Ramadan,* she chooses not to break her fast. She feels very anxious and is concerned about the possible consequences of not checking her blood sugar. Thomas informs Usma that blood sugar can be measured through a urine test and assists her in changing the timing of some of her daily tasks to take advantage of her change in eating patterns. Usma feels very grateful to Thomas for his help.

Establishment of Rapport

Here are a number of things that the occupational therapist has to consider and do to help him or her establish a good rapport with Arab American patients:

1. Identify one's own preconceptions and misconceptions, and to try to dispel them. This is an important step in understanding that your own worldview is shaped by your own culture and that recognition of these preconceptions is essential to understanding other people.

2. Avoid overgeneralizations that cause the therapist to "typify" a person:
   a. Remember that not all American Arabs are Muslims.
   b. Recognize that there are fundamentalist factions in all religions and outlooks and that most American Arabs are not fundamentalist Muslims.
   c. Be conscious of the misconception that Arabs and Arab Americans view men as being superior culturally and socially to women.
   d. Be conscious of the misconception that women are submissive and have no decision-making role in Arab and Arab American culture.
   e. Be conscious of the misconception that Arabs and Arab Americans support terrorism and terrorist activities.

3. Seek a better understanding of Arab Americans. Read articles and publications that provide a balanced and scholarly analysis of Arabs and Arab American culture (provide references).

4. One of the most important activities in building trust and rapport is to recognize the individuality of your patient. Talk to your patient, and ask about his or her culture to help you better understand.

5. Because many Arab cultures value socialization highly, a patient may be put on the defensive by an "immediately get down to business" approach. Start each session with a friendly talk.

Consider that the individuals may experience all of the fears and insecurities of illness and the inherent uncertainties of the healthcare system, so it is important to be empathetic.

The history, religion, and socio-temporality of Arab Americans can make the therapeutic relationship unusual at times. The events of September 11, 2001, have created a number of challenges that may have to be overcome in establishing therapeutic rapport gaining the trust of this population of patients. There are also distinct advantages that can be gained if the rehabilitation professional chooses to acknowledge and access the strong family and cultural bonds.

The next section briefly describes a selected number of Middle Eastern countries that include Kuwait, Iraq, Lebanon, Afghanistan, and Saudi Arabia. The authors hope that such background information on these selected countries can serve as a useful tool toward developing a better understanding of the rich cultures of the region.

History of Middle Eastern Countries

Kuwait

Kuwait is surrounded by desert sands and is known to have one of the largest oil reserves in the world. Since the discovery of oil in 1938 (Lerner Publications, 1989), Kuwait has moved its status from poverty to a new transformation into a wealthy state. By granting oil exploration rights to the British and the United States, the oil revenues brought a great deal of prosperity to the people and contributed greatly to the modernization of the country. As a member of the Organization of Petroleum Exporting Countries known as OPEC, Kuwait has played a very important role in regional and international affairs. The ancient history of Kuwait and the region dates back to 5000 B.C. where the roots of ancient Al-Ubaid culture have their origins and have cultivated Mesopotamia, whose people are known to have developed a very high culture of the ancient times. Between 4000 and 2000 B.C., the Dilmun civilization extended from present-day Kuwait to Bahrain in the south. The Dilmun civilization controlled the trade rout between Mesopotamia and the Indus River Valley in present-day Pakistan (Lerner Publications, 1989). Following the decline of the Dilmun commercial power, the Babylonians and later the Persians ruled this region. Alexander the Great of Macedonia conquered Mesopotamia in about 330 B.C. and established a colony for soldiers. After two hundred years, Greek rule was followed by the Roman Empire, which made Christianity legal in the region. In about A.D. 570, Muhammad was born in Mecca and later became the prophet for Muslims, who follow the monotheistic religion of Islam. During the early Islamic period, Kazima had become a very famous fertile area and served as a trading stations for travelers in the region. Because of its strategic importance, Kazima later became a station for Muslim armies. In Kazima the Arab Armies, under the leadership of Khaild ibn al-Walid, defeated the Persians. This battle is known as the Battle of the Chains since the Persian general had bound all his soldiers to a chain in order to prevent them from escaping. This event led to the death of every Persian soldier in the battle. The safe harbor of Kuwait has attracted inhabitants in the region that later became an important commercial center for the Persian Gulf. In fact, the golden age of shipping began in the eighth century when Muslim leaders after Muhammad, known as Caliphs, moved the political capital of Islam from Mecca to Baghdad.

The founding of modern Kuwait dates back to the 1722 drought that struck the Arabian peninsula, forcing many groups in the Nejd region to migrate northeast to the Persian Gulf in search of better pasture for their herds. A subgroup of the Anaiza tribe known as the Utub settled in a small town called Kuwait and mingled with the small population already in Kuwait. In 1756, Sabah bin Jabir was elected to be the first leader of the Utub people. Fearing the invasion of the Turks, Kuwait signed an agreement with the British seeking their protection and acknowledging their control over Kuwait's foreign affairs. The British provided the Sabah family an annual payment, and Kuwait remained a British protectorate until 1961 when Kuwait officially gained its independence. After World War I, Kuwait reached a border agreement with Saudi Arabia by establishing a neutral zone that later became a divided zone in 1969. Under this agreement, each country administers its own portion and shares the resources. The Kuwait border agreement with Iraq goes back to the Ottoman Empire in 1913. After gaining independence from Turkey in 1932, Iraq accepted this previously established line with Kuwait. Later in 1960s and 1970s, Iraq made claims to Kuwaiti territories. In 1990, Iraq invaded Kuwait, leading to the formation of the coalition forces that defeated Iraq and reversed their invasion of Kuwait in 1991.

There is a large population of other nationalities, such as Egyptians, Indians, Pakistanis, Palestinians, Iraqis, and Iranians who work in Kuwait. Kuwaiti citizens enjoy one of the most privileged and affluent lifestyles in the country. Some of the oil revenues is used to provide benefits for its citizens, resulting in a high per capita income. The social structure of Kuwaiti society is still based on traditional Arab customs of family connections and kinships. However, widespread economic growth and modernization have brought about some social changes in the country. The majority of people live in cities and have access to all necessities and conveniences of modern life. As a result of urbanization, most of the Bedouins have given up their nomadic lives and lead a more settled life in the cities. Family life serves as a strong unifying force in Kuwaiti society today. The traditional Kuwaiti family is extended and includes the husband, his parents, his wife, his sons and their wives and children, and unmarried sons and daughters. Traditionally, marriages are arranged by families, and it is not unusual to see unions between first cousins. Women in Kuwait enjoy a relatively greater degree of independence and freedom than in some other states in the region. The attitude of the educated men has changed toward women; however, traditional institutions still remain strong. Women are beginning to voice their political opinions and are active in social welfare and humanitarian programs. Islam is the dominant religion in Kuwait. The majority of people are of the Sunni sect, and the Shiite represent the minority, most of whom have come from Iran.

The health care in Kuwait has improved drastically since some of the revenues from the oil have been used to develop a sound health infrastructure in the country. The infant mortality rate and life expectancy have improved. Kuwait is divided into six health administration districts, each of which is located in different parts of the country. The Kuwaiti

Government has employed health care professionals from other countries while also trying to increase a cadre of Kuwaiti health professionals. The training hospital in Kuwait is focused on producing physicians who are Kuwaiti citizens. A good number of the nation's Kuwaiti doctors are women. Additionally, the Kuwaiti system provides the disabled, the elderly, families of students, widowed or unmarried women over the age of 18, orphans, the poor, and families of prisoners with a wide range of welfare programs unseen in most other parts of the world.

Education has received a great deal of attention from the government. Public education in Kuwait is considered to be one of the best in the Middle East. Education is compulsory for all children aged 6 through 14. Public education beginning in primary school up to university is free for all students. The government covers the cost of the books, meals, transportation, and uniforms. Additionally, the parents receive an allowance in support of educational expenses. The children aged 10 and older learn English as a second language in schools. The government of Kuwait provides scholarships for university students to study abroad in Europe, the United States, and other countries.

The National Council for Culture, Arts, and Letters was founded in 1974 in order to create awareness and support of the traditional artistic heritage. Bedouin arts such as weaving made of brightly colored wool on a loom, a "sadu," has been revived. Drums and tambourines accompany dancers who use swords with great agility. Popular folklore music is played in social gatherings, family meetings, and weddings.

Recreational activities are an important part of life in Kuwait. Because of its location on the Persian Gulf, water skiing, wind surfing, scuba diving, and yachting are popular activities in Kuwait. Soccer is the most popular sport in the country. The Kuwaiti National Soccer Team has performed well in regional and international competitions.

Iraq

The Republic of Iraq has served as a major power in the Middle East. The recent invasion of the United States and a few allies ousted Saddam Hussein and the ruling Baath party from power. The United States basically has the responsibility of controlling Iraq with the assistance of some allied forces and some involvement of the United Nations. There are many challenges facing the Iraqi people, the United States, and its allies in trying to bring stability and to build a democratic Iraq. History will judge the future of this great country that has been inhabited by various peoples who have left behind ruins of many ancient cities in the area. A great variety of cultures including the Sumerians, Babylonians, Chaldeans, and the Assyrian have left behind a great heritage and accomplishments in the form of trade, agriculture, literature, and science. The Arab empire began controlling Iraq in the seventh century when Islam emerged and has served as a cornerstone of the identity of Iraq and the rest of the Middle East (Lerners Publications, 1990).

After gaining its independence from the British in 1932, Iraq allowed foreign investors to develop its resources, and in 1972, Iraq took control of the extraction, processing, and export of the country's petroleum. The costly war with Iran between 1980 and 1988, the Gulf War of 1991 with the United States and its allies, and the most recent invasion of the country and ousting of Saddam Hussein from power have been very traumatic for the country and people of Iraq.

The two rivers the Tigris and the Euphrates have played a very important role in the economic life of the country, irrigating some of the most fertile soil in the region. Human settlements have had some impact on wildlife in the country. There are still bats, rats, jackals, wildcats, wild pigs, gazelles, and hyenas living in remote areas. Birds of prey, such as eagles, vultures, hawks, and buzzards, feed on these small mammals.

The shrine of Ali, one of the great leaders of the Shiite sect of Islam, is located in Al-Najaf. Each year thousands of pilgrims from Iran, Afghanistan, Pakistan, India, and other countries pay their respects to Al-Najaf. Karbala is another holy site where Imam Husayn, the grandson of Prophet Muhammad, is buried. He was killed in a revolt against the Sunnis. This tomb is considered to be a holy place, and followers mark the date of his birth with chanting and prayers. The Iraqi population of 27 million people represents various ethnic groups such as Arabs, Kurds, Turkomans, Assyrians, and Armanians. The Madan, also known as Marsh Arabs, live in tall reed homes in swamplands. People travel by boats from one location to another. The Bedouins are desert wanderers who travel through the hot zones searching for water and grass for their livestock. Each Bedouin family lives in a tent, and a number of these tents represent a clan. The Bedouins, who have a very strong sense of family loyalty and share strong clan identity, are well known for their courage and code of hospitality. The Kurds are a non-Arab minority group who lead a seminomadic life and are engaged in farming and herding livestock. The Kurds have strong ethnic ties with other Kurdish groups in Turkey, Syria, Iran, and the former Soviet Union. Iraqi Arabic is spoken daily, and modern standard Arabic is used in literary language. The Kurdish, Turkish, and Assyrians use their own languages.

The Iraqi literature shares common themes with the Christian Bible and sacred Jewish faith regarding creation, the Great Flood and the Garden of Eden. The Iraqi poetry and prose reflect the heritage of its culture and its people. The Thousand and One Nights is a well- known folktales in the western world. The government provides adequate health services to meet the needs of its citizens. However, the economic embargo imposed by the United Nations following the Gulf War has caused a great deal of suffering to the health and suffering of Iraqi children. The Iraqi art represents a wide range of cultural heritage from previous eras. The carved slabs of stone, mosaic tile work of mosques, delicate jewelry and geometric patterns are well known in the world. Beautiful hand made rugs, decorated metal items and other beautifully designed artistic styles and shapes are available in bazaars. Recently, the world community watched helplessly as these priceless arts and valuable pieces of history were looted from museums in Iraq during the United States led invasion.

Lebanon

This small country, which is about the size of the state of Connecticut, has a rich history dating back to 3000 B.C. when it was inhabited by the Phoenicians (Harik, 1987). The Phoenicians were well known as traders and navigators whose ships sailed as far as the Atlantic Ocean and South Africa. The Phoenician alphabet is well known, since it later became the source of the Greek and Roman alphabets. After the decline of the Phoenicians, other powers, such as Assyrians, Babylonian, Persians, and Greeks left a deep mark in the history of Lebanon. The Roman era is well known for its peace and prosperity in Lebanon. The magnificent city called Heliopolis with its splendid temples and huge race track and a famous law school in Berytus (Beirut) provided evidence of a very rich civilization (Harik, 1987). The Arabian conquerors were the next that swept through the area and established Islam as another religion next to Christianity, which was brought by the Romans. The Crusaders from Europe challenged Muslim control and built massive churches, castles, and towers in Lebanon. The Muslims resisted the invasion of the Crusaders, whose rule came to an end after 200 years. Turkish rule followed in Lebanon for 400 years. After the defeat of the Ottoman Empire, England and France as the dominant colonial powers divided the territory, thus leaving Lebanon under the mandatory government of the European power. After Lebanon's independence in 1943, the Maronite Christians, who had been supported previously by the French, maintained the most power in Lebanon. Lebanon had become a symbol of progress and freedom in the Middle East beginning in 1960s. Unfortunately, conflicts among different groups have devastated this beautiful country that once served as the gateway between east and west. Consequently, these bloody conflicts have forced many people to leave their homeland and live in other countries, including the United States.

The country's high mountain range between Israel on the south and Syria on the northeast, Mount Lebanon, is known for its beauty for thousands of years. The rich Beka'a Valley is located to the east of Mount Lebanon, providing wheat, grapes, and vegetables. Just like the mountains, another important part of Lebanon's history has been the sea that has connected the country to the rest of the world.

The first known Lebanese to come to the United States was named Antoun el-Bishalany, who arrived in Boston in 1854. In 1876 during the International Exposition in Philadelphia, Lebanese and Syrian merchants learned that their goods were in great demand in the United States. Soon Lebanese businessmen and others were leaving their country in search of the American dream. In 1985, *Harper's Weekly* published an article describing the New York Lebanese immigrants and their cultural heritage (Harik, 1987). Khalil Gibran, a well-known artist and poet, moved to the United States in 1985. There are many prominent Lebanese American politicians, business people, and other professionals who are well known in the United States.

Afghanistan

The citizens of Afghanistan who are not Arabs are called Afghans. Afghan culture and traditions are shaped by the country's geography, tribal code, ancient history, and political conditions. Centuries of invasion and conquests have brought many different people to the region, creating a multiethnic population. The different Afghan tribes are Pushtuns, Tajiks, Hazarahs, and Turkmens. The Afghan tribe is related to extended families and clans whose name the tribe shares. Tribal law and authority are a way of life that has evolved throughout centuries in order to exert authority, define rules of behavior, and maintain the unity of the people (Dupree, 1980). The resilience, toughness, fierce independence, love of family, honor, and defense of the homeland are deeply imbedded in every vein of Afghan life. All of these characteristics were shown during the freedom fighters' resistance against the occupying forces of the former Soviet Union. With the assistance of the United States and other Western countries, the Afghan freedom fighters forced the Soviet withdrawal from Afghanistan in 1989. During ten years of fighting, the Afghans paid a heavy price with over a million people dead and the country practically destroyed. Despite twenty-four years of turbulence in Afghanistan, the television images of people celebrating their renewed freedoms following the fall of the Taliban from power are unforgettable. The Afghans deep sense of hospitality and leisure are reflected in festivals and celebrations. One of the big festivals is Naw-roz, or the Afghan New Year. People in cities and towns celebrate by attending picnics, seeing family members, going to different public places, and enjoying life. Some farmers take their livestock to the show, whereas other people enjoy seeing kite fighting, dog fighting, egg fighting, and other cultural activities. The popular Afghan national dance called Aten is performed by a group of men in a circle. The tempo of the dance picks up and becomes very exciting as the dancers artfully jump and rotate their heads and bodies with the sound of the Afghan drums. Weddings are also very important to the Afghans. The ceremonies last from one to three days. It is not unusual to see anywhere from 300 to 1,500 guests attending a wedding.

Afghan hospitality dictates that guests are well fed and well treated. Both the quality and the quantity of foods are important in Afghan culture. Another important feature of Afghan culture is crafts such as woodworking, carpet weaving, leatherworking, pottery making, tile molding, embroidering, and silk weaving. Afghan fur coats were very popular items in the Western markets in 1970s. Goldsmiths and silversmiths have engaged in lapidary work for centuries.

Saudi Arabia

This nation, the largest in the Middle East, occupies 80 percent of the Arabian Peninsula. The Kingdom of Saudi Arabia is an extremely dry country with scorching hot rock and sandy deserts. Saudi Arabia is the birthplace of Muhammad and the home of Islam, hosting the two holiest cities of Mecca and Medina for more than one billion Muslims throughout the world. The first people in the country were the Bedouins, or desert people, who moved from place to place in search of pastures for their herds of camels and sheep (O'Shea, 1999). The country follows the Islamic lunar calendar, which marks the time of year when Muhammad in A.D. 622 fled from the city of Mecca to Medina. *Ramadan* is the holiest month for the Muslims when Prophet Muhammad received the sacred words of the Koran from the Angel Gabriel. During *Ramadan*, Muslims do not eat or drink from sunrise to sunset. The fasting philosophy is intended to establish self-discipline and control of the body, to learn the feeling of hunger, and to appreciate the gift of food given by God. *Ramadan* has a big impact on people and their sense of time and lifestyle. People develop a new routine in order to adjust to the demands of thirst and hunger. The fast is broken by the evening meal called *Iftar*. The last ten nights of *Ramadan* have a special significance for Muslims. Known as *Lailat-ul Qadr*, or the Night of Power, it is during this time that Muhammad received the first scriptures of the Koran. As a result, there is a stronger sense of devotion to the faith during the last ten days of *Ramadan*. Some people may spend the entire ten days praying in the mosque. After *Ramadan*, the Feast of the Breaking of the Fast, known as *Eid el-Fitr*, is celebrated in Islamic communities throughout the world. It is in Saudi Arabia where the sighting of the new moon is relayed to the rest of the Islamic world, marking the first day of the festivities. Families, friends, relatives, and members of the Islamic communities enjoy the festivities and thank God for giving them the fortitude for being able to make it through *Ramadan*. It is during the *Eid el-Fitr* that people exchange gifts and children receive money from the elders. Additionally, people donate some money to the poor.

As mentioned previously, Saudi Arabia is the home to the holy city of Mecca, the birthplace of Prophet Muhammad. The Grand Mosque of Mecca is big enough to hold close to a million worshipers. Every year, about two million Muslims from around the globe go to the city of Mecca for *Hajj*, a yearly pilgrimage that every Muslim can make at least once in a lifetime. The ritual of *Hajj* is one of the five pillars of Islam that should be performed by every able Muslim. The Saudi Arabian government provides an incredible quality of services in the area of transportation, shelter, food, water, and other logistics for two million diverse visitors speaking many different languages. On the first day of *Hajj*, men wearing simple white gowns and women with their faces unveiled enter the Grand Mosque and walk around the *Ka'bah* seven times. Then the pilgrims spend an entire day standing on the Plain of Arafat in prayers. On the third day, the pilgrims walk to the town of Mina for stoning of the pillars, a ritual that cleanses the evil. The last day of *Hajj*, people return to Mecca for a final circling of the *Ka'bah*. Some travel to the city of Medina as a pilgrimage to the Prophet's tomb. Needless to say, participation in the *Hajj* ritual has a very profound impact on each participant.

Eid el-Adha, or *Feast of the Sacrifice*, is a commemoration of Prophet Ibrahim's great sacrifice for God. Ibrahim's son was born near Mecca in Saudi Arabia. In order to test his faith, God ordered Ibrahim to make a fire and offer his son Ismail as a sacrifice. Ibrahim obeyed, and as he took his son to the altar for sacrifice, God intervened. God saved Ismail from his father's knife and made Ibrahim sacrifice a sheep intead. Ismail later helped his father build the *Ka'bah* or the house of worship in Mecca. As a reminder of Ibrahim's willingness to sacrifice his son in service to God, those Muslims who can afford to do so, sacrifice an animal during the Feast of Sacrifice. A third of the meat is given to the poor, another third to friends, and the remaining to themselves. During the *Eid el-Adha*, Saudi Arabia imports about six million live sheep for this occasion every year.

The *Festival of Jinadriyah* is an important occasion during which people have the opportunity to learn about their ancient heritage. The festival opens with a camel race and is followed by the traditional sword dance. Men dance in circles, carrying swords shoulder-to-shoulder while a poet is singing and the drummers use their musical talents. Other activities of the festival include folk music, concerts, craft workshops, and poetry reading.

Summary

The authors have provided an overview of Arab Americans in regard to patterns of immigration, demographics, and rehabilitation. Also, specific values and belief systems of the Arab culture, such as family structure, the impact of Islam as a religion, art, and vocational occupations, have been discussed throughout the chapter. In order to appreciate the rich histories of the diverse cultures of this region, information about a number of different countries in the region has been provided to the reader.

It is important for the rehabilitation practitioner to remember the following three points when working with an Arab American patient. First, the rehabilitation practitioner must become aware of his or her cultural perceptions about people of Arab Americans heritage. Second, it is important to validate the accuracy of these cultural perceptions with facts and to make necessary adjustments. Third, there is a considerable amount of diversity among Arab Americans, depending on age, gender, family background, religious orientation, and duration of stay in the United States. We believe that rehabilitation effectiveness will be achieved with cultural awareness, a positive attitude, and a genuine desire to help the Arab American patient.

Questions

1. Nidal is a patient who comes to the clinic with a severe laceration to his hand. Name three areas you would like to address in his initial interview.
2. Traditional Arabs follow what type of socio-temporal paradigm?
3. When you think about Arab Americans, what comes to mind (name your preconceived notions)?
4. Name three movies in which you have seen Arabs. How were they portrayed?
5. While working with an Arab American patient, name five cultural factors that you would consider as a rehabilitation practitioner.

References

Abraham, N., & Shryock, A. (2000). Arab Detroit: From margin to mainstream. Detroit: Wayne State University Press.

Al-Quaradawi, Y. (1980). *The lawful and prohibited in Islam*. Indianapolis. American Trust Publications.

Amir, A. and Ramey, D. (2000). Arab American Encyclopedia. Detroit: Arab Community Center for Economic and Social Services.

Arnold, Sir Thomas & Guillaume, Alfred (1931). The Legacy of Islam, Oxford at the Clarendon Press.

Barakat, H. (1993) the Arab world: Society, culture, and state/Halim Barakat. Berkeley and Los Angeles: University of California Press.

Barakat, H. (1994). *The Arab world: Society, culture and state*. Berkeley and Los Angeles: University of California Press.

Dupree, L. (1980). Afghanistan. Princeton, New Jersey. Princeton University Press.

El-Badry, S. (1993). *The Arab American market*. American Demographics. http://mgv.mim .edu.my/articles/002619601281.htm.

Friedman, T. (1989). From Beirut to Jerusalem. New York: Doubleday.

Hall, E. Gene, (1977) What context? Is in use? Research and Development Center for Teacher Education, University of Texas, Austin, Texas.

Harik, E. (1987). *The Lebanese in America*. Lerner Publications, Minneapolis, MN.

Hoogland, E. (1987). Crossing the waters: Arabic-speaking immigrants to the United States before 1940. Washington, DC: Smithsonian Institution Press.

Kurdahi-Zahir, L., Hattar-Pollara, M. (1998). Nursing care of Arab children: Consideration of cultural factors. *Journal of Pediatric Nursing: 13*, 6: 349–355.

Lerner Publications. (1989). *Kuwait in Pictures*. Minneapolis, MN.

Lerner Publications. (1990). *Iraq in Pictures*. Minneapolis, MN.

Levine, R. (1997). *A geography of time*. New York: Basic Books.

Lewis, Bernard. (1982). *The Muslim discovery of Europe*. New York: W. W. Norton & Company.

Malek, J., (1993). *Cradles of civilization: Egypt's ancient culture, modern land*. University of Norman, OK: Oklahoma Press.

Meleis, A. (1982). Arab students in western universities. *Journal of Higher Education: 53*, 439–447.

Moracco, J. (1983). Some correlates of the Arab character. *Psychology, A Quarterly Journal of Human Behavior: 20*, 3: 47–54.

Naff, A. (1980). Arabs. In S. Thernstrom, A. Orlov, & O. Handlin (Eds.), *The Harvard encyclopedia of American ethnic groups*. Cambridge, MA: Harvard University Press.

O'Shea, M. (1999). Festivals of the World. Milwaukee, WI: Gareth Stevens Publications.

Sadawi, Nawal (1983). Woman at point zero Zed Books, London, England.

Shaheen, J. (1984). *The TV Arab*. Bowling Green, OH: Bowling Green State University Press.

Shaheen, J. (2001). *Reel bad Arabs*. New York: Olive Branch Press.

Sheets, D., & El-Azhari, R. (1998). The Arab-American client: Implications for anesthesia. *Journal of the American Association of Nurse Anesthetists: 66*, 3: 304–312.

Thernstrom, S., Olov, A. & Handlin, O. (1980). *The Harvard encyclopedia of American ethnic groups*. Cambridge, MA: Harvard University Press.

Wesfield, G. (1990). Sociobiological patterns of Arab culture. *Ethology and Sociobiology, 11:* 23–49.

Young, R. (1987). Health status, health problems, and practices among refugees from the Middle East, Eastern Europe and Southeast Asia. *International Migration Review, 2193:* 760–782.

Zogby, J. (1991). *Arab Americans today: A demographic profile of Arab Americans*. Washington, DC: Arab American Institute.

10

Understanding Judaism and Jewish Americans

Marcy Coppelman Goldsmith

Key Words

Judaism	culture	rehabilitation
Jewish	religion	

Objectives

1. Describe how a rehabilitation professional might be able to assist with the religious needs that a Jewish client may have while in a rehabilitation setting.
2. Describe methods of incorporating dietary needs of the Jewish client into the rehabilitation plan.
3. Discuss communication barriers that a caregiver may encounter when giving care to a Jewish American client and his or her family.
4. Describe Jewish values, culture, and religious practices as they relate to rehabilitation.

Introduction

Judaism is as much a culture as a religion (Kolatch, 1985). Throughout history the community of Jewish people has been small and close-knit for both internal and external reasons. Religious principles and social values formed the internal ties, whereas the political environment shaped the external ones. Commonly, Jews were not given full rights as citizens and in turn not given full access to health care and other services. This difficulty resulted in the establishment of an infrastructure of businesses and health care services by and for the Jewish people regardless of the country of origin (Frommer & Frommer, 1995). Evidence of this arrangement is still visible in the presence of hospitals in a number of major cities around the United States, such as National Jewish Hospital in Denver, Colorado; Mount Sinai Hospital in New York City; and Beth Israel Hospital in Boston, Massachusetts. The United States was the first country to give Jewish people full rights as citizens (Karp, 1981). However, until the 1960s, Jewish doctors could practice medicine in only Jewish hospitals (Silbiger, 2000). This chapter is organized to describe the religion, customs, subdivisions within Judaism, and value systems. With that as a basis of understanding, the information pertaining to attitudes on health, health care, and medical ethics will be presented.

Arrival in the United States

Originally, all Jews came from the Middle East (Kolatch, 1985). Over time many Jews moved to Spain and Portugal. These Jews became known as *Sephardim. Sepharad* is the Hebrew word for Spain, and *-im* is the suffix used to make the word plural. Other Jews moved to Germanic countries, including France and other parts of Eastern Europe. This group was given the name *Ashkenazim*, the Hebrew word for Germany. Like Sephardim, this group of Jews became known for their new homeland. Through the centuries Jews have moved, but they continue to be classified by these two original roots. In 1492, Spain and Portugal expelled the Jewish people, so that many moved to North Africa (http://www.fordham.edu/halsall/jewish/1492-jews-spain1.html, retrieved 2/20/01). The first Jews to arrive in America came to New Amsterdam, later New York, in 1654 (Silbiger, 2000). They came from Brazil after the Dutch lost Brazil to the Portuguese. German Jews arrived in the early 1800s in larger numbers and spread out across the country, including the frontier. A later wave of immigration from Eastern Europe occurred in the 1880s. More recently, groups of Jewish people have immigrated to the United States from the Soviet Union. In America today, there are far more Ashkenazim than Sephardim. The overarching beliefs of the two groups, such as the belief in one God and in the Torah, are the same. However, the design of the temples and traditional foods differ.

Jewish Language and Communication

Jewish people primarily speak the language of the country in which they live. Thus, in the United States, the first language spoken is English; in Spain, the first language spoken is Spanish; and in Israel, the first language is Hebrew. The holy texts are written in Hebrew. Hebrew, unlike English, is a language written from the right side of a line to the left. Books are bound on the right side, so that they open from the American perspective of back-to-front. The letters are characters formed much differently than are English ones. Writing Hebrew words with English letters is called transliteration. Two Hebrew letters have sounds with no English equivalent. "Ch" is pronounced as if one is clearing one's throat, not as in the American equivalent of pronunciation as in "chair." "Tz" may sound like part of a plural English noun, such as "hats" or "cats," but this is a Hebrew letter that can appear in any position in a word. An example is *tzimmes* (pronounced as a two-syllable word tzim-mes), a sweet potato and carrot vegetable dish. In Hebrew, no cursive or printing style exists. Rather, there is a printed word format for books, newspapers, labels, and the like, as well as a handwritten version. It is the handwritten version that is called "printing." Children who attend religious school, called Hebrew School, learn to speak and write this language. Early elementary schoolchildren learn rote recognition of Hebrew words, and reading Hebrew is taught at approximately the third grade. Imagine the difficulties of a Jewish American dyslexic child trying to learn two languages, one that starts left-to-right and another that starts right-to-left. Having two sets of rules about reading adds confusion to an already difficult task. Also complicating the situation is the location of many of the Hebrew vowels. For the child who has spatial or perceptual difficulties, deciphering vowels that are placed in one of three positions can be quite confusing. Most Hebrew vowels are written below the consonant, and most are a series of lines or dots. As an example, think of the word *jar*. If this was written in Hebrew (and imagining the English letters were Hebrew letters), then starting right-to-left, the reader would see "rj" and the "a" would be placed under the "j."

Yiddush is an informal language blending German and other European languages with Hebrew. This folk language was used by the Jews of eastern and central Europe (Karp, 1981). The most famous written work encompassing the Yiddush language and the related culture is the story of *Fiddler on the Roof*. As in the story, the culture dissolved as the younger generation gave up the old ways and moved to America. Yiddush served to unite Jews first immigrating to the United States because they had common ground for a language. Common Yiddush expressions continue to be spoken today. Most notably "oy veh" is used as a term meaning "oh no." To be called a "mensch" is a compliment. It describes a person who has good character and humanity (Frommer & Frommer, 1995). Another informal language based on Spanish and Hebrew is called *Ladino* (Zimler, 1998), but it does not have commonly used expressions that have permeated English conversations.

Judaism and Its Sects

Common Elements

Within the religion of Judaism there are five sects including Orthodox, Conservative, Reform, Chassidism, and Reconstructionist. The common elements of the sects will be discussed first. All of these groups use the same holy texts, calendar, and holidays. The first important book is the *Torah*, which contains the instructions from God to the Jewish people (http://judaism.miningco.com/religion/judaism/library/intro/bl_intro_c.htm, retrieved 2/20/01). It contains the commandments describing how to live a Jewish life and stories about God's relationship to the Jewish people. Rather than being in book form, its form is a scroll handwritten in Hebrew and wrapped around two long wooden dowels. A special band holds the scroll together to keep it closed. Ornate cloth coverings protect the Torah, with metal filigree fittings decorating the tops of the dowels as well as a metal breastplate for the front. The Torah is stored in a special structure called an *ark* within the temple's sanctuary. The sanctuary is also the room where religious services take place. Each Jewish congregation has its own Torah, and some more established congregations have more than one. The two other important religious books are the *Haftorah* and the *Talmud*. Passages from the prophets are compiled in the Haftorah to complement portions of the Torah, whereas the Jewish laws are documented in the Talmud (Frommer & Frommer, 1995). The Talmud is divided into two parts. The Mishnah contains legal opinions and decisions, whereas the Gemorrah is the scholarly application of the law (Karp, 1981). A third book, called the *Shulchan Aruch*, contains practical application of the Halacha. This contains the Jewish health laws (Asheri, 1978).

Unlike the calendar of the United States, the Jewish calendar is based on a thirteen-month system reflecting the phases of the moon. Each month is 29 days and 12 hours long (Asheri, 1978). Since the days do not directly correspond to a twelve-month calendar, the Jewish holidays do not fall at the same time every year. For that reason, in some years Chanukah falls at the beginning of December, yet in others it could be after Christmas. Rehabilitation professionals who are not Jewish may find this irregularity a bit confusing, especially when scheduling staff work schedules and services for Jewish clients. Holidays always start at sunset. American calendars are not consistent in the notation used to describe the start of a Jewish holiday. "First day of Rosh Hashanah" means that the holiday begins at sunset the night before. American calendars may list only the name of the Jewish holiday, which most often translates to the notation of the holiday's first full day. Calendars printed by Jewish organizations are generally more specific when describing the start of a Jewish holiday.

Holidays

Jewish holidays vary in religious versus historical meaning as well as importance in daily life. Understanding the nature of the holiday and some of the related customs will help a rehabilitation professional develop or adapt treatment programs and home programs for his or her clients who practice Judaism.

The Sabbath starts on Friday night and extends until sunset on Saturday. In traditional families, this celebration is meant to honor the arrival of the Sabbath queen. It is a demarcation between the work done outside the home and a time to focus on both one's family and God. In the older view of the Sabbath, women are honored on Sabbath eve for their work and contribution to the home. Sabbath candles are lit, prayers are said over food and wine, and a loaf of braided sweet bread, called challah, is served. Some families attend a Sabbath service at the temple. In the Sabbath service, prayers are said, and each week a different portion of the Torah is read. Not all families continue the practice of observing the Sabbath. Some of the branches of Judaism follow additional traditions that would appear to be quite limiting to an outsider, such as the avoidance of driving or riding in a car. This aspect of Jewish life was made more public during the election campaign of 2000 when Senator Leiberman, a very religious Jew, ran as the Democratic Vice Presidential candidate (Higgins, 2000).

The most important major holidays in the Jewish year are Rosh Hashanah and Yom Kippor. These are the High Holidays, or High Holy Days, and take place in the early fall. People of Jewish faith will refrain from going to work or school during these important holidays. Rosh Hashanah is the start of the Jewish New Year. This is a two-day holiday, marking not only a new year but also the time in which the reading of the Torah starts at the beginning. Several different services take place at the synagogue, including ones in the evening, morning, and afternoon, but not all participants attend all services. At a family meal it is customary to serve challah, the braided sweet bread, and apples, each to be dipped in honey. This custom is meant to symbolize sweetness and good fortune in the New Year. Yom Kippor, the Day of Atonement, is a more solemn affair. It is the day to ask God for forgiveness for all one's sins from the past year. The religious services are quite beautiful, starting with the evening service of Kol Nidre. During the day of Yom Kippor, services take place all day. During the services, Jews reflect on their actions and ask God to be inscribed in the Book of Life. Being in the Book of Life is a request to live for yet one more year. A very poignant portion of Yom Kippor is the blowing of the *shofar*, or ram's horn. This is a very old tradition that was used to call the people of Israel to the temple of Jerusalem. Blowing of the shofar is no easy task; there is no reed or special fitting to help produce the sound. A prescribed set of calls is made. Included in the solemn acts of this day is one of fasting, which is to help the individual focus on God and repentance. A dinner is prepared and eaten prior to sundown of Yom Kippor. Enough food must be prepared such that sufficient leftovers need to be available for the breaking of the fast. No cooking or other typical daily work is to be done on Yom Kippor.

Rehabilitation professionals can include activities relevant to Rosh Hashanah and Yom Kippor. A speech and language pathologist could help a client be able to pronounce the Hebrew words of a short prayer. Sitting down and standing up from a low seat or a folding chair could become part of a physical therapists treatment because in parts of the religious service one must stand up. An occupational therapist may incorporate home management and meal preparation tasks that would be part of one of the holiday meals.

The Festival of Lights, or Chanukah, commemorates the occurrence of a miracle. This holiday coincides roughly with the Christian holiday of Christmas, although its meaning and significance are quite different. Chanukah celebrates the time in which the Jewish people reclaimed their synagogue in Jerusalem from the Roman people. The Romans had taken it over in 70 C.E. (Halsall, 2001) and placed symbols of their own religion inside the temple. A band of fighters, under the leadership of the family known as the Macabees, successfully fought the Romans. Upon reentering the temple, an important symbol of faith, the everlasting light, needed to be restored. This light, to signify the Jewish people's belief in God, needs to be lit at all times. The Macabees searched for oil to burn within the light but could find only enough to last one day. Acquiring more required a trip lasting eight days. By a miracle, the supply on hand lasted for the eight days needed to obtain more oil supplies. Hence, each year Jews celebrate this miracle, signifying the restoration of the temple and the lasting of a small supply of oil by lighting candles. A candelabra, called a *menorah*, is used, and it holds nine candles: one candle for each of the eight days and one candle used for lighting the others. At first, just one candle and the shamas (the lighter candle) are lit. Each night successively one more candle is lit until the end of the holiday. Traditions at Chanukah include eating potato pancakes (latkes) and playing with a top called a *dreidel*. Children are given small gifts, often one per night. If money is given, it is called *gelt*.

Application of these holiday rituals could be made in several ways. This is an important acknowledgment of Jewish customs at a time of year when the American culture places a very strong emphasis on Christmas. For example, when working with a special needs child, the therapist could recommend gift ideas of toys that improve sensory processing or motor skills. In classrooms where speech and language and occupational therapists provide services and multicultural holiday celebrations are part of the school culture, making latkes and playing with dreidels can be used for therapeutic activities. Latkes are simple to make; therefore, using the tasks for measuring, mixing, and sequencing could be beneficial for adults who have had a head injury. Additionally, using the lighting of a menorah with adults who need to practice upper extremity use because of a stroke or tremor may be a valuable therapeutic activity.

Passover is a holiday signifying the release of the Jewish slaves in Egypt by Pharaoh. It is a story that many are familiar with. To shed light on present-day Jewish customs, a brief account follows. According to history, Moses had gone to Pharaoh repeatedly to request freedom for the Jewish slaves (Passover Haggadah, 1995). Each time Pharaoh refused, and a plague sent by God resulted. For the last plague the firstborn male of each family was to be killed. To save the firstborn Jewish males, the blood of a ram was smeared on the doorpost. The plague killed Pharaoh's son, and in his grief Pharaoh allowed the Jews to leave immediately. They had no time to prepare, so in their haste they took flattened loaves of bread dough on their backs to cook in the sun. Pharaoh soon regretted his decision, and he had Egyptians chase after the Jews shortly after their departure. The Jews came upon the Red Sea. It would be difficult to cross, and the Egyptians were gaining ground. The Red Sea parted, and the Jews made it across, but the Egyptians were not so fortunate. The present-day celebration occurs over many days, is centered on activities within the home, and falls close in time to the Christian holiday of Easter. The importance of Passover is the time spent remembering how as a people, the Jews were once slaves but now live in freedom. For this purpose it is a joyous recounting of the story of Exodus from one generation to the next in the form of a *Seder*. The Seder consists of a religious service and a meal. Significant preparation is required for the Seder. All leavened bread in the house is removed. Symbols of the slaves' experiences are prepared and placed on the Seder plate. These include such items as bitter herbs as a reminder of the bitterness in the slaves' lives and a roasted lamb shank bone as a symbol of the final plague. Sweet kosher wine is used for many toasts and is liberally consumed. Children participate in these toasts and are allowed to drink the wine. Typical foods served at the meal include chicken soup with matzoh balls, gefilte fish, roast chicken or brisket, and tzimmes.

Seders are held the first two nights of Passover. The family continues the observance by eating matzoh and refraining from consuming leavened bread for a week. Furthermore, since many commercial food products contain yeast, some families replaced many foods with ones marked "Kosher for Passover." This process of preparing for Passover can serve as the rationale to do a spring cleaning. A traditional custom is to have separate utensils (plates, silverware, glasses, etc.) for use only during Passover, though only the most observant Jews may still do this. The final day of Passover is celebrated in some families. For this observance, these individuals refrain from usual daily routines such as work and school.

Incorporating Passover into therapy is possible by adapting foods used in any feeding or meal preparation activities. Also, bending, reaching, and cleaning could be incorporated into therapy programs by occupational and physical therapists. Usually participants at a Seder read passages of the religious service aloud, with some sections in Hebrew and others in English. Speech and language pathologists can use this material for therapeutic purposes.

Life-Cycle Events

There are other customs that are specific to Jewish culture, which center on how to live one's life and on rituals to mark life-cycle events. Not every Jew practices all of the rituals; however, most Jews are familiar with them. For this chapter, the rituals of Kashruth (dietary laws), circumcision, Bar/Bat Mitzvah, and death will be discussed. Kashruth, also called Kosher, limits the food that Jewish people eat (Asheri, 1978). The forbidden foods include those animals that are scavengers and are unclean. Fish must have scales. Examples of forbidden foods include shellfish and pork. Since the dietary laws were created in a time when food preservation methods were primitive, these laws served to protect one's health. Specific rules dictated how an animal was to be slaughtered and the blood drained prior to human consumption. The slaughtering was merciful for the animal, and the draining of blood was followed by salting of the flesh to prevent bacterial growth. According to the Kashruth, all foods are separated into categories of dairy or meat. Also, one is not to mix consumption of the parent animal with its milk. The outcome of this practice means that a Jewish person may not have a glass of milk with a meat entrée. In fact, if one consumes meat, then he or she is supposed to wait six hours before having milk. This is the time it would take to digest one item before consuming another. Even separate utensils are used for the two groups. As the names imply, dairy foods include cheese and milk. A "dairy" meal consists of foods such as blintzes (crepes with cheese or fruit stuffing), bagels, cream cheese, noodle pudding, and fruit. It is interesting that fish is not considered fish, so that smoked fish, such as lox (smoked salmon) and whitefish may be included as dairy foods. A "meat" meal, as one might expect, consists of beef or chicken. Foods that can be consumed with either milk or meat meals are called "parve." Many food packages, including cereal, canned vegetables, and dry pasta in grocery stores today are marked with a circle surrounding a white "U." The symbol Ⓤ is the insignia for Orthodox Union, the agency that certifies the Kosher status of commercial foods.

Individuals who follow the dietary laws and are in need of rehabilitation benefit from sensitivity by the professional when foods will be part of treatment. This may become an issue, with children receiving sensory integration-based therapy or adults receiving treatment incorporating meal preparation or feeding therapy.

Another manifestation of the personal health goal in Judaism is the custom of circumcision. It is both a ritual and a life-cycle event. Circumcision is not perceived as a medical procedure; rather, it is an important method for a man to maintain personal hygiene. In this custom a ceremony, with friends and family present, is held in the home when the baby is eight days old. The person performing the circumcision is called a *moile* (pronounced so that it rhymes with *toil*). Gauze soaked in wine is put in the baby's mouth to decrease the pain and discomfort. The procedure takes place in a matter of seconds.

Notice that this is the second instance mentioned in which children are given wine. At Passover, wine is for celebration, whereas in this situation it is medicinal, but the value is important to recognize. Alcohol is not a forbidden substance for children. It is provided in moderation at specific times. Thus, when children of Jewish descent become teenagers, consuming alcohol is not a foreign activity.

Many religions have an important ceremony to acknowledge a child's religious education and to mark his or her place within the religion. In Judaism, this life-cycle event is called a Bar-Mitzvah or a Bat Mitzvah. Historically, only boys were offered this opportunity, for which it was called a Bar Mitzvah. At a Sabbath coinciding with youngster's thirteenth birthday, the boy was called to read from the Torah on the Sabbath in the presence of his family, friends, and the congregation. This time in the child's life was to signify moving from childhood to adulthood. In the last forty years, American Jews included their daughters in this ceremonious event. Originally, this was called a Bat Mitzvah, though the sectors of Judaism now using gender-neutral language use only the term Bar Mitzvah. Another modern adaptation is the varying of age of the daughter's Bar Mitzvah between the ages of 12 and 13. Maturation between males and females differs, and Jewish custom is making allowances for this difference. Regardless of sex or specific age, the youngster must learn to recite a portion of the Torah and will stand up to read it directly from the handwritten scroll. If the ceremony takes place on Saturday, as opposed to Friday night, then the weekly Haftorah portion must be recited. Recall that the Haftorah is the words of the prophets, and this is chanted instead of read. No matter whether this ceremony takes place on Friday night or Saturday, it is a very proud moment for the whole family. A large party is held, which can be as simple as a brunch or as fancy as a black tie dinner dance. The Bar or Bat Mitzvah is an important rite of passage. Though the child is now seen as an adult in the Jewish community, there is no such correspondence with adulthood in American society.

Incorporating facets of the Bar or Bat Mitzvah into therapeutic activities could take many forms. Learning the Hebrew text, projecting one's voice, being able to sit still in front of an audience, and preparing a thank-you speech are all required by the adolescent who may be receiving rehabilitation. Alternately, a therapist may be working with a sibling of the Bar or Bat Mitzvah child who needs to be able to contain himself or herself on the sideline. An older relative of the Bar or Bat mitzvah child (mother, father, grandmother, grandfather, etc.) could be receiving therapy services at this important family time. Event planning and organizing could be part of a therapy regime, or something more physical such as standing for periods of time or walking longer distances.

The final life-cycle event to be discussed is that of death. Understanding these customs may help a rehabilitation professional who wishes to attend a funeral of a Jewish person. The ceremonies and rituals around the death of a Jew are quite different from those of other religious groups. In addition to the timing of events, there is a prescribed set of events and activities to help those who mourn the loss of a loved one. People of Jewish descent must be buried within 24 hours of dying. The exception occurs if a death occurs on Friday afternoon. The funeral cannot be held during the Sabbath, hence it would be postponed until Sunday. The funeral may take place either in a synagogue or a funeral home. No viewing of the body is done before, during, or after the service. In a traditional funeral, the dead person is buried not in his or her clothes, but in a plain piece of cloth called a shroud. The body is not left alone out of respect, so that a person from a special religious group called *shomerim* is hired to sit nearby and pray until the funeral (Rich, 2001). The service itself is similar in kind to the service in other religions. All persons familiar with the deceased individual are welcome to attend the funeral. An obvious difference in the funeral service is that some prayers are recited in Hebrew. One special prayer, called the Kaddish, is the prayer for the dead. The immediate family and any other participant who lost a family member in the previous thirty days stands for this prayer. After the service, the family and very close friends accompany the dead person to the cemetery, where another brief service is held. Tradition holds that Jews must bury their own dead. To accomplish this nowadays, after the casket is placed in the ground, immediate family members each take a shovelfull of dirt to put it in the grave. Often, other close family and friends will do the same, but not all attendees participate. The bulk of the dirt will be replaced after the family leaves. The family returns to either the home of the deceased or to that of a designated family member. A bowl of water is left outside the house for people to rinse off their hands on the return from the cemetery. Food is served and often consists of a dairy meal, with bagels, cream cheese, lox, whitefish, and fruit. A *Shiva* may begin either immediately or the following day. Shiva is Hebrew for seven, the number of days that the immediate family take visitors and receive condolences (Rich, 2001). This may be shortened to three days. Other customs still prevail. People drop in to express their condolences and have an opportunity to visit. The door is always left unlocked so that the doorbell never needs to be rung and visitors just let themselves in. The immediate family members are not to be thinking of themselves or in a position to have to do anything but mourn. In olden days, the family tore their clothes to demonstrate their grief. Mirrors in the house were covered. Nowadays the immediate family members wear a black fabric button with a torn piece of cloth attached. Mirrors may or may not be covered, though the immediate family will not look in one. Immediate family members are not supposed to cook for themselves. People who bring food and dishes into the home may not leave until the shiva is over. Each evening at dusk, a short service is held in which the Kaddish is recited. For this service there must be a minion that consists of at least ten people who have attained a Bar or Bat Mitzvah. Non-Jewish visitors do not participate in this service. After the Shiva is over, the mourners are supposed to begin to resume their usual routines. The structure for the immediate family continues for the next year. Every day for the first thirty days the family is to say Kaddish. After the shiva is over, immediate family members attend morning or evening services at a temple to say Kaddish. After the first month, it is prescribed to recite the Kaddish once per week. Again, this needs to be done in the presence of a minion and not done in isolation. Near the end of the first year, the headstone is placed on the grave. At this final point, a small family ceremony is held.

In summary, the major holidays of the Sabbath, Rosh Hashanah, Yom Kippor, Chanukah, and Passover have been described along with life-cycle events of circumcision, Bar and Bat Mitzvah, and death. These are customs that apply to all Jewish people. However, within the religion of Judaism, different sects exist that create variations in how some of the rituals are carried out.

Sects of Judaism

Orthodox Judaism is the sect that keeps most closely to the original interpretations of the Holy Books. People who consider themselves Orthodox continue to follow traditional lifestyles dictated by the laws of Judaism, including keeping kosher and not driving or working on the Sabbath. There are strong beliefs about gender-based behavior and roles. The men are given more education and can be on the first floor of the synagogue for services. Women wear wigs, keep their bodies covered, and must sit in the balcony for services. At weddings men and women do not dance with one another. The religious services are in Hebrew. Orthodox families usually live close to one another to support the lifestyle (Spero, 1978). Businesses that need to be close by include a kosher bakery and a butcher, whereas the social institutions are a school and a synagogue. As devout as this group is, an Orthodox family may visually blend into the environment, the only visible difference being the man's *yarmalkah* (small round cap) and the woman's wig and long clothing.

A subgroup of Orthodox Judaism is called *Hassidim*. This group is the least assimilated into American society and the rest of the American Jewish community (Spero, 1978). They keep a minimal economic relationship with the outside world. As a group, it is the Hassidic Jews who are very involved in the diamond business. The style of dress is quite different from that of mainstream America. The men wear tall black hats, black suits with white shirts, and grow long beards with long curled sideburns.

The *Reform* movement is at the other end of the spectrum in comparison with Orthodox Judaism. This movement has tried to assimilate the most with the society around it. Started in the early 1800s in Germany, it later spread to the United States. Reform services are a liberal mix of Hebrew and English. Services are led by the Rabbi (Martin, 1978) with many of the congregants making contributions and leading prayers. One emphasis of this sect is to use gender-neutral language when possible. Some congregations use a revised prayer book in which the traditional prayers have removed the pronouns "he" and "she." The education of both sexes is equal. Women can become rabbis. Reform rabbis can perform marriage ceremonies between Jews and non-Jews. Only Reform rabbis consider performing same-sex marriage ceremonies. The Reform movement strives to find ways to live as Jews within the current mainstream of society, including both lifestyle and scientific knowledge. Few Reform Jews keep a Kosher home.

In the middle is the *Conservative* sect. As the name suggests, this branch of Judaism is looking for a more traditional ground than Reform. More Hebrew is spoken in Conservative services, and there is a particular focus on the individual's method of praying to oneself, called "dovening." This group strives for more religious expression and "Jewish experience" than the Reform movement without being as confining as the Orthodox (Martin 1978). Men and women sit together in the temple, and women can become rabbis. In the early roots of Conservative Judaism, the evolution and adaptation of the religion to a society was acknowledged. Additionally, the role of the Jewish people was felt to be central to Judaism. Within this religious group, changes were intended to reflect the collective will (Martin, 1978). Hence, no one doctrine served all Conservative temples; rather, each Conservative congregation could decide on its own structure. Notice that one central leader or small circle of leaders does not dictate to the group; rather, the group influences its own direction under guidance by religious leaders. *Reconstructionism* started as an offshoot from Conservative Judaism. Created by one Jewish leader, it places its emphasis on Judaism as a civilization that includes religion with a unique history, literature, art, language, social organization, and norms of conduct (Martin 1978). Reconstructionist congregations build their Jewish community on the basis of the values of the members. It is a strong reflection of the current society blended with Jewish practices. Of all the different sects, there is probably more variability among Reconstructionist congregations than in any other group.

Given the variability among the sects of Judaism, there are many different ways a rehabilitation program can be devised to be sensitive to and inclusive of religious practices. With Orthodox Jewish life, two practices may be less visible, yet could play a role in therapeutic activities. The first, *tzitzit*, are thread fringes that are worn next to the skin and serve as a reminder of one's prayers (Higgins, 2000). A therapist working with a client to improve his or her independent dressing skills may include this as part of the article of clothing needing to be mastered. Second, on the Sabbath, Orthodox Jews refrain from working, driving, cooking, and the like. Thus, it may be important to ask rather than expect this individual to perform a home program on the Sabbath. Individuals who are members of the other sects may have fewer practices affecting daily life; however, respect for the holiday celebrations and any one particular family's religious expression is important.

Family Structure and Issues of Aging

In the culture, historically, men were given higher status as observed in the separation of sexes in Orthodox synagogues. More recently, women's roles have gained status by the addition of the Bat Mitzvah and inclusion of women in the role of rabbi. In Reform congregations, in general, there has been a move toward more equalitarian roles and gender neutral language. There is no specific gender bias that a rehabilitation professional would encounter when working with a Jewish family.

Within a family, Jewish child-rearing practices emphasize the importance of education and of the drive to succeed. To achieve this, the parents and culture set high standards for academic success, as well as to expose the children to many experiences and allow the opportunity for success and failure (Blau as cited in Silbiger, 2000). Not promoted are strict discipline and adherence of rules out of fear. Instead, a model of parental self-sacrifice and of provision to the child of the highest quality services and material goods is used to foster development. Freedom of expression and nurturing a strong ego and self-esteem are valued, ultimately yielding a parental style of permissiveness with protectiveness (Silbiger, 2000). Combining this parental style with the cultural factor of belief in self-determination for shaping one's destiny yields a family that will pursue avenues to foster the child's development

(Lipset & Raab, 1995). A rehabilitation professional working with a Jewish family may notice a push on the part of parents to obtain services for a special needs child and to express interest and worry in a very verbal way about the qualifications of the service provider.

No specific value is held about the aging process in the Jewish culture. By default, the emphasis of parents on their children's success results in families that can be geographically separated. Thus, this trend has fostered concentrations of older Jewish American communities in New York and Florida (Silbiger, 2000). Jewish family service agencies are affiliated with Jewish community centers in some parts of the country. These agencies offer services to help with the health issues related to aging as well as services to younger individuals. These can include social services, exercise programs, kosher lunch programs for seniors, and occasionally a kosher meals-on-wheels program.

Health Beliefs and Practices

The challenge of writing about Jewish health beliefs comes from the lack of explicit teaching of the topic within the culture. Within the religion, health is not considered a product of being a pious Jew, nor is it a result of a sin. Implicitly, or indirectly, Jewish individuals learn about how to be healthy through participation in life-cycle events such as a circumcision or by adherence to the kosher dietary laws. These types of preventative measures were introduced as early as the twelfth century. However, no single dogma exists for Jewish healing (Freeman & Abrams, 1999). The Jewish beliefs pertaining to health place a strong value on a person's life. Therefore, the goals of medical intervention need to be based on preserving a person's life, relieving his or her suffering, and offering any available treatment. Likewise, the person who is experiencing an illness is responsible for seeking medical care (Lavine, 2001, http://members.aol.com/Sauromalus/index.html, retrieved 7/29/04). Prevention of illness continues to be very important (Lavine, 2001, http://members.aol.com/Sauromalus/index.html, retrieved 7/29/04). The Halacha, or Jewish health laws, applies mostly to larger issues of life and death, of the physician-patient role, and the support of the community of ill individuals. Few of these laws have application to rehabilitation. However, a brief overview follows. The nature of Judaism to adapt to the environment means that rabbis and physicians look to examine the application of very old religious texts to current medical practices. Discussion and debates of these issues are not easily found in books and texts, but the most up-to-date information is obtainable via the Internet.

In relation to life and death issues, such procedures as abortion and organ donation are pertinent. Abortion is permitted when the mother's health is at risk (Kolatch, 1985). The organ donation debate within the Jewish community centers on the definition of death. According to Jewish law, death occurs when breathing ceases (Kolatch, 1985); thus, the medical definition of brain death does not meet the Jewish criteria.

The physician-patient role is extremely important. Physicians should not be constrained in their decision-making process regarding the most appropriate care for the patient (Lavine, 2001, http://members.aol.com/Sauromalus/index.html, retrieved 7/29/04). Thus, managed care policies are in conflict with Jewish medical ethics. Also, physicians should not take advantage of their patients by selling products or medication at a significant profit, but physicians may sell these items at reasonable prices (Lavine, 2001, http://members.aol.com/Sauromalus/index.html, retrieved 7/29/04).

Health care services are not limited to only those services that a physician provides. Other health care professionals are recognized and valued for providing optimal care for persons who are ill. Also, health care services may include alternative therapies if there is some evidence of efficacy and safety and if the alternative therapies are not used instead of a proven therapy (Lavine, 2001, http://members.aol.com/Sauromalus/index.html, retrieved 7/29/04).

Jewish laws describe visiting a person who is ill as a good deed, or "mitzvah," (Freeman & Abrams, 1999). The community at large is supposed to support its group members by going to see those who are sick. This is a circumstance in which the lifestyle of Jews is influenced but is not given a strict mandate about a meaning of becoming ill.

Health Risk Factors

Typical health risk factors for Jewish individuals are generally no different from those of the general population, at least in relation to possible rehabilitation. Genetic disorders occurring more frequently in Ashkenazi Jews include breast and ovarian cancer, Canavan disease, and Tay-Sachs disease (http://judaism.about.com/cs/health/index.htm, 7/27/01). Breast and ovarian cancers have been linked with the BRCA1 (breast cancer 1) and BRCA2 genes with three specific mutations being found in Ashkenazi Jews (Fergus and Simonsen, 2000). Canavan Disease (CD) and Tay-Sachs are rare and fatal genetic disorders affecting infants born to Ashkenazi Jews. Both diseases cause infants who appear normal at birth to lose functional abilities. CD appears between 3 and 9 months, whereas Tay-Sachs appears about 6 months. CD is a degenerative neurological disorder in which myelin is destroyed. The children with CD may live until 10 years of age (http://judaism.about.com/gi/dynamic/offsite.htm?site=http%3A%2F%2Fwww.canavanfoundation.org, retrieved 7/27/01). Tay-Sachs results from the absence of the enzyme hexosaminidase A. This enzyme is responsible for the breakdown of a fatty waste substance in the brain (http://judaism.about.com/gi/dynamic/offsite.htm?site=http%3A%2F%2Fwww.tay-sachs.org%2Fwhatista.htm, retrieved 7/27/01). Genetic testing is used to help in the prevention of the occurrence of these diseases.

Summary

Judaism is both a religion and a culture. By its nature, Jewish people can adapt to the environment in which they live, and the Jewish laws can be modified. Using holy books and its people's history, religious leaders take the Jewish teachings and interpret their application to the current issues and needs of the people. The balance of old traditions with modern ones varies with the sect within Judaism. Holidays and life-cycle events are important aspects of all the sects (Orthodox, Conservative, Reform, Hassidic, and Reconstructionist) and are different from the majority culture in the United States. Awareness of the differences will help a rehabilitation professional in understanding his or her Jewish colleagues and Jewish clients. Incorporating aspects of holiday and life-cycle practices into a rehabilitation program can serve to strengthen and generalize the goals of therapy into a client's life. One cannot assume that all Jewish people carry out the practices in the same way. A rehabilitation professional can start by asking a client, "How does your family celebrate _____ ?" (Hanukah, Passover, etc.). This question can open the discussion and provide information to help tailor a treatment program to the physical, spiritual, and cultural needs of a Jewish person. Also, simply showing awareness of when holidays fall, so that treatment will not conflict with Jewish religious practices, can strengthen the respect and working relationship between therapist and client.

Questions

1. How does your own culture differ from that of Judaism? How is it similar to Judaism?
2. Identify the two major ethnic groups within Judaism, and describe the origins of these two groups.
3. Identify and describe the five major sects within the Jewish culture.
4. Describe Hebrew, Yiddish, Torah, Haftorah, and Talmud.
5. Name some stereotypes about Judaism and Jewish people. What have you learned from this chapter that helps to better understand Jewish beliefs and practices?
6. If you, the reader, are Christian and celebrate Christmas, take a moment to think about life without the Christmas celebration. Next, imagine what it would be like to live in a culture in which a holiday you don't participate in (Christmas) permeates almost all aspects of life outside one's home.
7. Describe the following Jewish holidays: Sabbath, Rosh Hashanah, Yom Kippor, Chanukah, and Passover. As a rehabilitation professional, why should you understand these holidays?
8. Describe some cultural-specific activities that a rehabilitation professional might incorporate during therapy with Jewish clients.
9. Describe the structure of family life and some rituals and ceremonies discussed in this chapter.
10. What is the basis for the values of health and health care? How are these values taught to Jewish individuals?

Case Study

You are a therapist working with stroke patients, and one of your clients, Mrs. T, is Jewish. Mrs. T. is particularly concerned about making certain that her kosher diet is maintained while she is undergoing rehabilitation, and she is also expressing great anxiety over every aspect of her treatment by constant questioning. She is also expressing open distrust of many of her caregivers. Describe some of the methods you might use to allay her anxiety so that she is able to fully participate in her rehabilitation program.

References

Asheri, M. (1978). *Living Jewish.* New York: Everest House.

Bleich, D. J. (1998). *Bioethical dilemmas: A Jewish perspective.* Hoboken, NJ: KTAV Publishing House, Inc.

Dorff, E. N., & Newman, L. E. (1995). *Contemporary Jewish ethics and morality: A reader.* New York: Oxford University Press.

Fergus, K. and Simonsen, J. (2000). *Breast and Ovarian Cancer in the Ashkenazi Jewish Population.* http://judaism.about.com/. Retrieved January 25, 2005.

Freeman, D., & Abrams, J. (1999). *Illness and health in the Jewish tradition: Writings from the Bible to today.* Philadelphia, PA: Jewish Publication Society.

Frommer, M. & Frommer, H. (Eds.). (1995). *Growing up Jewish in America: An oral history.* Lincoln, NB: University of Nebraska Press.

Halsall, P. (n.d.). *Jewish history sourcebook: The expulsion from Spain, 1492* CE http://www.fordham.edu/halsall/jewish/1492-jews-spain1.html. Retrieved February 20, 2001.

Higgins, R. (2000, August 19). *Living their faith modern Orthodox Jews are blending best of both worlds. Boston Globe.* p. B1.

Karp, A. J. (1981). *Jewish way of life and thought.* New York: KTAV Publishing.

Kolatch, A. (1985). *The second Jewish book of why.* Middle Village, NY: Jonathan David Publisher.

Lavine, J. (2001). *The thirteen principles of Jewish medical ethics of Harofei Yaakov Ben Ben-Tzion Halevi.* http://members.aol.com/Sauromalus/index.html, retrieved July 29, 2004.

Lipsett, S., & Raab, E. (1995). *Jews and the new American scene.* Cambridge, MA: Harvard University Press.

Martin, B. (Ed.). (1978). *Movements and issues in American Judaism.* Westport, CT: Greenwood Press.

Oetter, P., Richter, E., & Frick, S. (1995). *M.O.R.E. Integrating the mouth with sensory and postural functions* (2nd ed.). Hugo, MN: PDP Press.

Passover Haggadah, deluxe edition. (1995). Produced by Maxwell House Coffee and Kraft General Foods. Northfield, IL.

Rich, T. (2001). *Judasim 101.* http://www.jewfaq.org/death.htm, retrieved February 19, 2001.

Silbiger, S. (2000). *The Jewish phenomenon.* Marietta, GA: Longstreet Press.

Spero, X. (1978). Orthodox Judaism. In B. Martin (Ed.), *Movements and issues in American Judaism* (pp. 25–78). Westport, CT: Greenwood Press.

Zimmler, R. (1998). *The last kabbalist of Lisbon.* Woodstock, NY: Overlook Press.

11

The Smorgasbord of the Hispanic Cultures

Toni Thompson and Eduardo Blasquez

Key Words

Hispanic   Chicanos   Cubanos
Hispanos

Objectives

1. Describe the diverse Hispanic cultural groups and their immigration patterns to the United States.
2. Describe the population distribution and demographic changes of these groups in the United States.
3. Describe patterns of communication among these populations.
4. Describe Hispanic traditional health beliefs and practices.
5. Provide specific recommendations on intervention techniques and strategies while working with clients of Hispanic backgrounds.

Introduction

People of Hispanic descent encompass persons living in or descended from the majority of countries in the Western Hemisphere. Distinct immigration trends span centuries and continue today, fueled by economic and political conditions. The Hispanic people encompass a variety of personal, national, regional, acculturation, and socio-economic differences that contribute to a true complexity of cultures. As the United States remains the melting pot for immigrants from all over the world, the Hispanic cultures exemplify a true smorgasbord of values and beliefs about family, health, pain, illness, communication, and spirituality.

Use of the Term "Hispanic"

People of Hispanic origin or descent generally do not like to be referred to as Hispanic. Comedian Paul Rodriguez chided, "I don't want to be called anything with 'PANIC' in it." The word *Hispanic* was developed by the U.S. government in the late 1970s (Castex, 1994, pp. 289, 293). This term refers to all people from Latin America, including people who do not have ties to Spain. "It reminds many persons so ascribed of the colonial exploitation of the Spanish state," reports Castex. In addition, the use of the term may be seen as the same type of imposition by the U.S. government. Many people prefer to be perceived as an individual rather than as a term used by the government, such as Caucasian, Asian American, mixed race. For purposes of continuity and for lack of a more appropriate term, Hispanic is considered standard terminology and will be used in this work (U.S. Bureau of the Census, 2001a, p. 1).

Most people tend to be proud of their national origin and exclaim, "I'm Cuban" or "I'm Mexican-American," or "My parents are from Argentina," just as non-Hispanics who talk about their roots say that they are "Italian-American," "Irish American," or "first-generation Japanese." Many people in the United States tend to identify with their favorite college or professional sports team with the same fervor that Hispanics use to identify with their country. Various Hispanic groups have immigrated into the United States at different times into a variety of regions, creating diverse Hispanic-American populations.

Immigration Patterns

Hispanos

Hispanos, Chicanos, Puerto Riqueños, and Cubanos represent immigrations that have become established in the United States. More recently, immigrants from over fifteen of the Central and South American countries seek a new home in the United States.

"Hispanos" are the original Hispanic settlers in the United States. Cortes, under the flag of Spain, conquered the Aztecs in 1521. Then the Spanish settlers moved northward into what are currently the states of New Mexico, Colorado, and California throughout the end of the sixteenth century. Roman Catholics from Spain established the city of Santa Fe

("Holy Faith"), New Mexico, in 1609 and came to be known as "Hispanos." The Pueblo Indians drove out the settlers around 1680, but the settlers returned thirteen years later. The settlers consisted of two distinct social classes. The lower socioeconomic group consisted of Spanish peasants, native Americans, "Mestizos" (mixture of Spaniards and native Americans), and "Genizaros" (mixture of various native American groups, sometimes with Spanish blood). Religious and aristocratic leaders of Spanish blood comprised the upper socioeconomic group.

After the formation of the United States of Mexico (EE.UU. México) in 1821, migration into this area of the United States continued steadily. A large migration of Anglos into the area in 1848 reinforced the use of the term "Hispano" for the people of Spanish descent.

Chicanos

"Chicanos" refer to a second northward wave of immigration of people of Spanish Roman Catholic background. The word *Chicano* comes from the Mexican Indian Nahuatl word *Mechicano*. After the 1810 Revolution, the Metizos drove many Spaniards from Mexico northward into Texas, Arkansas, California, Florida, and, to a lesser degree, Colorado, New Mexico, and Illinois. Many feel that strong influences on the movement include the presidency of Benito Juarez, a strong advocate for the Mexican lower class, as well as the California Gold Rush in the 1850s.

Until the passage of the NAFTA (North American Free Trade Act) during the Clinton Administration, an undisclosed number of Mexicans illegally crossed the border to work as migrant workers and as unskilled workers throughout the United States. Zuniga (1998, p. 211) states that Mexicans in this group comprise half of the estimated 3.5 to 4 million undocumented persons in the United States. This group continues to be the focus of ongoing debates and legislation on immigration status and on access to medical care and education even as the period of clemency for such immigrants has now been closed in spring 2001 (Spector, 1996).

Puerto Riqueños

"Puerto Riqueños" represent another major influx of Hispanics into the United States. The Arawak Indians occupied Puerto Rico, *La Isla del Encanto* ("The Island of Enchantment") up to 1493. The Spaniards then took over and by 1599 established a strong population base of 1,000 people. Puerto Rico then became a territory of the United States as a result of the Spanish-American War in 1898. Since the establishment of Puerto Rico as a commonwealth in 1952, debates continue over statehood.

After World War II, many Puerto Ricans immigrated to New York, the eastern seaboard states, and, to a lesser degree, the Chicago area. Often, migration is a one-way street with people bringing customs into a new area but with little influence of the new location on the old homeland. The unique role of Puerto Rico as a commonwealth and the postwar industrial boom may have been factors that contributed to bringing many U.S. mainland influences to the island. Currently, Puerto Ricans remain free to live in and travel to the United States with no notable strong immigration trends (Zuniga, 1998, p. 212).

In 1992, Puerto Rican families showed the lowest median family annual income in the United States at $20,000. Mexican families showed median family income of $24,000, and Cuban families showed median family income of $30,000. The highest poverty rates occurred in Puerto Rican families at 32.5% (Castex, 1994, p. 289).

Cubanos

"Cubanos" have immigrated into the United States in several steps and show the highest level of fervor over wanting to defeat the communist rule of Fidel Castro. In 1869, the Cuban Vicente Martinez Ybor migrated to Key West, Florida, to develop his cigar business. During that time, a small stream of Cubans also migrated for other purposes. Ybor took his workers north to Tampa, Florida, in 1886, where he established the area of "Free Havana." Ybor's domination of the cigar manufacturing industry continued to prosper until World War I, when cigarettes became more popular and machines replaced many workers. Another wave of Cubans came to Florida following the depression in the 1930s. A large influx of Cubans fled Fidel Castro's regime in the 1950s.

Currently, immigration to the United States is prohibited by the Cuban government, although a small number attempt to flee Cuba on makeshift floats. Many Cubans and Cuban Americans advocate the return of a free Cuba.

In the early 1980s, many Cubans came to Florida in the Mariel boatlifts, also known as the "Freedom Flotilla." Cuban psychiatrists in Melbourne, Florida, tell of their struggles to come to the United States in the 1950s to flee Castro's regime, leaving behind their homes and comfortable lifestyles. One doctor talked of waiting on tables while he learned English so that he could take the medical boards. As a waiter, he supported his wife and four children, who were accustomed to the upper-class lifestyle in Cuba. When the immigrants began to come from Cuba in the 1980s in the Mariel boatlift, the physicians wanted to offer a helping hand to their fellow Cubans. The doctors were quickly turned off by the high levels of expectancy from many of the refugees, claiming that they were not political prisoners, but rather criminals. Many immigrants from the 1950s were upset by the new refugees, who did not reflect the same attitudes towards work and self-help (Thompson & Blasquez, 1996, 1998c).

Dominicanos

Limitations on emigrations for "Dominicanos" from the Dominican Republic were lifted after the 1961 assassination of the leader Trujillo. Since then, Dominicans have entered the United States both legally and illegally. Many enter the United States via Puerto Rico. Many Dominicans occupy nonskilled and semiskilled jobs in the United States (Zuniga, 1998, p. 213).

Centraleños

"Centraleños" from Central America includes people from Guatemala, Honduras, El Salvador, Nicaragua, Costa Rica, Belize, and Panamá. About 1.1 million Central Americans have immigrated to the United States in the last 180 years, with 90% of those arriving since 1981. Refugees fleeing the civil wars in the countries of El Salvador, Nicaragua, and Guatemala frequently settled in Florida but less frequently in major cities throughout the United States (Zuniga, 1998, p. 213).

Sureños

"Sureños" includes people from the South American countries of Venezuela, Colombia, Ecuador, Perú, Bolivia, Chile, Paraguay, Argentina, and Uruguay. French Guiana, Suriname, and Guyana are often considered the non-Hispanic South American countries, whereas Brazil is a country with people of Portuguese descent. Immigrations, legal and illegal, from South American countries tend to follow patterns of economic difficulty in the respective countries. Statistics on the exact number of immigrants in this category tend to be sketchy. People from all socioeconomic levels make up this group, which is steadily increasing in numbers. Many South Americans have settled in Miami, originally the base of the first-wave Cuban immigrants who hope to return to a free Cuba one day.

Population Demographics

People of Hispanic descent include those from Spanish-speaking countries in South, Central, and North America, and from Spain. This comprises the ethnic group with the biggest impact on health care, employment, and the media in the United States over the past thirty years. In 1970, Hispanics made up 5% of the U.S. population. By 1990, this population rose to 10%, then to 15% by 1998. By 2050, the Hispanic population should make up just under 20% of the U.S. population, the largest minority group (U.S. Bureau of the Census, 1993a, 1993b, 2001a, p. 3; 2001b, p. 1; 2001c, p. 2).

According to the 1990 census, 60.4% of the Hispanic population in this country consider themselves of Mexican origin, 12.2% of Puerto Rican origin, and 4.7% of Cuban origin. The remaining 22.8% consist of people of origin from the other seventeen Latin American countries. According to the 2000 census, the Hispanic population rose from 22.4 million to 35.3 million, an increase of 57.9%. Currently, 12.5% of the U.S. population is Hispanic. More specific groupings were used in the 2000 census to determine that 58.5% consider themselves of Mexican origin, 9.6% of Puerto Rican origin, and 3.5% of Cuban origin. The remaining 17.3% of the Hispanic population consists of 2.2 % of Dominican origin, 3.8% of South American origin, 4.8% of Central American origin, and the remaining 6.5% of other Hispanic origin (U.S. Bureau of the Census, 1993a; 1993b; 2001c, p. 2).

Population Distribution

According to the 2000 census, the Hispanic groups represent 12.5% of the U.S. population. Nine states have more than 12.5% of Hispanics in their population, including California, Texas, Arizona, Nevada, Colorado, Florida, New York, and New Jersey. The remaining 41 states and District of Columbia have populations of less than 12.5% of Hispanics. It is interesting that 50% of all the Hispanic people in the United States live in the states of California and Texas. Persons of Mexican origin are the largest Hispanic groups in California, Texas, Arizona, Nevada, and Colorado, whereas those represented by the groups other than Mexican, Puerto Rican, and Cuban origin are the highest Hispanic population in New Mexico, Florida, New York, and New Jersey. The Hispanic population is distributed across these regional breakdowns: the West 43.5%, the South 32.8%, the Northeast 14.9%, and the Midwest 8.9% (U.S. Bureau of the Census, 2001b, p. 2; 2001c, pp. 2–3).

Diversities

The smorgasbord of Hispanic cultures is characterized by a variety of socioeconomic, personal, national, regional, and local differences in areas ranging from grammar and syntax to foods and work values. National, regional, and local rivalries flourish. In times of adversity, people overcome these rivalries to unite. For example, Argentineans living in other South American countries in the 1980s occasionally experienced informal social discrimination. In the early 1980s, England invaded the Falkland Islands (called Islas Malvinas in Spanish) to restake their claim to the islands. Many South Americans throughout the continent put their rivalry to rest to support the Argentineans in their fight with England. The dispute passed and many of the rivalries quickly returned to pre-conflict level.

Small but diverse, Ecuador boasts three major regions with diverse lifestyles: coast, mountains, and rain forest. Two areas are the most densely populated. People on the coast enjoy warm evenings, wear shorts, and refer to mountain residents as "serranos," meaning "mountaineers" and a pun for "closed off." The mountain lifestyle closes up early because of chilly evening weather. Wearing shorts is prohibited in government or religious buildings. "Serranos" refer to animated coastal residents as "monos," monkeys. The rivalry reflects differences of opinion on distribution of government funds between these two diverse metropolitan areas. When Ecuadorians play Peruvians in soccer, however, the country unites (Thompson & Blasquez, 1998b, 1998c).

Diversity in Immigration

The diversity of the Hispanic cultures combined with immigration of people over time leads to various levels of acculturation into the U.S. culture. People adopt cultural values along a continuum influenced by successful personal experience, socioeconomic levels, cognitive levels, educational level, exposure to other environments, psychological conditions, and age at which first exposed to the culture. The differences in acculturalization between parents and children are often compounded by normal developmental factors (Early, 2000, pp. 205–206).

In addition to Hispanic people coming to live in the United States, many Hispanics from Latin America come to this country for medical care. Sometimes, one's perception of the United States abstracted from movies and television that proclaim "miracle cures" and treatments can create high, even unrealistic, expectations for people living in other countries. A woman sold her car and her home to take her ten-year-old son to the United States for treatment. The child had severe spastic quadriplegic cerebral palsy and was totally dependent in all feeding, dressing, transfers, and toileting, and he was not able to communicate with words or gestures. The woman listened patiently to the results of evaluations by the orthopedic surgeon, neurologist, pediatrician, physical therapist, occupational therapist, and speech pathologist at a major pediatric hospital. The team made suggestions of a gait trainer, prone stander, wheelchair, adequate positioning during activities of daily living, and a communication device. The woman became distraught and hysterical, screaming, "No, I don't want a wheelchair. We sold our house and our car and spent all our money for you to cure my son—so he can be normal and walk and talk like other kids."

Cultural Differences

Even within each culture, the acceptance and practice of cultural values vary over a wide continuum (Andrews & Boyle, 1994, p. 24). Hispanic people represent a wide range of cultures, religions, and previous immigrations. Jewish immigrants who fled Europe during the time of Hitler, as well as many other Europeans, settled throughout many parts of Latin America. Groups from Asia have immigrated to various cities throughout Latin America.

Six-year-old Manuel and five year-old José received Speech Pathology services from a bilingual speech pathologist in the school system. The therapist noticed that when she spoke to the boys in English, they laughed, talked, and made eye contact with her. When she conducted sessions in Spanish, the boys bowed their heads, made no eye contact, and barely spoke to her. In English, they took on the roles that they had learned from their peers in school. In Spanish, they took on the roles of the children of humble migrant workers that they learned from their parents.

North Americans and Europeans have immigrated to Latin America for many reasons, including serving in the diplomatic corps and finding employment with international industrial and petroleum companies.

Language

The Spanish language that predominates in Latin America is fairly easily understandable from country to country, from social class to social class, and from region to region. Each area and each socioeconomic class are characterized by their own specific words, idioms, and accent. Some Latin Americans speak another language as a first language, including native Indian languages such as Quechua, Mayan, Aymara, and Guarani, the Creole-based Garifuna spoken in coastal Honduras, French, Dutch, English, and Portuguese (Castex, 1994, p. 291).

The Influence of Socioeconomic Differences

Social-class differences may influence a person's behavior even more than may ethnic background. Isaza (1991) addressed the differences between Hispanic women in various socioeconomic groups and said that throughout the world, most members of the lower socioeconomic groups tend to live a hand-to-mouth or paycheck-to-paycheck existence. According to Isaza, lower-income Hispanic women are concerned about getting food on the table for the children and for daily survival, whereas upper- and middle-income Hispanic women are concerned about keeping themselves physically and mentally in good condition as a means to preserve their marriage and home life.

Socioeconomic difference extends into health care. "Innumerable barriers restrict access to health care systems, but the major such obstacle is poverty." (Spector, 1996, p. 108.) Persons with inadequate health care coverage, regardless of their cultural or ethnic background and beliefs, may seek out other health options. People subscribe to cultural values and beliefs along a continuum, molded also by socioeconomic factors, personal beliefs, cognitive levels, emotional factors, and psychological conditions.

A case manager with a fair understanding of Spanish took charge of the case of a 21-year-old Mexican male with an incomplete lumbar spinal cord injury. The case manager sought the help of a staff member more fluent in Spanish because "I cannot understand his dialect." The case manager spoke Spanish as a second language, with native Mexican Triqui as his primary language. He spoke Spanish with an accent, but did not speak a dialect. This situation should remind health care workers to be aware that some clients speak Spanish as a second, not a first, language. In addition, health care workers should recognize their own limitations in dealing with issues of language and culture.

Cultural Values, Cultural Stereotypes

Health care workers would do best to ride the fine line between being aware of cultural values and using them as cultural stereotypes. A well-known Hispanic cultural value is familial proximity. Extended families are usually close, especially for the females. Often, grandmothers and aunts take care of the younger children. Often the main caregiver, usually the mother or other female relative, continues to feed and dress her children until early school-age years. This tendency to nurture continues into the care of persons with a disability or illness. It is not uncommon for the U.S. values and therapy goals for independence in self-care to conflict with this Hispanic cultural characteristic.

By the same token, many elderly family members remain in their home or their children's home rather than being placed in assisted living facilities. Ties to the extended family are often strong in many Hispanic families. Most young adults live in their parents' home until—or even after—they marry. An area of conflict for second- and third-generation Hispanics is that of how to care for elderly family members with assisted living facilities and other options in the United States.

Health care workers should recognize this cultural tendency but avoid assuming that all Hispanic clients have a united, dependable family unit for emotional and physical support.

High-Contact and Low-Contact Patterns of Communication

Cross–cultural communication is influenced by whether one's culture tends to be high-contact or low-contact (Hecht, Anderson, & Ribeau, 1989, p. 168). Hispanic communication tends to be high-contact, characterized by the use of facial expressions, subtle facial movements, rate and speed of interaction, and other subtle nonverbal components with less focus on specific words and precision (Hecht, Anderson, & Ribeau, 1989, p. 169). The low-contact cultures tend to focus on precise, logical, verbal communication (Hecht et al., 1989) with less attention to the nonverbal behaviors. Anglo-European American and northern European cultures tend to be low-contact. In general, high-contact cultures appear more formal, change slowly, and are based on tradition to offer more stability and consistency. Low-contact cultures tend to value change, appear more informal, and offer less connection with the past. High-contact cultures may be more oriented to gestures, use of touch, and indirect communication, whereas low-contact cultures want to verbally express direct, concrete instructions (Zuniga, 1998, p. 226).

The differences between the high-contact Hispanic cultures and the low-contact U.S. Anglo cultures often highlight differences between recently arrived immigrants and immigrants who have been in this country for one generation or more. This same conflict often reflects additional difficulties between older generations and younger generations in the same extended family than seen in mainstream U.S. families. Most often, the older members of the family, especially those who immigrated as adults, might tend to maintain more adherence to traditional cultural values and communication styles, whereas younger members of the family might tend to adapt more values and communication styles of the U.S. Anglo cultures.

One example of the high-contact tradition of touch and proximity is the rituals that Hispanics often use to greet each other: handshakes, hugs, and cheek kisses. These actions are simultaneously warm, high-context gestures and formal, structured rituals. Low-context cultures tend to get down to business and avoid physical contact beyond a firm handshake.

Tradition-Based Cultures

Another aspect of the high-contact cultures is the tendency to maintain traditions. Although people of various religions have immigrated to Latin America, many of the more traditional countries tend to maintain a hold on Roman Catholicism. Ceasar (2000, p. 2-C) related that Spanish conquerors tore down the Bolivian city of Tiwanaku to build the first Catholic church almost 500 years ago. This Catholic stronghold continued in Bolivia until 40 years ago. More than 200 non-Catholic religious associations have registered in Bolivia since 1960. These organizations include Baptists, members of the Church of God of Prophecy, Lutherans, Baha'i, Zen Buddhists, and Mormons. In the 1990 census, 80% of Bolivians considered themselves Catholic, and 10% evangelicals. Sociology professor and Bolivian religious expert Hugo José Suárez ties the recent change of "a huge migration from rural to urban areas" with a "new social structure in evangelical churches" (Ceasar, 2000, p. 2-C).

Indirect Patterns of Communication

Another cultural characteristic of the Hispanic cultures is to utilize techniques of indirect communication. One of these is *personalismo*, characterized by a short period of small talk before getting down to business. These personalized questions show an interest in the other person without asking for truly personal information. The ritual usually consists of exchanging general, superficial information about family, friends, and interests without delving into personal concerns or problems.

Many Hispanics consider the typical American tendency of "getting down to business" to be rude. It is important to begin a contact with a few moments of polite yet personal questions about the family, common friends, and how-are-yous before approaching the main issue. The tendency to build up to the point is called talking with flowers (*flores.*) In contrast, many Americans feel that someone who tries to be nice before getting to the point is just "closing in for the kill." In fact, a sales tactic in the United States is to ask a potential client several questions and then to use that information to form a contact with the goal of making the sale.

The Hispanic "No"

Often, it is considered rude to tell someone "No" directly. Although Americans tend to want a direct answer, Hispanics might view using a refusal or negative expression as rude. Much care is taken to soften negative answers, a characteristic that can frustrate the low-context communicator.

A young woman got lost looking for a new office in Quito, Ecuador. She asked four different people for directions. Each person gave totally different, often very elaborate, directions. Frustrated, she returned to the main office to get directions. She found that she had been right in front of the office when asking for directions, but the new sign had not yet been put up. Several coworkers in the office told her that she should be happy that the people made up elaborate directions—it meant that they liked her enough to go to all that trouble. It would have been rude to tell her, "I don't know where the office is."

The Hispanic "Yes"

Another area of communication difference is the use of the word "Yes." For Anglo-European Americans, "Yes" usually means a positive answer to a question. To many Hispanics, nodding or saying "Yes" can mean "I am listening" and sometimes means "I am looking at you and listening, but I really do not understand." This habit often represents a great source of miscommunication and frustration in carrying out therapy (Thompson & Blasquez, 1998a).

A frustrated therapist described her interaction with presenting a home program to a youngster and his caregiver: "I had the feeling that she didn't understand a word I was saying. I kept asking, 'Do you understand?' and she kept saying, 'Yes, yes, yes!' I kept going. When the translator came in, he said that the caregiver didn't know what I was doing. Why did she keep saying 'Yes'?"

"Cariños" (Small Gifts)

It is common for patients to bring small gifts or food items called *cariños* ("affections") to the staff. Refusing a small gift can easily offend the giver. Many facilities have strict policies prohibiting staff from accepting gifts from patients. Other facilities that frequently provide services to Hispanic patients and families have modified their policies to accommodate this tradition.

A mother brought her twins to a pediatric hospital for a two-week admission. She brought small gifts from her country as tokens to the staff. The scheduling secretary became upset and refused her gift, stating, "She just wants me to do something for her." The secretary was upset because she felt that the mother was trying to get her to do something outside of her job. The mother's feelings were hurt because her gift was rejected.

"Palanca"

Another cultural value present in most Latin American countries is the concept of *palanca*. A *palanca* is a wedge or lever used to push open a door, that is, a lever to help someone navigate a difficult path. The U.S. version of this concept is "You scratch my back, I'll scratch yours." A client or caregiver may offer to provide a needed contact or materials in order to gain a favor for needed health care information or services in return. Sometimes a client may ask to speak to several people at different levels in the chain of command or in different departments in order to get special services.

Concepts of Time

The concept of time varies in cultures. Many Hispanics tend to be present-oriented and focus on the current interaction. Often it is considered rude to tell the present person or group that one must go on to an upcoming appointment or event. This difficulty may be the source for the tendency for the use of the term *Latin time*, meaning "not running on time." Anglo-European Americans tend to focus on being on time for the next event, and it is not considered rude to say, "I have to get going" or "I have to go to a meeting." Even the language reflects this difference. In Spanish, "the clock walks" (*el* reloj anda) whereas in English, "the clock is running" and "my biological clock is ticking."

"Machismo"

Machismo is a concept with a variety of definitions. One end of the continuum sees a *machismo* as the man who takes care of his family by providing for them and being a loyal, devoted, hard-working role model. The other end of the continuum views a *machismo* as the man who asserts his masculinity by doing what he wants when he wants. This concept and its enactment are subjects of perpetual discussion, research, and conflict (Macklin, 1997, p. 18). The conflict over *machismo* parallels the conflict in the United States called "the battle of the sexes."

Last Names

The use of last names can be confusing to U.S. residents who use one last name or use hyphenated last names composed of the wife's maiden name and husband's surname. Many countries in Latin America use the custom of giving each person the use of the father's last name followed by the mother's maiden name. For example, in Latin America, the name Chris Gomez Johnson means that Chris's father's surname is Gomez and her mother's maiden name is Johnson. Traditionally in the United States, that person's name is Chris Gomez. After getting married in this country, Chris Gomez might retain her maiden name, might be Chris G. Rodriguez, or might use both last names to be Chris Gomez-Rodriguez. Upon marriage in Latin America, a woman could keep her name Chris Gomez Johnson or take on the husband's surname with the word *de* meaning "of." Use of the mother's maiden name is optional. Chris Gomez Johnson could then become Chris Gomez Johnson de Rodriguez or Chris Gomez de Rodriguez.

Health Care Options: Hot-Cold Model

Most Hispanic cultures utilize the hot-cold model of disease, based on a simplified version of four humors of Hypocrites. These four humors are blood (hot and wet), phlegm (cold and wet), yellow bile (hot and dry), and black bile (cold and dry) (Spector, 1996; Villaruel & Ortiz de Montellano, 1992). The hot-cold model categories all conditions, diseases, and disorders into either the "hot" group or the "cold " group. All medicines and most foods are also categorized as either "hot" or "cold" by type of food, not by temperature. A "hot" condition is treated with a "cold" food or liquid. "Hot" conditions include visible ailments, skin problems, pregnancy, ulcers, and heart problems. Examples of "cold" foods are whole milk, bananas, coconuts, and beer. In traditional medicine, a doctor may advise someone with a heart condition related to high blood pressure and high cholesterol to avoid high fat products such as whole milk and coconuts. This advice conflicts with the hot-cold model of care.

"Cold" ailments encompass conditions that are invisible or that include immobility or pain, such as arthritis, menstrual problems, and colds. "Hot" foods include evaporated milk, chocolate, onions, and liquors. Penicillin is considered a "hot" medicine. The client's desire to use the hot-cold model to cure ailments can conflict with principles of traditional medicine. Some foods, such as chicken, barley water, honey, and some fruits, are considered variable. Health care providers should consider each person's adherence to the "hot-cold" system in considering food preparation activities and feeding activities.

Food and Nutrition

In addition to the importance of food in the hot-cold illness system, food plays an important role in the implementation of some therapy activities. In a food preparation activity, a therapist might assume that a Hispanic client prefers black beans, rice, and pork. These foods are frequently found in many, but not all, Hispanic cultures, but many people prefer other types of food for religious, dietary, or ethnic reasons.

To begin therapy for meal preparation, a therapist asked a young adult what she would like to prepare. Expecting the client to select black beans, pork, and rice, the therapist was surprised to find that the client was a vegetarian and a member of a religious organization that refrains from eating pork products. Some people focus on Latin food as tacos, burritos, black beans, and "anything with hot sauce."

The Hispanic populations include people from a wide range of ethnic and religious backgrounds. Several groups do not eat pork, and vegetarianism is on the rise. Many Hispanic males tend to be lactose-intolerant. Ironically, the Latin fast foods found in the United States, such as tacos, burritos, and enchiladas, have recently been introduced into Mexico as "USA fast foods."

Some foods are influenced by environment. Tropical regions benefit from local tropical fruits such as pineapple, papaya, banana, platano, passion fruit, guava, mango, soursop, sweetsop, starfruit, grapefruit, oranges, and *nispero*. The southern parts of South America are home to apples, grapes, peaches, and pears. Each country and region has typical entrees, soups, and desserts.

Medical Conditions Unique to the Hispanic Cultures

Villaruel and Ortiz de Montellano (1992) and Zuniga (1998) find that some medical conditions prevalent throughout Latin America have been traced to a mixture of Spanish and Indian cultures. *Caida de la mollera* (fallen fontanel) refers to the sinking of the fontanel, and sometimes soft palate, of an infant. Traditional medicine relates this falling to dehydration or other cerebral problems. The folk system relates this falling to a loss of the soul. Folk treatments range from turning the infant upside down, shaking him or her while holding the feet, to pushing up on the soft palate.

Another cultural condition is *empacho*, or extremely upset stomach. Herbal remedies and putting the body in certain positions can help to relieve this condition. *Susto* is a series of behaviors resulting from extreme fright or distress, perhaps after viewing an emotional situation or event. Symptoms might include anorexia, weight loss, decreased interest in self-care and interactions, disturbed sleep, and decreased generalized strength. (Early, 2000; Zuniga, 1998). These behaviors are often viewed and treated as a psychiatric condition in traditional medicine.

Mal de ojo is the belief frequently called "evil eye." Parents may feel that excessive visual or verbal attention paid to their children can cause them to fall prey to the *mal de ojo*. One way to ward off the "evil eye" is to gently touch the forehead of a child after complimenting or paying attention to the child.

A little girl from South America accidentally turned over a pot of boiling water on her face and hands. Under pressure from family members with good experiences at a local hospital, she abandoned the local *curandero* to seek out traditional medicine. In the hospital, she underwent daily whirlpool treatments in a whirlpool that was not cleaned thoroughly. Her fingers became infected and gangrene set in. She eventually had to have all her fingers amputated. Her mother developed a distrust of hospitals, doctors, and traditional medicine.

Alternative Health Care Options

Alternative medical systems are frequently available to Hispanics of a variety of social class levels. Natural healers may be more readily available, both in terms of geography, beliefs, and finances, to lower-income families. The popularization of alternative medical practices in the mainstream of the U.S. culture has offered many alternative options to Hispanics who frequent traditional medical practitioners. Various natural healers, techniques, and rituals are available in many parts of Latin America and in the United States Natural healers, or *curanderos*, and spiritualists, or *espiritualistas*, both focus on the use of natural products for healing. The *espiritualistas* tend to focus more on the spiritual aspects with elaborate rituals, including the offering of pictures of saints, flowers, and other items to drive out evil influences and seek protection (Zuniga, 1998).

Optimally, alternative treatments and traditional medicine can work together, even in mutually exclusive events.

With the merger of Roman Catholicism and the religions practiced in the Caribbean, *Santeria* has evolved into a distinct faith (Perez, 1995, p. Metro-9). About 100,000 *Santeros* live in South Florida, with a total of 1,000,000 in the United States who worship seven deities that correspond to different forces of nature. *Santeros* use herbs, colognes, and ani-

A young Mexican girl slept in a crib protected by a *mosquitero* (mosquito netting). The candles that the parents burned every night all night long for protection set the *mosquitero* on fire. The child suffered burns on one arm. The father, following instructions from the *curandero* (folk healer), burned a dried gourd and rubbed the ashes into the fresh burn. The scar healed beautifully. Six years later, the child's wrist started to tighten into flexion as a result of growth, not because of the burn scar itself. He sought help from the pediatrician, who referred him to an occupational therapist. He and his daughter followed the OT program of splinting and of active and passive range of motion. She was quickly able to achieve full range of motion.

A woman waited as her 18-year-old son underwent a routine MRI under anesthesia. A housekeeper cleaned the young man's room, removing a glass of water, some fruit, and flowers that the mother had left on the bedside table. Even though the procedure was a simple, routine one, the boy had an allergic reaction and died. The woman became hysterical when she returned to the room to find that someone had removed the water, fruit, and flowers. The staff tried to comfort her to no avail. The woman believed that the death occurred because the housekeeper had removed the items. She believed that the items would have protected the boy from harm and from evil forces.

mal sacrifices to the gods to effect improvements in a variety of life situations, including health conditions. The practice of *Santeria* reinforces the comples intertwining of spirituality and health care in several Hispanic cultures.

Often, people believe that rituals and small gifts serve to protect and to heal. Frequently, people wear jewelry as a source of protection and healing. Gold bracelets, earrings, necklaces, and small gold or coral charms can serve to protect people of all ages.

Intervention Techniques and Strategies

Consider the following information during communication and intervention with a client, the client's family, or caregiver of Hispanic background. In each intervention, the therapist should be aware of all nonverbal communications. Many people of Hispanic cultures tend to use high-contact communication and rely on nonverbal behaviors. Use this information as a guideline, being careful to avoid stereotyping. People may subscribe to values and behaviors listed to different degrees.

- Focus on positive facial expressions. Avoid neutral and negative facial expressions such as a flat affect and frowning. A smile that expresses warmth and concern is frequently the best nonverbal behavior.
- Keep the arms relaxed at the sides rather than crossed to express openness.
- Good eye contact conveys interest and concern. However, avoid intensive eye contact with members of the opposite sex. Many Hispanics of lower socioeconomic status

"There are two things you want to do in your first language: get your hair cut and get medical care."

Anonymous.

avoid eye contact, on the basis of the customs of the social hierarchy. In an interaction with someone who looks away or down and does not maintain eye contact, the health care worker should continue to make eye contact with the person being addressed.

- Shake hands, and speak first with the male patient or caregiver.

- Whether the health care provider speaks Spanish or uses an interpreter, begin each contact with small talk. The few minutes of small talk will pay off in a more open communication.

- If one cannot communicate verbally with the client, take a few brief seconds to smile and focus on the client before proceeding with the examination.

- Avoid rushing or giving the impression of being in a hurry.

- Avoid laughing or joking in front of those who do not speak or understand English. In the absence of verbal language understanding, people may interpret the laughter as laughing at them.

- Discussion of issues that result in frowning or negative facial expressions can cause those who do not understand the language to feel that something is wrong.

- Speak slowly and clearly without being condescending.

- Repeat important ideas, concepts, and terms.

- Utilize photographs, clear drawings, and models as much as possible, especially if someone appears to be unable to read. These items can be more helpful than graphs and statistics.

- Present ideas one at a time, especially when using an interpreter.

- Be sure that the interpreter is competent and nonjudgmental. Sometimes using a family member to interpret might help the client feel comfortable. On the other hand, the use of a family member might affect the client's intimate communication with the therapist.

- Be sure that the interpreter, whether a family member or a professional, is accurate. Without knowledge of exactly what the interpreter says, it is extremely difficult to determine that the information is accurate. Signs that the interpreter is accurate are that the interpreter talks to the client after each presentation of small amounts of information. Look also at the client's nonverbal behavior for looks to indicate understanding or confusion. The translated answers should correspond to the questions asked. On the other hand, if the translator tells the family little information, if the family appears confused, or if the information returned by the translator is not in line with the original information given, consider using another translator or another option.

- Make sure that the interpreter translates after each small bit of information.

- Make sure that the interpreted questions and statements of the client and the caregiver(s) match the questions and comments made by the family.

- After complimenting a child, lightly touch the child on the forehead or top of the head. This is a long-standing tradition to prevent *mal de ojo*, evil eye.

- Try to say "¿Me explico?" instead of "¿Me entiende?" or "¿Entiende? The former means "Do I explain myself?" and is not as direct, and also encourages one to state areas of doubt and to ask questions. The latter expression is strong and more direct, and asks "Do you understand?" often making someone feel dumb for not understanding.

- Shaking the head up and down and saying "yes" and "sí" are acknowledgments of attention to the speaker. They do not reflect a true positive answer to or an understanding of an explanation or a question.

- Try to ask questions so that "No" is a positive answer. For example, ask "Does your child stay home alone after school?" rather than "Is your child supervised by an adult after school?"

- Ask questions at least two times. Some families are reluctant to share information about alternative health care interventions. Also some families may have higher boundaries about what constitutes private family information. Moreover, some families fear deportation if they offer too much information about funding, immigration status, and other services.

- Encourage questions. Many Hispanics, especially of a lower socioeconomic level, are not used to asking questions directly to medical personnel. The persons might be more likely to direct questions to different medical personnel at a later time to avoid direct communication. This outcome can make accurate communication of information more difficult and more time-consuming.

- To some people, questioning medical personnel may be seen as offensive. An effective technique is to state that the medical personnel are flattered when asked questions. State that "it is considered polite to ask questions now" or that the health care worker is flattered when someone asks questions. This step can decrease the discomfort level of both the clients and the caregivers in asking questions.

- Occasionally people are reluctant to discuss pain when asked, "¿Tiene dolor?" ("Do you have pain?") or "¿Donde le duele?" ("Where does it hurt?"). It might be more helpful to ask "¿Donde le molesta?" ("Where does it bother you?") in these situations.

- Be aware of each person's background. Also, be aware of religious and other ethnic influences on food preferences.

- Be aware of the importance of the hot-cold system of conditions, diseases, and foods for each person. Do not assume that the person is anorexic, or noncompliant because of food refusals. Explore food refusals more closely, and determine a method to offer acceptable alternatives.

- Be aware of alternative medical beliefs and practices that are utilized, and try to work with such practices. Alternative systems sometimes involve rituals or herbs in dealing with health care.

Intervention Strategies Specific to Therapy

Use the following strategies in situations involving therapy.

- Jewelry may be very important in preventing illness and in providing protection. Be aware that people may be reluctant to remove jewelry for fitting hand splints or to perform therapy procedures. Work to accommodate jewelry during therapy in ADLs, splint construction, transfers, ambulation devices, and communication systems.

- In therapy, conflicts can occur between the family and the therapist when the latter focuses on independence in ADLs. The therapist might refocus therapy goals to improve trunk control, to improve fine motor skills, or to increase strength instead of to increase independence in dressing.

- Another area of conflict might be the tendency to avoid the role of the caregiver. Traditionally, the family may perform self-care for the patient with a disability or an illness. Therapists should find a specific role for the caregiver who is used to taking care of the patient. For example, the caregiver who carried someone to the restroom might have the role of spotting the person during ambulation to the restroom.

- Sometimes it is helpful to show how weight-shifting across the pelvis and trunk control used while dressing on a bench can facilitate ambulation (Thompson & Blasquez, 1998a).

- The therapist might explain that independence in transfer skills also addresses improved general and upper extremity strength that contributes to improved ambulation skills.

- Speech pathologists might change focus from increasing the child's communication abilities to a change in the role for the caregiver to that of facilitator for the child in new communication activities. Instead of talking for the client, the caregiver may take on the role of setting up a communication board or system.

- Foods vary by country, region, religion, additional ethnic influences, and medical concerns, such as diabetes, as well as by socioeconomic level. In interventions and events involving food, ask what foods the person likes. Use these foods to make a list of possible selection to use in the situation.

Summary

The Hispanic cultures encompass a vast number of people with a history of migrations into the United States over the past 500 years and that continue on a daily basis. The Hispanic people espouse personal, cultural, and personal values, beliefs, and customs along a broad continuum. Today, the Hispanic people comprise a growing segment of the population of the United States with a profound impact on media, education, employment settings, and health care services. Health care workers should be aware of the customs and values that comprise the Hispanic culture to be able to provide the best quality of care and to meet the needs of this population.

The important element in health delivery is to consider everyone as an individual. Each person, on the basis of personal beliefs, values, and habits, encompasses cultural norms at different levels along a continuum. Focus on finding out what is important to each person to determine that individual's needs, strengths, valued occupations, and goals. Intervention is best when based on seeing and treating each individual as just that, an individual.

Case Study

A ten-year-old boy from Puerto Rico started prosthetic training, and an 11-year-old girl, also from Puerto Rico, was receiving hand therapy. This was a perfect opportunity to utilize a small therapy group setting for exercises, board games, and functional skills. The girl's mother, from a prominent area of the capital city, and the boy's parents, from a small town, started chatting. Within ten minutes, the parents were not speaking to each other. The girl's mother displayed facial expressions of disgust, and the boy's parents bowed their heads. Although the children got along well, the parents did not.

Questions

1. What do you think was communicated during the initial conversation between the two parents?
2. What are some of the reasons for the girl's mother to show disgust in her facial features?
3. How would you facilitate positive interaction and experiences between the two clients in a small group therapy?
4. How would you handle the situation if either one of the parents objected to allowing his/her child to participate in a small therapy group with the other child?

Questions

1. State three nonverbal behaviors to demonstrate and to be aware of during an evaluation or intervention session.
2. Name two behaviors that are more related to socioeconomic level than to cultural background.
3. During the contact, the patient and the family do not make eye contact with the therapist. What should the therapist do?
4. State three components of a high-context culture and three components of a low-context culture. Discuss ways that differences in the contexts of the therapist and of the client and family might cause conflicts.
5. Discuss three characteristics of appropriate translations in a clinical setting. Discuss three ways that a health care worker may determine that a translator is doing an inadequate job of conveying information.
6. A client says "yes" and shakes his head up and down at every explanation but cannot duplicate the presented information. What can the health care worker do to ensure understanding?

7. What would be the best way to engage the caregiver in self-dressing skills when the caregiver prefers to dress the child?

8. What should health care workers do when someone offers a small token gift?

9. Discuss three areas to explore when a client continues to refuse certain foods.

10. Name three alternative health care options for Hispanic clients and families.

11. Discuss the actions to be taken when a client says that she is receiving treatment from a *curandero* or an *espiritualista*.

12. Name three steps that a therapist should do to design a meal preparation activity for someone who is taking a variety of medications.

Suggested Readings

Arguijo, Martinez, R. (1978). *Hispanic culture and health care.* St. Louis, MO: C. V. Mosby.

Abdel-Moty, A. R. (1997, September 2). Cultural sensitivity. *Vital Signs*, pp. 6–7.

Angel, R. J., & Worobey, J. I. (1991). Intragroup differences in the health of Hispanic children. *Social Science Quarterly, 72*(2), 361–377.

Becerra, J. E., Hogue, J. R., Atrash, H. K., & Perez, N. (1991). Infant mortality among Hispanics. *Journal of the American Medical Association, 265,* 217–221.

Bender, D., & Leane, B. (Eds.). (1997). *Illegal immigration: Opposing viewpoints.* San Diego, CA: Greenhaven Press.

Center for Health Economics and Policy. (1991). Health status among Hispanics: Major themes and new priorities. *Journal of the American Medical Association, 265,* 255–257.

Cocking, R. R., & Greenfield, P. M. (1994). *Cross cultural roots of minority child development.* Hillsdale, NJ: Lawrence Erlbaum Associates, Publishers.

Cornelius, L. (1993b). Ethnic minorities and access to medical care: Where do we stand? *Journal of the Association for Academic Minority Physicians, 4*(1), 16–25.

Council on Scientific Affairs (1991). Hispanic health in the United States. *Journal of the American Medical Association, 265,* 248–252.

Cushner, K., & Brislin, R. W. (1996). *Intercultural Interactions* (2nd ed.) Thousand Oaks, CA: Sage Publications.

Dresser, N. (1996). *Multicultural manners: New rules for etiquette in a changing society.* New York: John Wiley & Sons.

Farley, R. (1996). *The new American reality: Who we are, how we got here, where we are going.* New York: Russell Sage Foundation.

Fernandez, E., & Robinson, G. (1994). *Illustrative ranges of the distribution of undocumented immigrants by state.* (Bureau of the Census, Population Division, Working Paper 8). Washington, DC: U.S. Government Printing Office.

Fernandez, R. C. (1991, October 7). [Lecture at University of South Florida Psychiatry Center, Tampa, FL]. Clinical issues in psychotherapy of Hispanics and their families.

Flasherud, J. H., & Hu, L. T. (1992a). Racial/ethnic identity and amount and type of psychiatric treatment. *American Journal of Psychiatry, 149*(3), 379–384.

Flasherud, J. H., & Hu, L. T. (1992b). Relationship of ethnicity to psychiatric diagnosis. *American Journal of Psychiatry, 180*(5), 296–303.

Harry, B. (1992). Developing cultural self-awareness: the first step in values clarification for early interventionists. *Topics in Early Childhood Special Education, 12,* 333–350.

Harry, B. & Kalyanpur, M. (1994). Cultural underpinnings of special education: implications for professional interactions with culturally diverse families. *Disability and Society, 9*(2), 145–165.

Harwood, A. (1981). *Ethnicity and medical care.* Cambridge, MA: Harvard University Press.

Helman, C. (1985). *Culture, health, and illness.* Bristol, England: IOP Publishing.

Henderson, G. (1999). *Rethinking ethnicity and health care: A sociocultural perspective.* Springfield, IL: C. C. Thomas.

Henderson, G., & Primeaux, M. (1981). *Transcultural health care.* Menlo Park, CA: Addison-Wesley.

Hewitt, N. A. (1991, October 7). [Lecture at University of South Florida Psychiatry Center, Tampa, FL]. Race, class, and ethnicity.

Joe, B. E. (1989). Chilean OTs keep steady course amid political changes. *Occupational Therapy News, 1,* 1–16.

Joe, B. E. (1990). Serving the underserved. *Occupational Therapy News,* pp. 28–29.

Kerr, T. (1994, November 14). Cultural differences can have high impact on treatment success. *ADVANCE for Occupational Therapists,* p. 10.

Loranger, N. (1992). Play intervention strategies for the Hispanic toddler with separation anxiety. *Pediatric Nursing, 18*(6), 571–577.

Lynch, E. W., & Hanson, M. J. (1998). *Developing Cross-Cultural Competence.* (2nd ed.). Baltimore, MD: Paul H. Brooks Publishing Co.

Marmer, L. A. (1991, September 9). Lack of info, role models hampering minority recruitment. *ADVANCE for Occupational Therapists,* p. 6.

Mastrangelo, R. (1991, September 9). Minorities: How are they faring in OT? *ADVANCE for Occupational Therapists,* p. 14.

Mauras-Neslen, M. (1990, December 13). An Hispanic perspective. *Occupational Therapy Week,* pp. 10–11.

Montgomery, P. A. (1994). The Hispanic population in the United States: March 1993. (Bureau of the Census, Current Population Reports, Series P29-475). Washington, DC: U.S. Government Printing Office.

Mormino, G. R. (1991, October 3). [Lecture at University of South Florida Psychiatry Center, Tampa, FL]. The Columbian exchange: The consequences of Columbus.

Novello, A. C., Wise, P. H., & Kleinman, D. V. (1991). Hispanic health: Time for data, time for action. *Journal of the American Medical Association, 2,* 253–255.

Parry, K. (1994, October). Culture and personal meaning. *PT Magazine,* pp. 39–45.

Perez, L. A. (1991, October 4). [Lecture at University of South Florida Psychiatry Center, Tampa, FL]. Cubans and the United States.

Reitz, S. (1990, December 13). Report highlights disparity in health conditions. *Occupational Therapy Week*, p. 11.

Rorie, J. L., Paine, L. L., & Barger, M. K. (1996). Primary care for women: Cultural competence in primary care services. *Journal of Nurse-Midwifery* (41) 2, 92–100.

Saltz, D. L. (1990, December 13). Different ethnic origins mean different types of therapy. *Occupational Therapy Week*, pp. 6–7.

Sayles-Folks, S. (1990, December 13). University curriculum includes sensitivity training. *Occupational Therapy Week*, pp. 8–9.

Thompson, T., & Blasquez, E. (1998b, June 2). [Presentation at World Federation of Occupational Therapy, Montreal, Canada]. You don't have to speak Español to work with Hispanic families.

Thompson, T., & Blasquez, E. (1998c, February 22). [Lecture at Florida Association of Child Life Professionals, Orlando, FL]. Working with the Hispanic population.

Thompson, T., & Blasquez, E. (1996, October and November). [Lecture series at Shriners Hospital for Children, Tampa, FL]. Implementing health care services with the Hispanic child and family.

Thompson-Rangel, T. (1992). The Hispanic child and family: Developmental disabilities and occupational therapy intervention. *Developmental Disabilities Special Interest Section Newsletter*, pp. 2–3.

Tridas, E. (1991, October 7). [Lecture at University of South Florida Psychiatry Center, Tampa, FL]. Learning and attention problems of Hispanic children.

Vilaubi, A. (1990, December 13). Cultural influences: Rehabilitation, treatment, and outcome. *Occupational Therapy Week*, pp. 4–5.

Winn, K. (1994). On cultural diversity, anthropology, and physical therapy. *PT Magazine*, pp. 46–48.

References

Andrews, M., & Boyle, J. (1999). *Transcultural concepts in nursing care*. Philadelphia: Lippincott, Williams, & Wilkins.

Castex, G. M. (1994). Providing services to Hispanic/Latino populations: Profiles in diversity. *Social Work, 39*(3), 288–296.

Ceasar, M. (2000, August 27). Bolivia journal: Evangelicals gaining ground. *Sun-Sentinel, South Florida*, p. 2-C.

Cornelius, L. (1993a). Barriers to medical care for white, black, and Hispanic children. *Journal of the National Medical Association, 85*(4), 281–288.

Cornelius, L. (1993b). Ethnic minorities and access to medical care: Where do we stand? *Journal of the Association for Academic Minority Physicians, 4*(1), 16–25.

Early, M. B. (2000). *Mental health concepts and techniques for the occupational therapy assistant* (3rd ed.) Baltimore, MD: Lippincott, Williams, & Wilkins.

Fuller, M. A. (1991). Occupational and physical therapy services for disabled children in the developing world. *Physical and Occupational Therapy in Pediatrics, 11*(2), 67–81.

Hecht, M. L., Andersen, P. A., & Ribeau, S. A. (1989). The cultural dimensions of nonverbal communication. In M. K. Asante & W. B. Gundykunst (Eds.), *Handbook of international and intercultural communication*, pp. 163–185. Beverly Hills, CA: Sage Publications.

Isaza, M. H. (1991, October 21). [Lecture at University of South Florida Psychiatry Center, Tampa, FL]. Psychological stressors of the Hispanic woman.

Macklin, W. R. (1997, July 6). Hispanics debate machismo. *The Tampa Tribune-Times.*

Mendoza, F. S., et al. (1991). Selected measures of health status for Mexican-Americans. *Journal of the American Medical Association, 265*(2), 227–232.

Perez, E. (1995, November 12). Sacrificial practice emerging from shadows. *The Tampa Tribune*, p. Metro-9.

Shapiro, J., & Tittle, K. (1990, April). Maternal adaption to child disability in Hispanic population. *Family Relations, 39*, 179–185.

Spector, R. (1996). *Cultural diversity in health and illness* (4th ed.) Norwalk, CT: Appleton & Lange.

Thompson, T., & Blasquez, E. (1998a). Overcoming English-Spanish language barriers. *OT Practice, (3)*4, 23–26.

Thompson, T., & Blasquez, E. (1996, October and November). [Lecture series at Shriners Hospital for Children, Tampa, FL]. Implementing health care services with the Hispanic child and family.

U.S. Bureau of the Census (2001a, March 2). *Overview of race and Hispanic Origin* [PDF] (C2KBR/01-1). Washington, DC: U.S. Government Printing Office.

U.S. Bureau of the Census (2001b, February 2). *Population change and distribution* [PDF] (C2KBR/01-2). Washington, DC: U.S. Government Printing Office.

U.S. Bureau of the Census (2001c, May 10). *The Hispanic Population* [PDF] (C2KBR/01-3). Washington, DC: U.S. Government Printing Office.

United States Bureau of the Census (1993a). *Hispanic Americans Today* (current populations reports, population characteristics, series P-23, No. 183). Washington, DC: U.S. Government Printing Office.

United States Bureau of the Census (1993b). *Population projections of the United States by age, sex, race, and Hispanic origin* (current populations reports, series PS-25, No. 1104). Washington, DC: U.S. Government Printing Office.

Villarruel, A. M., & Ortiz de Montellano, B. (1992). Culture and pain: A Mesoamerican perspective. *Advances in Nursing Science, 15*(1), 21–32.

Zuniga, M. E. (1998). Families with Latino roots. In E. W. Lynch & M. J. Hanson, *Developing cross-cultural competence* (2nd ed.). Baltimore: Paul H. Brooks Publishing Co.

12

Pacific Island Peoples and Rehabilitation

Katherine Ratliffe

Key Words

Pacific island   cross-cultural studies   rehabilitation

Objectives

1. Describe cultural values that may influence the rehabilitation of Pacific Islanders.
2. Discuss communication style differences in this population that may cause difficulties for those outside the culture.
3. Identify differences in time orientation between those in this culture and those with a more Western time orientation.

Introduction

Neileen's parents want her home. She has spent all of her life in the hospital. She was born with arthrogryposis, an orthopedic disability in which many joints and some muscles are malformed. She is not able to breathe well on her own, and she needs to use a mechanical ventilator to help her. She is a bright little girl who has learned to use some sign language to communicate. Neileen frequently uses the sign for "hug" to encourage physical interaction with her nurses and therapists. Her family is from the Republic of the Marshall Islands. They moved to Hawaii before Neileen was born. Her father has learned to speak a little English, but her mother, although able to understand a little, must rely on interpreters to express herself to Neileen's English-speaking caregivers. The parents live on a neighbor island and must save up their money for infrequent trips to see their daughter in the hospital on the island of Oahu. Hospital staff members are reluctant to send this medically fragile, ventilator-dependent child home to a small, rural house with 13 people living in it. Her discharge is delayed over and over.

Viliamu is a big man with tatoos on his arms and legs. He is from American Samoa and traveled to the Rehabilitation Hospital of the Pacific in Honolulu so that he could learn more independence in his life skills after a spinal cord injury. Two years earlier when he was 20 years old, he was involved in a car accident after partying with his cousins. He broke his neck and sustained a C-5 level of quadriplegia. It took him a year after the injury to accept his condition and begin to look forward in his life. He is eager to learn how to care of himself.

Satrick looks wistfully at his tricycle. He would like to ride it in school, but this skill is not in his Individualized Educational Plan (IEP). Satrick has hemiplegic cerebral palsy, as well as mental retardation. He is a large 10-year-old boy with no verbal language skills. His family, who are from Pohnpei in the Federated States of Micronesia, moved to Hawaii in order to obtain better services for Satrick. His mother is frustrated. She is educated, and understands the IEP system and the services that Satrick has a right to have. But she cannot express herself well enough in the IEP meetings, and no one seems to listen to her. The goals she has for her son have not been translated onto his IEP.

Alana is just emerging from a coma. A bus hit her as she was crossing the street in Waimanalo on the island of Oahu in Hawaii. Alana's family is proud of their Native Hawaiian culture. But her mother is frustrated in a California rehabilitation hospital where Alana was sent because of limited opportunities for pediatric rehabilitation in Hawaii. Besides the mother's fatigue and stress about her daughter's recovery, the hospital staff won't listen to her concerns. Annie is afraid that Alana, who is combative as she emerges from her coma, will fall out of bed. The staff wants to tie her in, but that is not acceptable to her mother. She wants a bed with high rails to protect her daughter, but the staff say that she will have to move to an adult floor in order to get that kind of bed. Also, Alana won't eat. She doesn't like the food that the hospital is offering her. Annie doesn't know where to get the Hawaiian foods that she knows Alana loves, and the hospital has been so difficult about everything else, she doubts she'd be allowed to bring it in.

This chapter will follow the stories of these four individuals, each from a different cultural background in the Pacific Islands and in different life circumstances. We will explore how to practice rehabilitation services in a culturally competent manner and learn about Pacific Island people and their geography, history, and culture through the stories of Neileen, Viliamu, Satrick, and Alana.

Cultural Proficiency

Although other chapters in this book explore more fully the idea of cultural proficiency, it is important to reiterate some concepts here. Cultural proficiency is achieved not only by learning facts about other cultures. Every rehabilitation professional must examine his or her personal cultural perspectives and biases in order to appreciate others' perspectives. Suspending personal viewpoints and "trying on" those of others can lead to greater understanding and acceptance. Respecting the attitudes of others, even if they contradict personal beliefs, can lead to greater empathy. And finally, adapting professional practice to accommodate the values and beliefs of others will lead to more culturally proficient care. These steps are not easy, and they take practice.

Many families who have immigrated to the United States have become partially acculturated to the dominant culture. Other families participate in cultures that existed in the United States prior to the advent of the European American culture, such as the Native Hawaiian, Native American Indian, or Native American Eskimo cultures. It is up to the service provider to determine which values influence their decisions and outlook. Each family is unique in its perspective. Stereotypical ideas about the background culture may not represent the family's true viewpoint. It is up to each therapy provider to assess the family's perspectives and adapt his or her practices to accommodate these.

This is not a passive undertaking. It takes conscious thought and action. Skills such as active listening, suspending beliefs, brainstorming, researching, questioning, cooperating, collaborating, and adapting are essential to this task. If we find ourselves frustrated, we must ask why, and then look into our own actions and underlying beliefs. If we find ourselves pleased, we must ask why, and then question whether the result achieved fits our own perspectives or those of the family with whom we are working. It is not an easy process.

This chapter provides you with information about some Pacific Island cultures. The family stories and perspectives portrayed here are unique, and they represent some of the perspectives of Pacific Islanders. It is hoped that this is just a starting place for you. The facts mentioned here about Pacific Island cultures will help you understand the perspective of families who come from these cultures. But it is up to you how you use this information to change your own perspective. Each of us must learn to practice our profession and to live our personal lives in a culturally competent manner.

The Pacific Islands

For two years after his injury, Viliamu struggled to get the American Samoa government to pay for extended rehabilitation in Honolulu. There were no comparable services in American Samoa, and he wanted to learn how to be more independent. His parents advocated for him also, and finally an agreement was reached to provide one month of residence at the Rehabilitation Hospital of the Pacific in Honolulu.

Nele, a staff member at Fatu'o'aiga, a Catholic long-term care facility in American Samoa, was supported by the American Samoa government to accompany Viliamu to Hawaii so that she could learn the skills that she needed to work with him and the two others at Fatu'o'aiga with spinal cord injuries. She spent almost every day at the hospital.

Viliamu had spent six months learning to paint by using his mouth after his accident. He initially was not interested, but he was encouraged by the sisters at Fatu'o'aiga and by Viki, another man with quadriplegia who lived at the Catholic center and was an accomplished artist. Viliamu had gotten quite good at painting "siapo" patterns.

Siapo is the Samoan name for tapa cloth, made of the bark of the mulberry tree. The bark is stripped off and pounded flat in such a way that it spreads into a cloth. The off-white cloth is traditionally decorated with two colors, brown and black. The brown dye is made of clay, found in the mountains of the Samoan islands, mixed with the sap of a tree. The black dye is made from the roots of the coconut tree. Viliamu used regular paints to produce traditional designs.

He enjoyed painting in his room at the hospital, but he was reluctant to join the art recreation offered on Saturday afternoons at the hospital. After failing in multiple attempts to get him to come, the recreation therapist began bringing materials up to Viliamu's room.

The Pacific is an area of millions of square miles, stretching from California to Asia and from Alaska to Australia. In this large area of ocean, over 3,200 large and small islands dot the Pacific. Over 200 of these islands are inhabited. At least 40 distinct cultural groups live in the Pacific Islands, most making their homes in small island states or nations. Because of a complicated and varied history of colonization, these island groups are organized politically and economically in different ways, and they are associated with at least six Western nations. These are summarized in Table 12.1.

Some political lines cut across cultural groups. For example, American Samoa and Samoa (formerly known as Western Samoa or Independent Samoa) are close to each other geographically and have the same language and culture, but one is an independent political entity recently emancipated from New Zealand, and the other is politically tied to the United States as a territory.

The Pacific is frequently divided ethnically and geographically into Polynesia, Micronesia, and Melanesia (see the map in Figure 12.1). Polynesia, the eastern group of islands stretching from Hawaii in the north to Pitcairn Islands in the south, encompasses native people from Hawaii, the Samoan islands, Tonga, French Polynesia including Tahiti, Pitcairn and Cook Islands, Norfolk, Easter Island, and others. Political associations are indicated on the map in Figure 12.1. The influence of the United States in this area is limited to American Samoa and Hawaii.

Micronesia is the largest area with the smallest islands. It includes Guam, the Commonwealth of the Northern Mariana Islands (CNMI), Palau, the Republic of the Marshall Islands (RMI), Federated States of Micronesia (FSM), Nauru, and Kiribati. Political associations are indicated in Table 12.1. The United States is affiliated with many of the island groups in Micronesia.

Melanesia includes the most western of the Pacific Island groups. It is known as the "dark islands," referring to the dark skin of the Melanesian people. These islands are some

TABLE 12.1 Political Affiliations of the Pacific Islands

Commonwealths

Definition: A political unit having local autonomy but voluntarily united with the U.S.

- Commonwealth of the Northern Marianas Islands (CNMI)

Unincorporated or Overseas Territories

Definition: A part of a nation not included in any state but organized with a separate legislature.

- Guam (US)
- American Samoa (US)
- New Caledonea (France)
- Wallis and Futuna (France)
- French Polynesia (France)

Dependencies

Definition: A territorial unit under the jurisdiction of a nation but not formally annexed by it.

- Tokelau (New Zealand)
- Pitcairn Islands (Britain)
- Easter Island (Chile)

Freely Associated States

Definition: States with partial independence, with control over local affairs and internal government, but with military control by another nation along with assistance with money and defense.

- Palau (US)
- Republic of the Marshall Islands (US)
- Federated States of Micronesia (US)
- Niue (New Zealand)
- Cook Islands (New Zealand)

Independent

Definition: A self-governing country.

- Nauru
- Kiribati
- Papua New Guinea
- Solomon Islands
- Vanuatu
- Fiji
- Samoa
- Tonga
- Tuvalu

of the largest in the Pacific and therefore have more natural resources, including more land. Melanesia includes Papua New Guinea, the Solomon Islands, Vanuatu, New Caledonia, and Fiji. Political associations are indicated in Table 12.1. The United States has few affiliations in Melanesia.

Although there are many cultural groups across the Pacific, each one is unique and rich in its heritage and practices. This chapter will be able to focus on only a few groups. The chapter will provide references for you to research other groups that are not explored

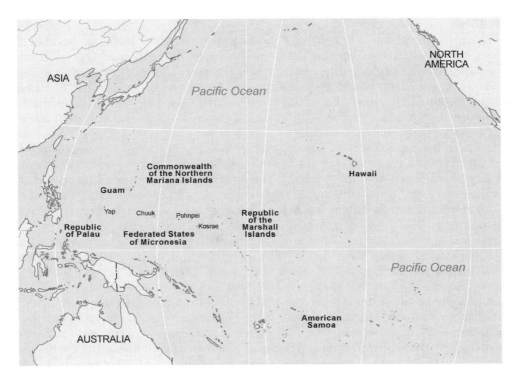

FIGURE 12.1 Pacific Islands
Source: This material has been reproduced with the permission of Pacific Resources for Education and Learning (www.prel.org). Copyright PREL (2001).

here. Because of their ties to the United States, as well as the subsequent ease and volume of immigration to the United States, this chapter will focus on the American Samoan and Hawaiian people of Polynesia, and on the Micronesian and Marshallese people of Micronesia. People from Melanesia do not have direct political ties to the United States and are less frequently encountered in United States rehabilitation service systems.

Polynesia

Alana's family are of mixed races, but a large percentage of their blood is Native Hawaiian. They live in a largely Hawaiian neighborhood on the east side of Oahu. Alana attends public intermediate school. Her mother works as a civilian employee for the military. Her father lives in California, and she doesn't see him much. Her stepfather farms taro, a leafy plant with a starchy root that is a staple of the traditional Hawaiian diet. Alana's maternal grandmother lives just down the road, as does her mother's two sisters and their families. When Alana's mother can't find Alana or her sister, she checks at Tutu's house.

GEOGRAPHY

Although the history and geography of Polynesian peoples differ from one another, their common ethnic heritage means that there are more cultural similarities than differences. The geographic area of Polynesia can be found primarily in the triangle among Hawaii, New Zealand, and Easter Island. Polynesian people tend to be taller than the Micronesians and lighter-skinned than their Melanesian counterparts. Most large Pacific islands are volcanic in origin, with many smaller and flatter islands formed by coral atolls left when ancient volcanoes receded into the ocean.

American Samoa is east of Samoa. Its main island, Tutuila, is the most populated of the seven islands in the group and has the best sheltered deep-water bay in the Pacific, Pago Pago Bay (pronounced "Pahngo Pahngo"). The total land area of American Samoa is about 79 square miles, and the population is fairly dense at approximately 58,000 people. The American Samoan islands include lushly forested mountains with most of the livable space along the coast.

In contrast, Samoa just to the west has nine islands with a land area of approximately 1,133 square miles. Its population is 172,000. The main city, Apia, is located on the island of Upolu. The largest island, Sava'i, is also known as the "Big Island." Samoa has more land mass that is flatter and less forested than American Samoa.

Hawaii, the last state admitted to the United States, is located in the middle of the Pacific Ocean and is the northernmost group of the Polynesian islands. Hawaii has eight main islands, seven of which are inhabited. The islands are volcanic in origin, with several dormant and active volcanoes. The most populated island is Oahu, home to the capital city of Honolulu. The largest and most western is the island of Hawaii, also known as the "Big Island." This island is still forming and has two active volcanoes, one of which, Kilauea, has been erupting almost continuously since 1973 and has added hundreds of acres of new land to the island. In 2000, the population of the Hawaiian islands was approximately 1,212,000, with almost 1,000,000 people living on Oahu. Hawaii reflects the natural beauty of the Pacific, an eclectic combination of ethnic groups, and has all of the modern conveniences of American life.

All of the Pacific Islands, including Hawaii to a much lesser extent, have problems related to limited natural resources, poverty, isolation, depressed economies, confusion related to the changing of social controls, draining of local talent through emigration, and dependence on outside money. They also have strong cultural traditions, strong family ties, and improved access to modern conveniences and knowledge because of increased involvement and access to the United States and other developed Pacific Rim countries. Lifestyles in the Pacific Islands are changing as a result of rapid modernization and exposure to outside information and services. People who move or travel to the U.S. bring with them cultural practices that may or may not be effective in the mainstream of American life. However, Pacific Island people are adaptable and forward thinking. With a little help, they can succeed in establishing new lifestyles to support their extended families and a new way of life.

LANGUAGE

Samoans all speak the same language, Samoan, and Hawaiians mostly speak English. In American Samoa, early grades are taught in Samoan, but English is introduced early, and children in later elementary years and in high school are learning in English. Most American Samoan children go to a Samoan school in their village to learn the Samoan language and Bible studies from their pastor. In Hawaii, the resurgence of interest in the Hawaiian language and culture is causing public schools to create immersion schools where children can be educated in their native language (Ratliffe, 1999; Yamauchi, Ceppi, and Lau-Smith, 1999).

Although they are different languages, similarities among Samoan, Tongan, Hawaiian, and Tahitian have enough in common that many of these peoples can understand each other. For example, *Aloha* (meaning "love/hello/goodbye") in Hawaiian is *talofa* in Samoan. *Aina* in Hawaiian (meaning "land") is *aiga* in Samoan ("g" is always pronounced "ng" in Samoan). *Aiga* is translated frequently as "family" in Samoan, reflecting the close ties between the people and the land in both cultures. Frequently only a few letters need to be changed to translate a word into the other language.

All of these cultures have strong oral traditions of storytelling and singing. Certain individuals are designated as "speakers" in their political systems and are responsible for using appropriate language and forms of language to express group sentiment and ideas. This tradition is common throughout the Pacific.

HISTORY AND POLITICAL RELATIONSHIPS

Both American Samoa and Hawaii have had interesting and varied political histories and relationships with foreign powers. In the late 1800s, the United States, Britain, and Germany were all interested in controlling Samoa, now politically split into American Samoa and Samoa (originally called Western Samoa, then Independent Samoa, and now just Samoa). Originally the traditional chiefs controlled different villages and fought among themselves for power. Tutuila, the main island of what is now known as American Samoa, was an island of refuge for chiefs who had been exiled from Savai'i and 'Upolu in what is now known as Samoa. When several chiefs fought to become the high chief of all Samoa, foreign powers backed different chiefs in an effort to improve their own political control. In order to finance the wars, the chiefs sold land to foreign governments. The huge typhoon (hurricane) of 1889 quelled some of the unrest by sinking both American and German ships. Only a British ship survived the typhoon, but the British relinquished their claim on Samoa to Germany for control in other parts of the Pacific. Germany and the United States divided up Samoa, with the United States taking the eastern islands and Germany taking the western islands. During World War I, Germany lost control of the western islands to New Zealand, which administrated the islands as a United Nations trust territory after World War II and prepared them for their eventual independence in 1962.

The United States maintained political control of the eastern islands by getting the chiefs to sign treaties of cession giving the islands to the United States. Currently, American Samoa is an unincorporated territory of the United States. Its citizens are able to travel freely and work in the United States and are considered U.S. nationals, but not citizens. This status means that they cannot vote in U.S. elections. The government of American Samoa is quite autonomous from that of the United States. The people elect their own government officials and maintain almost complete political control over their own islands. They receive generous grants from the United States to assist with health, education, welfare, and other social and economic programs. Treaties with the United States guarantee the continued supremacy of the *Fa'asamoa*—the Samoan way of life. Currently, only American Samoans own land. Residents who have American citizenry or who are American nationals with at least a year of residency can vote in elections along with American Samoans.

Hawaii, originally settled by sojourners from Tahiti and other places in the southern Pacific, developed in relative isolation for hundreds of years before being "discovered" by Captain James Cook in 1779. The initial and subsequent contact with Westerners introduced diseases that killed much of the original population and gave Westerners a stronghold on island economy. King Kamehameha conquered and united the major islands of the group by 1795, and his family ruled from Oahu. American sugarcane planters initiated a strong sugar industry in Hawaii that was threatened by an American tariff on foreign sugar implemented in 1893. Queen Lili'uokalani, the reigning monarch, was not as responsive to the American planters as they would have liked, putting the sugar industry in jeopardy. She and other Native Hawaiians resisted the urging to allow annexation of Hawaii to the United States. In order to install a provisional government that viewed annexation favorably, white settlers arrested the Queen and took over the government with some help from the U.S. military. The Spanish-American war five years later gave the U.S. government incentive to annex Hawaii as a territory, and in 1959 the legislature voted to make Hawaii the fiftieth state, and President Eisenhower signed the Hawaii Statehood Bill. Ironically, the sugar industry is greatly reduced in the islands, but the animosity produced by the actions of the sugar planters and early American settlers still causes racial and ethnic difficulties in Hawaii.

PATTERNS OF IMMIGRATION

Prior to World War II, very little immigration to the United States occurred from American Samoa. After World War II, political affiliations, exploding birth rates in American Samoa, and poor economic conditions at home led many American Samoans to emigrate to the United States. In 1951 the Naval headquarters that had governed American Samoa for fifty years moved to Hawaii, bringing with it over 1,000 Samoan workers (Ridgell, 1995). American Samoans have been underemployed in American Samoa because of a lack of jobs, causing young people to emigrate to find employment opportunities (Ward, 1999). As of 1990, almost 63,000 Samoans were living in the United States. More people than the entire population of American Samoa are living outside the islands. Most settled in Hawaii, California, New York, New Jersey, and other "gateway" states. Thirty-two thousand were living in California, and 15,000 in Hawaii. But even less populated states had small communities of Samoans. In the decade since the 1990 census, the populations have increased significantly. The 2000 census shows that Samoans living in California numbered almost 38,000. Those in Hawaii numbered over 16,000. Samoans abroad tended to have lower incomes and fewer jobs than Americans, causing poverty and stress. The term "chronically unemployed" was used regarding Samoans who had emigrated to Hawaii by the Samoan Service Providers Association Census (1990).

Since statehood in 1959, Hawaiians left Hawaii to find better jobs and educational opportunities and to follow family members who had moved to the continental United States. More than 80,000 Native Hawaiians were living in Hawaii in 2000, but an equivalent number were living in other states as well. California was home to 20,000 Native Hawaiians, with Texas having almost 3,500, and even Illinois had 1,000 Native Hawaiian people living within its borders. Young Hawaiians continue to leave the islands for educational and job opportunities in other states. The cost of living in Hawaii is among the highest in the United States, pushing young people to search for opportunities elsewhere.

Micronesia

In Pohnpei, Satrick's family lived in their own house, with other family members living nearby. Satrick, with a disability since birth, was cared for by all of his family members. His cousins and brother played with him, and everyone watched out for him. He went to school, but his mother was not satisfied with the services that he was getting. There was no physical therapist, occupational therapist, or speech-language pathologist in Pohnpei for the children in school. Satrick went to the hospital sometimes to see the physical therapy technician there who was trained primarily to work with people with orthopedic disabilities. He had attended workshops and training sessions in Hawaii and in the Pacific, but he did not receive training specifically geared toward children with disabilities. He did his best but was not able to work with the teachers to help them optimize Satrick's education.

GEOGRAPHY

Micronesia, meaning "small islands," spreads across the northwestern Pacific. Four island groups are represented, including the Northern Marianas Islands; the Caroline Islands; the Marshall Islands; and the Gilbert Islands, now called Kiribati. Other islands included in Micronesia are Guam and Nauru.

The northern Marianas Islands string north of Guam in a chain of fourteen volcanic and raised coral islands. Most of the 78,000 people live on Saipan, the capital, with fewer people living on Rota and Tinian. Only a very few people live on the far northern islands. Important historical events took place in the Northern Marianas Islands during World War II. Saipan was the site of major battles between the United States and the Japanese, causing huge loss of life on both sides. Later in the war, the *Enola Gay* took off from Tinian to drop the atomic bomb on Hiroshima. Japanese tourists visit these islands today to remember the war and commemorate their fallen relatives. The total land area of the islands is 184 square miles, and the climate is warm.

The Caroline Islands include the four island states of the Federated States of Micronesia (FSM), Kosrae, Pohnpei, Chuuk, and Yap. Each of the island states includes at least one main island and many smaller inhabited islands and atolls. The Caroline Islands also include the Republic of Palau and Nauru. Most of the larger islands (Pohnpei, Yap, Kosrae) are high volcanic islands, but many of the smaller islands are coral atoll islands. Very simply, these islands were formed when a precipitating volcano and its volcanic island sank beneath the sea and the live coral reefs that were left behind continued to grow, forming small, low islands around a deep central lagoon. The low islands are particularly vulnerable to the vicissitudes of Pacific weather, including tsunami (tidal waves) and typhoons (hurricanes). The four states of FSM are spread across a wide area of the southwestern Pacific Ocean bordered by Palau on the western end and Nauru on the eastern end. The population of FSM is 108,000. Yap, the westernmost state, is known as the most traditional state in the FSM. Chuuk state includes a series of islands around a huge lagoon. Its history is remarkable for the number of Japanese ships sunk by the United

States that are still intact on the bottom of the lagoon. It is also the largest and the most populated state. Pohnpei is the site of the capital of FSM in Palikir. Kosrae is the smallest state on the eastern end of the islands.

Satrick's mother watched him walk into the kitchen, holding onto the wall for support. Her goals for Satrick were for him to walk without help, dress himself, and to be able to express his needs to others. She moved her family to Hawaii in order to get Satrick the help he needed to meet these goals. She had planned for a two-year stay, but already they had been in Hawaii three years, and Satrick had not yet achieved the skills she had hoped for. His walking was better, but he still needed help. He was able to put his shirt on when really motivated, but the one time he accomplished this it took him 20 minutes and the shirt was inside out. He was using a few signs, but he still had no words for communication.

With the help available in Hawaii, she had dreamed for him to learn how to use a computer so that he could eventually hold down a job. She found herself revising this dream too. Life in Hawaii was more difficult than she had envisioned. Both she and her husband had to work, and the cost of living was high. Although her niece lived with them and helped care for Satrick and his brother, it was not the same as in Pohnpei where many family members helped each other. She wondered how moving back to Pohnpei would affect Satrick and his brother.

The Marshall Islands, which are in the northeast portion of Micronesia include two chains of coral atoll islands running south to north. Twenty-four islands are inhabited, and all are low, flat islands. The total land area is only 66 square miles with a population of 58,000 people. The climate is dry and warm, with some northern islands having problems with water shortages, and all of the islands having limited food production. The United States military has built a large base on Kwajalein, the largest atoll in the world with a lagoon that stretches 80 miles across in places. The native population was moved to Ebeye, a smaller island in the atoll, which now is densely overpopulated and known as "the slum of the Pacific." The American military also ruined Bikini and Enewetak through atomic testing, causing overpopulation on several of the smaller islands by moving whole populations off the uninhabitable islands to islands with areas and natural resources insufficient for the new population.

LANGUAGE

Each state and republic has its own primary language, and even within each state different dialects or languages are spoken, usually between the inner and the outer islands. In Yap, for instance, the outer islands were originally populated by a different people than the four main islands, and inhabitants speak different languages. In the state of Pohnpei, Pohnpeian is the primary language, but Pingalapese is spoken on Pingelap, Kapinga is spoken on Kapingamaranga, both outer islands of Pohnpei state. Mortlockese from the Mortlock Islands of Chuuk have settled in Pohnpei, as well as other groups bringing in their own languages. Languages between the islands differ because they were peopled by sojourners from different places. Even the languages of Pohnpei and Kosrae, islands that are close to each other, show evidence that their origins are different (Segal, 1995).

English is the official language nationally in FSM and the Marshall Islands, and all secondary and postsecondary instruction is given in English. English is a second language for all of the educated residents of FSM. However, only those lucky enough to have gone through high school have much command of English. Because there are so many languages, people frequently speak three or more fluently.

Neileen's family immigrated to Hawaii just before she was born. They came from Ebeye, a small island in the Republic of the Marshall Islands, near the American military base of Kwajalein in the Kwajalein atoll. Ebeye has a land area of only 78 acres and a population of 10,000 people. It is considered the slum of the Pacific, because of the high population density, the poverty, and unsanitary conditions. There is inadequate water on the island, and children take the ferry to Kwajalein daily during the dry season with plastic containers to bring back water for drinking, bathing, and washing. The island's population grew large after the United States moved native Marshallese off Kwajalein to Ebeye, and then extended family members followed for the opportunity to work on the military base. Neileen's family was able to leave after saving their money. It was a risk to leave, but they hoped that they and their children would have more opportunity in Hawaii.

Living near Hilo, on the Big Island of Hawaii, Neileen's parents, two uncles and their wives, and seven children lived in a small house near several other Marshallese families. On Ebeye they had lived in a smaller house made of cement and corrugated tin with their extended family, including Neileen's grandparents and several other aunts, uncles, and cousins. In Hilo, they felt that they had lots of room. They didn't understand why the doctors at the hospital would not let Neileen come home.

HISTORY AND POLITICAL RELATIONSHIPS

Micronesia has had relationships with the Spanish, Germans, Australians, Japanese, and Americans over the last few centuries. Until 1868 many Micronesian islands were under the control of Spain. The Spanish wall and church in Pohnpei are a testament to both the Spanish rule and their introduction of Catholicism. Germany then controlled most of the Pacific until after World War I, when Japan took control. Since World War II, the United States has controlled most of the islands. When the United Nations was formed after the war, its General Assembly formed the Trust Territory of the Pacific Islands to administer the Pacific Islands and to prepare them for eventual independence. The United States, New Zealand, Australia, and others were designated the custodians holding the islands "in trust" for the time when their people were able to take the responsibility of self-administration.

The United States successfully proposed to the United Nations Security Council that the islands become Strategic Trust Territories instead of just Trust Territories. This arrangement meant that the United States, which considered the islands to be of strategic military importance, could control their development for the foreseeable future. Unfortunately, the United States ravaged some of the islands through building military bases and testing nuclear devices on Bikini and Enewetak in the Marshall Islands. Nuclear fallout contaminated people on nearby islands and ruined many islands for habitation. It was not until 1961 that the United States increased its efforts to substantially develop the economy, education, and services for the people who lived in the Pacific (Hezel, 2001).

The Federated States of Micronesia has been recognized as a freely associated entity through a compact of free association with the United States since 1986. Thus, this nation controls its own internal affairs through an independent government. They accept funding from the United States, which is also responsible for defense of the islands and controls all military matters. The compact was recently renegotiated in 2003 with amendments addressing funding and military involvement. The Republic of the Marshall Islands is also a freely associated entity whose compact was renegotiated in 2003. This compact includes cleaning up the islands that are contaminated with radioactivity and financing medical intervention for the people who were exposed.

Palau is a freely associated entity with its compact finally agreed to in 1994. The Palauans refused to join the FSM and negotiated on their own with the United States. Disagreements hinged on issues around nuclear material being brought into Palau. The population of Palau is 20,000, and it is known as the most progressive of the Micronesian islands.

Nauru is an independent nation, which is quite wealthy because of phosphate mined in the center of the eight-square-mile island. Most of the American interactions with Nauru are around international investments that it has made to support the economy once the phosphate runs out.

PATTERNS OF IMMIGRATION

Prior to 1961, there was little attention from the United States and little travel to and from Micronesia. In 1961, the U.S. presidency changed, and funding doubled for development of hospitals, airports, roads, education, and government throughout Micronesia. By the early 1990s, 2000 Micronesians were emigrating to the United States and Guam each year (Ridgell, 1995). Early migration patterns are difficult to ascertain because the first U.S. census to document Pacific Islanders was done in 1980. The 1990 census showed almost 7,000 Micronesians and almost 50,000 Guamanians living in the United States. Hawaii was home to almost 2,000 of the Micronesians and to a little over 2,000 of the Guamanians. California was home to 25,000 Guamanians and over 1,500 Micronesians. Other states reported from only a few to up to 1,000 Micronesians in residence. These numbers have increased significantly during the 1990s as Micronesians have seen the opportunities available to them in the United States and Guam, and have had the opportunity to freely travel to and from the United States. Figures from the 2000 census show almost 400,000 Native Hawaiian and Pacific Islanders living in the United States. This is an increase from almost 250,000 in 1990 (Grieco, 2001).

Three-quarters of all the Pacific Islanders in the United States live in the West, with half living in just two states, Hawaii and California (Grieco, 2001). The census also showed that the Pacific Island population is relatively young compared with other ethnic groups. The proportion of divorced Pacific Islanders is one-half that of non-Hispanic whites, and the majority of Pacific Islander households are family households (Reeves & Bennett, 2003).

Most Micronesian jurisdictions send their seriously ill or injured citizens to Guam, Hawaii, the Philippines, or the continental United States for treatment. Therefore, a disproportionate number of Pacific Islanders may be seen in some hospitals and rehabilitation facilities in the United States, especially those in Hawaii and California.

Because of the importance of extended family among all Pacific Islanders, the availability of education and jobs in the United States and the ease of travel from the Pacific to the United States, it is clear that immigration continues at a relatively high pace among Pacific Islanders. As the Compacts of Free Association were renegotiated in the early 2000s, more Pacific Islanders, afraid that travel will not be as easy with the new agreements, moved to the United States. Census figures will likely document this influx to Hawaii, to California, and to other areas of the continental United States.

Cultural Practices

Cultural practices in the Pacific include many commonalties around the importance of the ocean, the prevalence of a subsistence lifestyle, the way that people live with others, the role of the extended family, and magic and spiritual beliefs. The influx of Western practices, foods, economics, and political structure are altering how many people live, but pride in their history and culture and their strong affiliation with their islands pervade life in the Pacific. How people perceive family life, education and work, time and situation, religion and spirituality, and communication can portray a sense of their values, and the way that their values are similar, yet different, among the different island groups in the Pacific. These cultural considerations will be explored through the stories of Viliamu, Alana, Satrick, and Neileen.

Family Structure

Family is perhaps the strongest cultural component of the Pacific Islands. In the past, and in the present in traditional societies, families provide total support to their members, including those with disabilities. All individuals are members of their nuclear family, extended family, clan (matrilineal or patrilineal), village municipality, state, and nation. Although these entities have responsibilities to each of their members in different ways, the most important social element is the extended family. Families are interdependent, each member contributing what he or she can.

Some hospital visitors saw Viliamu's artwork displayed and asked to purchase it. They paid him several hundred dollars for several of his paintings. The following week Viliamu's mother visited him in Hawaii, her only visit since his injury. She had heard about Viliamu's success in selling his paintings. When she left, she had some of Viliamu's money with her.

A therapist who worked with Viliamu heard about this situation and approached him about it. "How could you let her take your money, Viliamu?" she asked him. "Your mother doesn't take care of you, she hardly comes to visit you, and yet you give her your hard-earned money. You should keep it, Viliamu. You earned it!"

Viliamu smiled and said, "In my culture, giving back to the family is a matter of pride. I grew up in a more Caucasian-oriented household, so I am not as obligated to give my earnings to my family as a person in a more traditional household. But it makes me feel good to give some!" He thought for a minute. "My parents give me freedom to do what I want to do, and they support me as much as they can. They helped me fight for this rehabilitation, and they helped me fight with Vocational Rehabilitation to get my power wheelchair. I respect my parents, and I love my family."

Traditionally, related families tend to live with or adjacent to each other, in the same house, compound, or village. Nuclear families may live in their own house or hut, but usually they share common living space with extended family members in adjacent houses. It is common to have three generations living in one household or compound. When Pacific Islanders immigrate to the United States, they may live in more nuclear family groups for a time, but frequently other family members join them and form more extended family groups.

With the change from a subsistence economy to that of a cash economy and with the availablility of Western material possessions such as televisions and canned food, open communal homes are changing into more nuclear family homes. This change especially affects families who immigrate to the United States where fewer family members are available. This change affects all aspects of family life, decreasing the support of the extended family and adding stress to young parents. Abuse and neglect are on the rise because of less community support (Hezel, 2001).

Families who have moved to the United States tend to congregate in Micronesian, Marshallese, or Samoan communities. Even in Hawaii, where there is a mix of cultures, Pacific Islanders tend to live together in extended family households and in culturally homogenous communities.

The nahs (Pohnpei) or open fale (Samoa) is an open structure where much day-to-day living is shared in Micronesia and Polynesia, and is usually centrally located among the various family houses. In Hawaii where a Western style of houses prevails, open garages have taken the place of these communal structures. Extended families tend to gather in the garage or carport to spend weekend afternoons or evenings with each other, playing games, listening to music, watching television, and "talking story."

Family needs come before individual needs. Many young people from Pacific Island cultures have had their own dreams changed abruptly when family needs mandated that they return home to care for ill parents. The culture of sharing with family also puts a financial damper on young people trying to make it in the United States. Money and goods must be sent home to help with births, weddings, funerals, and other family and community expenses.

Although the clan system is matrilineal in most areas of the Pacific Islands, meaning that extended family is traced back through female members, male elders of the family tend to make most family-related decisions. In most cultures, younger family members must abide by the decisions made for them. In many Pacific cultures, although a Western-style government is in place, political decisions also occur through the village hierarchy, using traditional systems.

Traditional systems are institutionalized in American Samoa where the legislature is divided into two houses. One house is for leaders elected by popular vote. The other is for leaders elected by the Matai—the chiefs of the extended families. The Matai control all of the land of the family, as well as who lives where and who farms which land. They also are involved in local and island politics. They epitomize the *Fa'asamoa* way of life and also perpetuate it through maintaining control and direction of families. Even family members who have moved away consult the Matai and come under their direction when making life decisions. This structure provides a sense of security but also some limitations on freedom for young members of the community.

Relationships and Social Structure

Neileen's parents were able to come to see her every few months with occasional help from charitable organizations for plane fare. When it became clear that Medicaid wanted her out of the hospital, her parents said that they would take her home. They did not want her to go into a foster care placement. The nurses agreed to train them to do her care when they were visiting, in preparation for taking her home.

The nurses were frustrated because the family did not come when they said they would. Sometimes they were late, and some weekends they did not come at all. The nurses and therapists were angry at Neileen's parents for not keeping appointments. When the nurses talked with them about this, Neileen's parents smiled and nodded.

Neileen's mother learned to suction through her tracheostomy, to feed her through the gastrostomy tube, and to check her oxygen saturation values on the monitor. She learned to give her medications through the tube and to help her learn to sit up and use her hands to play with books and blocks. Neileen's father smiled and said "yes" whenever the nurses asked him whether he understood, and he translated for his wife. But the nurses never saw him do any of her care. Sometimes he would wander off to the cafeteria or to the playroom, taking their older daughter to play, and would leave his wife to do Neileen's care. At other times the nurses would see him sleeping next to Neileen's crib while his wife was caring for both children. They talked among themselves about the lazy Marshallese man who let his wife do all the work.

The nurses resisted final preparations for sending Neileen home, feeling that the family were not ready. Her father had not yet demonstrated that he could do the care, and they had no idea what the support structure was at home for Neileen's mother.

People on Pacific Islands live, work, and play together. Everyone is linked within a family network in the community, with food, shelter, and material wealth shared freely (Cheng, Nakasato, & Wallace, 1995). The population tends to be heavy in more developed areas and to be sparse in less developed areas where there are also fewer resources. In order to survive, people have had to work closely with each other, even in the face of difficulty. Therefore, much of the work is shared. It is less difficult to build a house with many people working on it than if one family tries to do it alone. A subsistence economy relies on working together. Cooperation and working together were the primary means of learning from each other prior to the advent of Western-style education.

Harmony between people is important when people depend on one another. Therefore, most Pacific people will not say anything offensive, disagree with those in authority, or show their true feelings. This behavior is sometimes difficult for people in Western cultures to understand. Islanders will say what they think that someone wants to hear, rather than what they think or feel. This conduct may be difficult when assisting someone with needs related to the person's rehabilitation. It is important to get to know the family well and to earn their trust, so that appropriate questions can be asked and so that the family members will feel more comfortable expressing what they really need.

Social structure varies among the islands, but status is recognized and is important. In some communities, such as Yap, a strict caste system is in place. Caste is dictated by birth and cannot be changed. In other communities, there is more social openness; however, people usually marry others of similar status. Therefore, social mobility is fairly restricted in most Pacific cultures. Traditional leaders are respected, and people work hard to do what is expected of them. They care very much what others think. For example, when asked why the villagers did not eat the plentiful, nutritious, and wild-growing kang kung plant when they did not have enough rice or fish, an outer island teacher replied that a family would be seen as "poor" if they ate what was perceived as a weed. They would rather go hungry.

The opportunities that education and travel to the United States present is challenging the social structure among Pacific Island people outside their own communities. When employing a translator for Pacific Islanders in Hawaii or in the continental United States, it may be necessary to ascertain the social hierarchy of the participants to assess the effectiveness of the translation, and also the comfort levels of the participants. A translator of a lower social status than the family may find it impossible to translate certain information. Other cultural traditions that are fairly universal in Pacific Island cultures include certain behaviors between siblings and other close relatives of opposite gender. Women must observe certain behaviors when in the presence of male relatives. These behaviors could include always sitting lower than the men or not crossing in front of men. Men also must observe specific rules regarding their close female relatives, including not using bad language and always showing respect to the women. In some cultures, men and women relatives should never be alone in the same room together. These customs may be tempered in families who live outside their traditional communities; however, certain prohibitions will continue to affect how people interact with each other. For example, men cannot talk about personal subjects such as menstruation or female body parts with sisters or female cousins. This may cause difficulties if a family member is asked to translate in medical situations. It is important for service providers to be aware of the potential for discomfort if these prohibitions are challenged, even inadvertently.

The concept of independent living is outside the traditional values of interdependence. No one lives completely independently in the Pacific Islands. Everyone depends on family and community for support and sustenance. People with disabilities are accepted as they are, and they are cared for by family members without question. Therefore, the idea of independence is an anathema to Pacific Islanders. Why would an individual with a disability *want* to live alone without family support? Western society emphasizes intelligence and work skills, whereas the Pacific worldview emphasizes relationships to family, village, and church.

Sometimes children with disabilities are not enrolled in school. "Shame" is the reason most often attributed to this behavior. Another explanation is that parents may feel that they can protect and provide the best care for the child. One Samoan mother exclaimed, "My child is unable to walk and talk. If he goes to school, how will he tell me that someone did something bad to him? How would I know if the teacher hit him? How would I know that everyone will love and care for him the way his family does?" (Mamea, 2002, p. 64).

Religion and Spirituality

Satrick's mother and father stood in front of the many boxes they had packed to take back to Pohnpei. Satrick's tricycle that he loved was packed in its own box. His new walker with the built-in seat was in its original packing material. Satrick could go on walks now that he had that walker. Before he had the walker, he tended to get tired and sit down on the ground, and his mother didn't have the strength to lift him up again. So to take him on walks, she used to have to scope out the route, finding appropriate places where he could sit down and rest every 20 feet or so.

She was able to advocate getting him a walker with a seat to take back to Pohnpei. She was proud that she learned to navigate the system well enough to accomplish that. It was too bad that the same services were not available in Pohnpei. The discretionary funds from the Hawaii Department of Health that paid for the walker would not be available. Respite money would not be available, but they would not need it because family were there to help. She checked the envelope where she had put all of Satrick's papers. His completed IEP was there. That would help the special education staff in Pohnpei. The specifications and warranties on his walker and tricycle were there in case anything went wrong with them.

She watched Satrick playing with his brother. He held onto the wall as he made his way along the house. He was laughing. It would be good to get him back to the family, she thought. It would be good for her to get back to her family. She thanked God that they were finally going home.

When the Spanish and the Portuguese first began exploration in the Pacific in the 1500s, they "discovered" many island groups and brought their religion of Catholicism to the islanders. The outside religion was easily assimilated because the islanders usually accepted what they felt were the stronger religions of conquerors. In the later 1500s and 1600s, the British and the French began exploring and brought Protestantism to the islands. Missionaries from Spain (Jesuit), London (Protestant), Boston (Protestant), and France (Catholic) also had strong influences in the Pacific. They competed on different islands, but eventually all of the islands converted to Christianity of one sort or another. Primarily Catholic areas include the Northern Marianas and Guam, the Marquesas, New Caledonia, and Wallis Island. Primarily Protestant areas include most of Micronesia and Hawaii. American Samoa has a mix of Protestantism and Catholicism.

In modern times other Christian religions have taken hold in Micronesia, particularly the Church of the Latter Day Saints (Mormon), which has a strong presence on most islands. Other religions include the B'hai, Jehovah's Witnesses, and Assembly of God, which are established on many islands. Immigrant workers from China, Korea, and Japan brought Buddhism to Hawaii, and in smaller measure, to some of the other Pacific Islands.

As Frances Hezel, a prominent Jesuit priest and scholar in Micronesia, recounts, "The church in the Pacific is in a truly privileged position. Religion has always been an essential element of life for islanders, and the churches are tightly woven into the fabric of these societies. The church enjoys a position of respect and influence that probably is equaled in few other regions of the world." (Hezel, 1993, p. 7)

Indigenous polytheistic religions included belief and worship of different gods, spirits, and ghosts. Different islands worshipped different gods. Magic was important in most island cultures, enabling people to tell the future, cause physical or mental illness, cure illness, or cause someone to fall in or out of love (Ashby, 1993; Oliver, 1989). Because these beliefs and practices were discouraged or even prohibited by missionaries, they moved underground. Although most people today outwardly practice Christianity, and the church pervades local life and culture, indigenous religions continue to have an effect on cultural beliefs and practices, including health practices, on all of the islands.

Economy and Lifestyle

Most of the political entities in the Pacific Islands that are affiliated with the United States receive huge grants and other subsidies for creating and maintaining infrastructure. The U.S. government has spent millions of dollars developing transportation, education, and health systems, and other infrastructure to encourage political and economic development. In most islands, more than one-half of the population who work, work for the government. Other activities that support the economies of the islands include exporting dried coconut meat (copra), fish, and handicrafts, and sustainable lifestyles such as fishing, hunting, and agriculture. Tourism is an important contributor in some areas, especially Guam, Saipan, and Hawaii. The military presence of the United States is also a contributor to island economies, especially in the Marshall Islands, Guam, and Hawaii, where there are established military bases.

Most people in the Pacific Islands live very simply. Subsistence lifestyles have, in most cases, given way to a moneyed lifestyle by which goods are purchased rather than collected (Hezel, 1993). For many families, only a few family members work to collect wages, most working for the minimum wage, which is less than $2.00 an hour in FSM and RMI and ranges to over $4.00 an hour on Guam. These family members support others who care for the home and the family, or who hold other roles. Many families supplement their incomes with handicrafts that are sold to each other or to tourists. Families with more education generally have more members working and are wealthier than those with less education. Some families, especially those in more rural or outer island areas, continue to live a subsistence lifestyle, fishing, farming, and gathering to meet their needs.

Work opportunities for people with disabilities on the Pacific Islands are significantly more limited than for those without disabilities. People with disabilities frequently have less education and fewer English skills than people without disabilities, making the prospect of finding employment even more difficult. Pacific Island people with disabilities outside their own island communities may have the additional handicaps of low levels of English proficiency and of lack of education and/or skills necessary to succeed in the workforce. Also, their own cultural mores do not place high value on assertiveness and a Western work ethic that may be necessary to succeed.

Most Pacific Islanders moving to the United States have some basic education and skills, but they cannot easily compete in the job market against more-educated Americans. They may hold unskilled jobs, hold seasonal jobs, or rely on the few family members who have been able to get more highly paying jobs to support the rest of the family. People from Guam, CNMI, and American Samoa have the highest levels of education and may be more able to continue their education and get higher-paying or even professional jobs.

Education

Hawaii's educational system is similar to that of other states, except that the entire state makes up one centralized school district. The diversity of cultures and languages and the high levels of poverty among some ethnic minorities negatively affect the quality of education in the state. Many of the wealthier and more educated families send their children to private school, causing a drain of community resources away from the public schools.

Annie sat at the table looking at all of the professionals around her. Not one of them had actually met Alana, yet they were trying to get Annie to sign off on Alana's IEP. On the basis of therapy reports from California, they recommended physical therapy, occupational therapy, and speech-language pathology once per week for 30 minutes. This proposal wasn't right. Alana's skills were changing every day.

They had returned from California two weeks ago. Annie thought about the admonition that the physiatrist gave her. "Get Alana into school right away. The first year is the most important regarding her rehabilitation from a traumatic brain injury. She needs to get services immediately. Don't wait!"

She struggled with her confusion and frustration. Not one of the therapists or doctors who had started treating Alana on their return was at this table. Where was the communication between the health and the education people? What was wrong with this picture? Was it her job to make sure that happened? Well, she would just have to take it on.

Alana was at home now. She could not walk, she could not talk, and she drooled all of the time. Annie was sure that her daughter could learn her skills again. But she needed help to get her there. Once-per-week therapy was not enough. This time was critical.

Most local parents would have gone along and accepted what was offered. But Annie refused to sign the IEP.

All Pacific Islands have American style education available for elementary age children. High schools are also available, but in many places, only to a limited number of students who qualify through testing. Public schools are taught in the local vernacular through third or fourth grade, and in English thereafter. English is introduced to elementary school students as a second language, and by high school most are expected to be able to learn entirely in English. Private religious schools are also available in most Pacific jurisdictions where English is the language of instruction from kindergarten through twelfth grade. The cost of private education, although much lower than in the United States, is prohibitively expensive for most of the population.

Nowhere in the Pacific is the quality of education the same as in the United States. Teachers are not as highly trained; many have only a high school diploma or an associate degree. Some areas, such as American Samoa, are increasing their educational requirements for teachers. Other areas, such as Saipan, recruit teachers from the continental United States. Most areas have limited preschool or Head Start programs that cannot accommodate all children. In 2004, the U.S. government rescinded Head Start grants in all Pacific Island jurisdictions, and the programs were taken on by the local departments of education, but with less funding and serving even fewer children. Other jurisdictions begin schooling in kindergarten or first grade. Higher-education opportunities vary widely as well. Most major islands have a local community college offering vocational training. The University of Guam and the University of Hawaii as well as several California-based universities have affiliations with local colleges to provide four-year degrees and a few Masters level programs.

Individuals immigrating to the United States from the Pacific Islands have a lower level of formal education than have most Americans because of the lack of educational tools and skills in their home jurisdictions and the differences in language and culture. People immigrating to the United States with a disability may be at even more of a disadvantage entering the educational system.

Time and Situation

Neileen's family were finally taking her home! Her mother had passed the hospital training, and home care nurses had been trained to help care for her at home. Her parents took an earlier flight home so they could do last minute preparations. They were waiting at their door with Marshallese maramar (circlets of flowers and shells for the head) for the nurse, respiratory therapist, doctor, and paramedic who wheeled Neileen from the ambulance. The house was full of children. Cousins and aunts and uncles were lined up to greet Neileen, whom they had never met. She was put on a blanket on the floor, sitting up, while her equipment and crib were set up. Little children hung back, watching her, wanting to approach. Neileen signed "Come here!" and "Play with me!" to her cousins, but they didn't understand. Neileen scooted herself across the floor toward her cousins, stretching to the end of her ventilator tubing. The nurse moved the ventilator to allow her more room. Finally, one cousin approached, prompted by an adult, and gave her a kiss on the cheek. Other cousins then approached, and finally the children were interacting with her, handing her toys and books. Neileen bounced up and down in excitement, signing phrases that her cousins tried to understand.

At noon, Neileen's father looked at his watch and said, "Lunchtime?" The nurse nodded and was amazed to see him prepare Neileen's meal and medications without any help or prodding. He suctioned her, fed her through her gastrostomy tube, washed her face and hands, and set her back down on the floor to play. He talked directly to Neileen and paid only the necessary attention to the machines that helped to keep her alive. Apparently he had learned her care perfectly while watching his wife being trained at the hospital and was not intimidated by the machines.

When the nurse later asked him about his behavior, he explained that he was often exhausted on his visits to the hospital, having worked long hours in the weeks before to afford their plane tickets. He explained that he was her father, so he learned what he needed in order to care for her safely at home.

The hospital team left at the end of the afternoon, feeling confident that Neileen would blossom in her development at home and would be cared for safely by her family.

Concepts of time in Polynesia and Micronesia are different than in the United States, mostly because the pace and style of life are different. Rather than trying to get a lot done in a little time and compartmentalizing life into work/home/recreation/church, Pacific people work together to accomplish tasks over a period of time. They may work for a short while on one task, then turn to another, then return to the first. Family needs always take precedence over work requirements. If a family member needs to be taken to the doctor or if a family member dies, is born, or is married, people will always attend to those issues rather than go to work. Even in Hawaii, children may be absent from school because of family obligations that range from taking care of younger siblings, preparing food for a family gathering, or doing chores around the house (Ratliffe, 1999).

In the Pacific, being late is called being on "Hawaiian time," "Micronesian time," or "Samoan time." Time is plentiful in the Pacific; traditional people are more in touch with today than with the future (Ratliffe, 1998). This outlook is changing as the pressures of modern society encroach, but "Pacific time" still paces much of life in the Pacific.

Communication

Theresa handed Viliamu his home program. She had just gone over with him how to do the ten exercises on the paper. At the urging of an American Samoan coworker, she had illustrated each exercise with stick figures showing direction and amplitude of movement. "You need to do these every day so you don't lose the gross motor skills you gained while you were here. It's important that you keep your strength in the muscles you still have." She looked at him. "Viliamu, I want you to teach me how to help you transfer from your wheelchair to your bed. I need to make sure you know how to do that."

Viliamu looked away. That had been one of the hardest things—to learn to teach others how to help him. "Okay," he said reluctantly. He wanted to go home.

"What do you want me to do?" asked Theresa.

"Come over here," Viliamu mumbled. "Take off the footrests and slide me forward in the chair." He didn't look at Theresa.

"Viliamu, you need to look at me to make sure that I'm doing it right. Is this how you want me to do it? I didn't hear you clearly."

After ten minutes Viliamu was safely on the bed, and Theresa was satisfied that he knew the steps well enough to teach other caregivers. "Viliamu, you did that well! You need to have more confidence in yourself. You know how to do this, and others don't."

Viliamu sighed. "I know. I'm not comfortable telling other people how to take care of me."

"If you don't tell them, they may do it wrong and hurt themselves as well as you."

Viliamu sighed again. This was going to be hard. But he was going home tomorrow, and he would have to do it.

Although English is the language of commerce and instruction throughout the Pacific Islands, local languages reflect the culture and the community of the people. At least a dozen different languages are spoken throughout Micronesia.

Communication in the Pacific is not only through spoken language. Nonverbal communication is also very important. Because cultural mores dictate that people not always say what they think, nonverbal cues are essential to assess what someone is truly saying. Body language, facial expression or lack of expression, and actions can be more telling of what a person is thinking than his or her words. A health care provider should be aware of nonverbal communication cues and not be dependent only on verbal language when working with a person from the Pacific Islands. When a person acts differently than his or her words lead one to believe, this behavior does not mean that the person is lying or deliberately trying to mislead. Rather, it means that not enough attention was paid to nonverbal cues. The message is usually quite clear to the experienced listener/observer.

Some examples of "face talk" include the following:

1. Raised eyebrows mean "yes" or "agree."
2. Furrowed brow with little eye contact can mean "don't agree" or "don't understand," regardless of the words used.
3. Looking away with minimal or no response means "I'm not comfortable with this conversation/idea."
4. A direct gaze signifies strong feeling about the topic of discussion.

Health Beliefs and Practices

Roger sat on the plinth, looking at Alana. She refused eye contact and refused to participate in her therapy. "Come on, Alana, can't you just stand up for a minute?"

"Alana, I want you to stand up for Mr. Chin." Annie wasn't sure how to help. This was the third therapist she'd tried. Alana's stubbornness had caused both of the previous therapists to discharge her, saying that when she was ready to work, they'd be happy to see her again.

"What motivated her when you were in California?" Roger asked.

"She wouldn't eat until we brought in some poi (a paste made from pounded taro root) from Hawaii and froze it. Then we mixed it with everything. As long as there was poi in it, she would eat it. And rice. We had to give her rice with every meal. The speech therapist was amazed at how much she ate!" Annie laughed, remembering how frustrated she was at the time.

"There must be something. What does she like that's not food?"

Annie thought about it. She was determined to make this work. Her determination had worked for her so far. In California Alana was finally given a bed with rails. She had to move to an adult floor, but at least she was safe. The IEP was finally signed after each therapist assessed Alana and increased their recommendations on the basis of her progress since she had left California.

Roger saw the round cardboard discs that the local children collected and called POGS that were taped onto Alana's backpack on the back of her wheelchair. "Alana, do you like POGS?"

Alana raised her head. Roger walked over to her. "Oh, I have this one too," he said, pointing to one. "Do you want to see my collection?"

Alana nodded. "Okay, if you stand up, I'll even give you one." Alana struggled, but she stood up with Roger's help.

Annie smiled. This would work.

HEALTH CARE SYSTEMS

Health care in the Pacific Islands is influenced by their relationship to the United States and by their economies. In Hawaii, the health care systems are similar to most around the country with both fee-for-service and managed-care programs covering those with health insurance, and managed-care programs for those served under Medicaid. There is some choice of health care programs, but many managed care programs do not provide extensive rehabilitation or long-term care should it be necessary.

In the FSM, health coverage is mandated in their constitution and is viewed as an entitlement by the people. A December 1999 report on the status of health care in the FSM states the following:

> Recent surveys in the FSM have shown that most health consumers have a very low opinion of health services in the FSM, including the providers, the equipment and availability of supplies. However most still feel health services should be delivered without charge. Additionally, there is very little "ownership" of health services and responsibility for one's healthcare remains the government's business. (Development Associates, Inc., 1999, p. 104)

This perspective of health care decisions being left to the professionals and payment for it to the people in authority is also seen in sojourners to the United States. People travel to the United States to obtain what they perceive to be higher-quality health care than is available to them at home, and they are mostly happy to leave difficult decisions up to the medical personnel.

In FSM, primary health care is provided by health assistants working in dispensaries located in rural areas and on outer islands. Health assistants are trained on the job and provide triage, deciding who needs to be seen at the hospital and who can receive services at the dispensary. They also dispense medications. On the main islands, people either use a few health dispensaries or travel to the hospital for services (Development Associates, Inc., 1999). Some health assistants work as a team with doctors, and some work independently, but under a doctor's supervision. Doctors, called medical officers, are available in all areas of the Pacific Islands; however, the training that doctors receive may be different from that of American physicians. Many of the doctors have graduated from the Medical Officers School that was located in Pohnpei, FSM, and has relocated to Fiji. Most are trained as primary care physicians, not as specialists. As a result, there are few or no specialists in areas such as pediatrics, psychiatry, gerontology, or rehabilitation.

In American Samoa primary health care is provided by physicians at the LBJ Hospital in Pago Pago. Some specialists are available in limited areas such as pediatrics, but not for rehabilitation. Consultation is sometimes available from Hawaii and other areas of the United States, and patients who need tertiary facilities and rehabilitation can be sent to Hawaii, California, or New Zealand. Limited telemedicine services are available on Tutuila. However, cultural and social practices, as well as limited medical, social, and other resources still influence the outcomes for any person with a disability in American Samoa.

Service systems such as the Division of Vocational Rehabilitation are available in Hawaii, American Samoa, Guam, and CNMI, and can assist some people with disabilities to live more fully in their communities. Accessible housing, supported or even unsupported employment for individuals with disabilities, and assistive technology are not often available, or are limited, outside of Hawaii and Guam. The level of acceptance for individuals to pursue living more fully in their community is low because the expectation for people with disabilities is to live in the supportive environment of their families.

Disabilities Common to the Pacific Islands

Illnesses and disabilities seen more frequently in Pacific Island jurisdictions than in the United States include various forms of malnutrition. The change in diet resulting from the move from a sustainable lifestyle of gathering, hunting, and fishing, to a moneyed economy has led to malnutrition and undernutrition, especially in children. The governments have made efforts to provide supplements and educate people about necessary nutrition, but more work needs to be done. Vitamin A deficiency, common throughout the Pacific, leads to diarrheal diseases, night blindness, and otitis media, among other problems. Chuuk state in the FSM was found to have the highest percentage of Vitamin A deficiency in the world in 1988 to 1989 with 96% of children between two and seven years affected (Elymore, 2000). Other nutritional problems include a high incidence of lead poisoning and iron deficiency anemia. Both of these disorders can lead to mental retardation and other disabilities.

Other diseases leading to disability include a high incidence of otitis media leading to hearing impairment and deafness. A high incidence of meningitis is the leading cause of cerebral palsy and mental retardation. Meningitis is frequently not diagnosed in time to treat it effectively. Hydrocephalus cannot be treated because of the high costs and lack of neurosurgeons to place and monitor shunts, so that children are treated with supportive care rather than reparative care. This treatment leads to high incidences of disability and death in children with hydrocephalus.

Other disorders encountered with higher frequency include some genetic disorders with a high prevalence in certain areas of the Pacific Islands. For example, achromatopsia, a rare disorder of color blindness and lack of visual acuity resulting from a lack of cone cells in the eye is common on the island of Pingelap, an atoll off Pohnpei (Sacks, 1996). Achondroplasia, sometimes known as dwarfism, is relatively common on the island of Enewetak in the Marshall Islands.

Other disorders seen in high numbers among Pacific Island populations include diabetes, heart disease, and stroke. These diseases and their resultant disabilities are often the result of a poor diet, obesity, and genetic predisposition.

Alternative Health Care Practices

Most Pacific Islanders use local health care practices including herbs, massage, and magic. Herbal lore has been passed from generation to generation; however, much of the knowledge is being lost as Christianity "teaches" people to disrespect their own cultural knowledge and practices, and the older generation dies without passing on their knowledge. Herbs, locally available plants, and other substances are made into pastes and poultices through cooking; they are infused to make a tea; or they are ingested (Judd, 1997). Some are mixed with coconut milk or juice prior to being eaten. Massage is also practiced as a remedy for many ailments. Coconut and other oils are used as lotion.

Depending on the level of acculturation to Western ways of life, some families trust more in local medicines, whereas others trust more in Western medicine. Many families use both, and they may not tell the Western health practitioner about their use of local practices. Since Western medicine is available to most people in the Pacific, most are already familiar with basic preventative medicine such as immunizations and antibiotics when they come to the United States. The concept of rehabilitation is not yet widely understood.

BELIEFS REGARDING CAUSES OF DISABILITY

Perceived causes of disability relate primarily to the family's relationships internally within itself, externally with others, and with God (Cheng, Nakasato, & Wallace, 1995; Marshall, 1994). This attitude is especially true of families who have a child with a congenital disability. One perception is that a person with a quarrel or a grudge against the family put a curse or spell on them, or that a family member worshipped an evil spirit. Ghosts or spirits who live in the house, on the beach, or outside can cause illness or disability. Others believe that the cause relates to the behavior of the parents themselves. Parents may even blame each other, citing spousal abuse, excessive drinking, or sexual promiscuity as causes. Other common beliefs include environmental factors such as taking drugs, eating the wrong kinds of food during pregnancy, or going outside at night causing disability in children. The "meningitis shot" is frequently thought to cause the disability if children have cerebral palsy or deafness from meningitis infections. The "meningitis shot" may refer to the spinal tap or to the shot administering antibiotic used to treat the illness.

Causes of acquired disabilities are also ascribed to the individual or the family. For instance, a person who has a stroke may be perceived to have done something wrong in some way, to have offended God, and thus to be responsible for the disability.

In many traditional communities in the Pacific Islands, families who have children with disabilities are shunned; they are blamed for their own situation. Some families of typically developing children do not allow their children to go to school or to play with a child who has a disability. As people become more educated about Western medicine and about disabilities, these views are changing, and communities are becoming more accepting of children who are different.

Within families, in many cases, children with disabilities are considered the "most loved one." Others perceive that the child is "a gift from God." The life of the family revolves around the child with the disability. Yet, families frequently avoid bringing their child to social gatherings because of shame and because of social rejection. In some families, the mother may be blamed for the problem and bear the full burden of caring for her child. This outcome can cause rifts in families, leading to the neglect of the child in some cases or the stepping in of other relatives to care for the child.

BELIEFS REGARDING REHABILITATION

Rehabilitation is a concept that has not arrived in the Pacific Islands for the most part, except for Hawaii and Guam. The Division of Vocational Rehabilitation is funded in CNMI and American Samoa, so that many there are becoming more familiar with the concept. The strong belief that providing care and love are the fundamental priorities of families leads to the common conception of a person with a disability as someone to care for. The expectation that an individual with a disability can learn to care for himself or herself or can be productive in society is not yet common, although education and awareness activities are slowly changing attitudes.

The level of health care is secondary at best on the less developed islands. Local hospitals have only basic laboratory facilities, no intensive care units, few medical specialists, and few, if any, rehabilitation specialists (Developmental Associates, 1999). Care in the hospital is basic, with the family taking care of most daily needs. A family member usually stays in the hospital with a sick family member, sleeping near the person who is sick or injured. Once a person is discharged from the hospital, outpatient care is available for ongoing medical needs, and in some areas, for basic physical rehabilitation needs.

In American Samoa, the Marshall Islands, and The Federated States of Micronesia, physical therapy technicians were trained in the late 1980s to provide basic assessment and rehabilitation services through a Rehabilitation Research and Training Grant. Ten physical therapy technicians were trained, and some of them continue to run the physical therapy departments affiliated with hospitals. Some treat children with developmental disabilities as well as adults with acute and chronic orthopedic or neurological disabilities. The level of expertise is fundamental; however, many of the technicians have been practicing for over ten years and have developed more advanced skills in certain areas. Some hospitals have equipment such as parallel bars, crutches, mat tables, walkers, and wheelchairs, whereas some have very little equipment. Contracted therapists occasionally are hired for short periods of time, especially in American Samoa, and are able to set up procedures and written programs for assessing and treating people that can be carried on after they leave. In Guam and Saipan, many of the licensed therapists are contracted from the continental United States and stay for only a few years.

The Related Services Assistant (RSA) program is a relatively new program in FSM, the Republic of the Marshall Islands, American Samoa, CNMI, and Palau. Individuals (mostly special education teachers) have been trained since 1994 in a one-year educational program to work with children with severe disabilities at home and at school. RSAs assess motor, communication, academic, nutrition, and basic health needs of children, and also plan interventions. They liaison with health services and advocate for families and children to get needed services. They work with families and children on an ongoing basis to address their developmental needs and teach the children and families needed skills and strategies to benefit from their educational programs.

These two categories of personnel—the physical therapy technician and the related services assistant—are bringing the concept of rehabilitation to the Pacific Islands. However, many needs are still not being met. The community assumption about an individual with an acquired disability is that the family will care for him or her. In most cases, the individual is not expected to relearn skills. If the person with a disability chooses to relearn skills, the family will help by making minor adaptations such as making a cane or tying a rope between trees, and if they have time, helping the individual to walk. Assistance for the family in developing a rehabilitation plan is not usually available. It is up to the ingenuity and resourcefulness of the family to rehabilitate their family member. Concepts such as accessible housing, independent living, and supported employment are not yet part of the culture except in Hawaii, and to a lesser extent, on Guam. These concepts are not yet applicable to the cultures of the Pacific Islands. In the Pacific no one lives alone, work opportunities are limited for everyone, and everyone works together to surmount obstacles to daily living, or learns to accommodate to them. Some families choose to relocate to Guam or Hawaii where services are more readily available.

A recent emphasis on disability awareness on some Pacific Islands is educating people about the causes of disability and the potential for rehabilitation. This knowledge is beginning to change perceptions and to open the way to more effective rehabilitation of persons with disabilities.

Pacific Islanders in the United States

Service providers working with Pacific Island families in the United States will need to assess the families' level of acculturation to the American culture. Respect for the culture of the family, respect for the role of the extended family in decision making, and being aware of nonverbal forms of communication can assist the service provider to work more effectively with persons from Pacific Island cultures. The service provider needs patience to allow a relationship to develop with the family, to allow the family to process spoken and written information, and to allow the family to develop thoughts and questions. Finally, it is important to resist judging families negatively on the basis of American values, especially when the families' actions do not fit into the service system expectations (e.g., being late, not following directions, ignoring advice, not communicating effectively, not following through). These behaviors usually have their root in conflict between languages or cultures and will take patience and understanding to sort out. The effort taken to understand behaviors will result in the individual's and the family's receiving appropriate services and having the best chance at optimal rehabilitation.

Working with People from the Pacific Islands

The following list contains suggestions and ideas to help the service provider in working with people from the Pacific Islands.

Family Structure

1. Identify the decision makers in the family and ensure that they are included in important communications and decisions. Even immigrants to the United States may have a respected, older, or more educated person to assist in making decisions. It is important to identify this person and to speak to him or her prior to initiating a treatment plan.

2. Speak to the eldest person, the father, the mother, or the closest relative before you interact with a child. Obtaining permission to interact with the child is expected.

3. Don't ask about the background of the family; for instance, if the child is accompanied by an aunt or a grandmother, do not ask directly about the role and the whereabouts of the biological mother or father. The family is taking care of the child, and the specific information is considered private. This information will have to be asked if guardianship or consent to sign is an issue. Adoption of or fostering of related children is common in Pacific Island families and does not usually imply abuse or neglect.

Relationships and Social Structure

4. Develop a relationship with the family to engender trust and more open communication. Be patient and allow enough time for all interactions.

5. Carefully assess what the social status of interpreters and families is and how they interact with each other before relying on this form of communication.

6. Be persistent.

7. Parenting is a shared responsibility of the extended family. Trust that the family has the best interests of their family member in mind.

Religion and Spirituality

8. Expect that families may be using local methods of healing and that they may be reluctant to share this information with you.

9. Respect the strong religious affiliations that many families have.

10. Explore the family's understanding of causes of the disability.

Time and Situation

11. Call to remind the family about appointments. Get the phone number of an English speaking relative or neighbor to call. Schedule creatively to allow family priorities to be met.

12. Be clear about your expectations. Give information (phone numbers, addresses, directions) as often as needed.

13. Be mindful that other events may take priority for the family, and try not to negatively judge lateness, missed appointments, or lack of follow-through. Family obligations are many, and you do not know what the issues are for a family.

14. Assist families to navigate through the health care system. They may not understand the services that they are entitled to or how to access them.

Communication

15. Allow time to develop a relationship with a family. Shyness compounded by language difficulties can impede appropriate communications until a level of trust is built. The concept of "shame" includes embarrassment, shyness, and reluctance to be assertive. Only personal trust developed through the relationship can overcome shame to enable true communication.

16. Women service providers may have an easier time communicating initially with women of the family. Men may have an easier time communicating initially with men of the family. The authority of the medical personnel is always respected, whether male or female.

17. Pay attention to nonverbal communication cues. These might include body language, facial expression, lack of eye contact, silence, quick acquiescence, or avoidance of a direct answer to a question.

18. Do not assume that when a person tells you that he or she understands or agrees, that it is true. Assess understanding and perceptions of families in multiple ways such as asking for practical demonstrations of skills, asking them to repeat back to you what they heard, or asking their opinion about the matter from another perspective.

19. Allow silences to occur. People need time to collect their thoughts and sift through information, especially in a second language. Listen patiently.

20. If a family seems overly negative regarding the potential for rehabilitation for a family member, availability of resources, or their ability to cope, maintain a positive attitude, and encourage them to express their concerns.

21. Never raise your voice to a family. Deal with your frustration on your own. Expressing it verbally or nonverbally may damage any developing relationship.

22. Provide information using pictures or very simple written form if possible. For example, draw a stick figure with arrows indicating movement of limbs instead of verbally describing an exercise. This advice applies especially for home activities or exercises. Even families whose spoken English appears good may have difficulty reading English or understanding written documents.

23. Create a chart or poster documenting exercises and including photographs or drawings. This material can help a family understand the importance and the content of the home program.

24. Offer alternatives and encourage choices. Avoid yes/no questions.

Summary

The Pacific Island cultures compose a relatively small number of people but a varied array of beliefs and values. This chapter described the history of these peoples and many of the cultural values and beliefs that may influence their rehabilitation. Included in these values and beliefs are the importance of the family structure and how children are often raised by extended family members, the importance of being patient and developing a relationship with the family of the person receiving rehabilitation, and of respecting the likely strong religious and spiritual values of Pacific Islanders. The chapter also discussed and identified some of the cultural expression of communication and time orientation—expressions typically very different from mainstream Western cultures. As stated earlier, it is hoped that this chapter is just a starting place for exploring the richness and variety of Pacific Islander cultures, and the starting place for developing cultural proficiency in providing rehabilitation services to this population.

Annotated Bibliography of Useful References

Ridgell, R. (1995). *Pacific Nations and Territories: The Islands of Micronesia, Melanesia, and Polynesia* (3rd ed., Rev.). Honolulu, HI: Bess Press.

Riley Ridgell applies his considerable experience and knowledge about Pacific Islands to this well-organized and amply illustrated textbook. Geared toward advanced high school and college students, this text briefly summarizes in an easy-to-understand way the geology, geography, history, economy, and culture of the Pacific Islands. It is an excellent reference to have on hand, and it provides a balanced view of the inherent problems as well as the richness of culture in the Pacific.

Hezel, F. X. (2001). *The New Shape of Old Island Cultures: A Half Century of Social Change in Micronesia.* Honolulu, HI: University of Hawaii Press.

Father Hezel, a long-time resident and Jesuit scholar of Micronesian culture, history, and government, has shared his perceptions of and research into the social changes taking place in Micronesia since World War II. Presented in a very readable form, his research and insights into changes in family, land, gender roles, birth, marriage, death, sexuality, political authority, and population and migration over the last fifty years includes personal vignettes and statistics of social trends and changes, offering some understanding of the directions and the reasons for significant changes with implications for Micronesians living in the United States.

Cheng, L. L., Nakasato, J., & Wallace, G. J. (1995). The Pacific Islander population and the challenges they face. In L. L. Cheng (Ed.), *Integrating Language and Learning for Inclusion: An Asian/Pacific Focus (Culture, Rehabilitation, and Education)* pp. 63–103). San Diego, CA: Singular Publishing Group.

Hawaii, Guam, and American Samoa are the featured cultures in this chapter outlining history and demographics, lifestyle, and educational implications for students with disabilities. The discussion includes the overrepresentation of children in special education, implications of their limited English proficiency, and ideas for intervention. The treatment of each of the cultural groups is not balanced well, but the chapter gives a good overview of the cultures in relationship to children receiving special education services.

Questions

1. How does the Western perception of disability compare with that of people from the Pacific Islands?
2. Why do children of Pacific Island descent (including Hawaiian) qualify for special education services in a higher proportion than their representation in the community?
3. How does the tendency to "do for" individuals with disabilities, as opposed to "teach them to do for themselves" relate to Pacific cultural values?
4. What is the relationship between "natural" or "local" healing and more Western styles of medicine among Pacific Island people?
5. What is your belief about "natural" healing and the Western style of medicine?
6. How are your beliefs about "natural" and Western medicine influenced by your cultural background?
7. How has the history of colonization affected the relationship of Pacific Island people to Americans?
8. What are some of the differences in communication styles and strategies, and how can a rehabilitation professional accommodate or work with these differences?
9. How can a rehabilitation professional accommodate differences in the sense of time and of priority between himself or herself and a person from the Pacific Islands?
10. Discuss teaching strategies to use with a client who cannot read well.

References

Ashby, G. (Ed.). (1993). *Micronesian customs and beliefs* (Rev. ed.). Eugene, OR: Rainy Day Press.

Cheng, L. L., Nakasato, J., & Wallace, G. J. (1995). The Pacific Islander population and the challenges they face. In L. L. Cheng (Ed.), *Integrating language and learning for inclu-*

sion: An Asian/Pacific focus (Culture, rehabilitation, and education), pp. 63–103). San Diego, CA: Singular Publishing Group.

Development Associates, Inc. (1999). *Human resources study for ADB* (Rep. No.3165). Federated States of Micronesia: Development Associates, Inc.

Elymore, J. (August 23, 2000). Personal communication.

Grieco, E. M. (2001). *The Native Hawaiian and other Pacific Islander population: 2000.* U.S. Census 2000 Brief Series C2KBR/01-14, Washington, DC.: U.S. Census Bureau. Available: http://www.census.gov/population/www.cen2000/briefs.html.

Hezel, F. X. (May, 1993). Culture in crisis: Trends in the Pacific today. *The Micronesian Counselor* (Occasional Papers-No. 10). Pohnpei, Federated States of Micronesia: Micronesia Seminar-FSM Mental Health Program.

Hezel, F. X. (2001). *The New shape of old island cultures: A half century of social change in Micronesia.* Honolulu, HI: University of Hawaii Press.

Judd, N. L. K. M. (1997). *Laau Lapaau: A geography of Hawaiian herbal healing* (Doctoral Dissertation, University of Hawai'i). UMI Microform, 9733608.

Mamea, T. (2002). *It takes a village to raise a child: The acceptance of disability within the Samoan culture.* Unpublished Master's Thesis. University of Hawaii.

Marshall, M. (January, 1994). Social isolation, cultural competence, and disability in the Carolines. *The Micronesian Counselor* (Occasional Papers-No. 13). Pohnpei, Federated States of Micronesia: Micronesian Seminar-FSM Mental Health Program.

Oliver, D. L. (1989). *Native cultures of the Pacific Islands.* Honolulu, HI: University of Hawai'i Press.

Ratliffe, K. T. (1998). *Clinical pediatric physical therapy: A guide for the physical therapy team.* St. Louis: Mosby.

Ratliffe, K. T. (1999). *Perceptions of special education on Moloka'i* (Doctoral Dissertation, University of Hawai'i). UMI Microform, 9925290.

Reeves, T., & Bennett, C. (2003). *The Asian and Pacific Islander Population in the United States: March 2002,* Current Population Reports, P20-540, Washington, DC: U.S. Census Bureau.

Ridgell, R. (1995). *Pacific nations and territories: The islands of Micronesia, Melanesia, and Polynesia* (3rd ed., Rev.). Honolulu, HI: Bess Press.

Sacks, O. (1996). *The island of the colorblind.* New York: Vintage Books.

Samoan Service Providers Association Census (1990). *Needs Assessment Study.* American Samoa: Samoan Service Providers Association.

Segal, H. G. (1995). *Kosrae: The sleeping lady awakens.* Kosrae, Federated States of Micronesia: Kosrae State Tourist Division.

Ward, S. P. (1999). *Exploring the place of "Tautua" in the 21st century: A descriptive study of Samoans at work in their culture and in the marketplace* (Doctoral Dissertation, University of Hawai'i, 1998). UMI Microform, 9913970.

Yamauchi, L. A., Ceppi, A. K., & Lau-Smith, J. (1999). Sociohistorical influences on the development of Papahana Kaiapuni, the Hawaiian language immersion program. *Journal of Education for Students Placed at Risk (JESPAR),* 4(1): 27–46.

13

Cross-Cultural Meaning of Disability

Ronnie Linda Leavitt

Key Words

cross-cultural studies	disability	illness beliefs
ethnography	illness meanings	illness behaviors

Objectives

1. Examine the meaning of disability from a cross-cultural perspective.
2. Define strategies to foster cultural proficiency in clinicians.
3. Discuss the importance of using appropriate research tools for any given cultural group.

Introduction

Disability exists in all societies, yet how much does the casual observer (or even the rehabilitation practitioner) understand about the meaning of disability? How does one ever understand the lived experiences of people with disabilities (PWD)? Clinicians rarely appreciate the reality of disability and usually have no more than a passing familiarity with the prevalent "appearance" of disability. Is disability even a universal phenomenon?

This chapter will examine the meaning of disability from a cross-cultural perspective. Specifically, for a range of cultures, such issues as disability subcultures, beliefs and behaviors associated with disability, attitudes toward PWD, the macro (societal and community) and micro (individual and family) level responses to the presence of disability, and some strategies to increase cultural proficiency will be addressed. The underlying goal is to add to the cultural knowledge base of clinicians, while acknowledging at all times the need to consider both *intercultural* diversity and *intracultural* diversity. Information and examples given within the chapter may be extrapolated to other cultures. Generalized lessons (with varying details) may be applicable to more than one context. If the notion of culture is a construct always held in high regard, rehabilitationists will likely practice in a more culturally proficient manner.

In reality, the concept of disability is not a cultural universal. That is, disability as we know it is not a concept found in all known cultures. Sometimes PWD are expected to follow the same life cycle as everyone else. Disability does not define their status in the culture and thus does not serve as the identifying and unifying characteristic of a subculture. As Ingstad and Reynolds (1995) state: "In many cultures, one cannot be 'disabled' for the simple reason that 'disability' as a recognized category does not exist. There are blind people and lame people and 'slow' people, but 'the disabled' as a general term does not translate easily into many languages. . . . The concepts of disability, handicap, and rehabilitation emerged in particular historical circumstances in Europe" (Ingstad & Reynolds, 1995, p. 7).

If disability does exist as a recognized category, there is variation in its meaning. In individual cultures that have defined what constitutes a disability, its significance for the individual and their family depends upon each society's values. Attitudes toward individuals with a disability; concepts of rehabilitation; the sociocultural, biological, and economic implications of disability; and policy affecting individuals with a disability also vary.

The study of the meaning of disability is relatively new, and much of the research has historically occurred in the developed world. For individuals from a Euro-American culture, it is more likely that a subculture based on disability exists. Although many other variables, such as ethnicity, religion, or socioeconomic status, may be important determinants in helping to define an individual, disability may be paramount. For example, people with hearing impairments often identify primarily with "the deaf community" (culture). In Euro-American cultures, the following conditions are more likely to be present and contribute to a subculture of disability:

1. Medical treatment makes survival with disabilities common.
2. Culturewide concepts of normality and disability exist.
3. Cultural values stress individualism and achievement, and PWD are likely to strive for independence and autonomy.

4. Disability is an overriding determinant of status and identity.
5. PWD have opportunities to meet and interact with one another.
6. PWD have access to education and technology that facilitate their interaction with others.
7. PWD have access to a modern infrastructure such as transportation and communication systems. (Loveland, 1999)

The presence of a disability subculture within Euro-American communities has several implications for the rehabilitation practitioner. Most obvious is the greater likelihood of a fully developed program for the client, encompassing the physical, vocational, psychological, and social components of rehabilitation. Also, it is possible that the clinician will more readily become involved in the existing disability rights movement in an effort to ensure full participation of PWD in society.

In contrast, most of the world does not have these conditions, and the presence of a disability subculture with an associated disability-rights movement or patient advocacy group are absent or in the early stages of development. There are few rehabilitation professionals or lay people, and the barriers to accessing rehabilitation are at best difficult to overcome, and at worst, insurmountable.

Acculturation

To get a better understanding of "where one is coming from" when assessing disability and associated beliefs and behaviors, an assessment of acculturation—the degree to which an individual has taken on the characteristics of the normative culture—is necessary. Although other key variables may again play an important role, level of acculturation is particularly relevant to health status and the way that one interacts with the health care delivery system.

One may be fully assimilated (whereby boundaries between two cultures are erased), bicultural (whereby one has "a foot in each door" and is comfortable intermingling in both the "old/ethnic" society and the normative society), or traditional (whereby one maintains strong emotional and cultural ties to the original ethnic group). Many factors, such as migration history, age, socioeconomic status, place of residence, and more, affect the level of acculturation. Acculturation measures have been developed, relying primarily on the degree to which one speaks a first or preferred language at home, the media one relies on, and the degree of social interaction outside one's cultural group. Other instruments use scales to evaluate worldviews, values, and perspectives on individualism and collectivism.

Cultural Beliefs About Disability

The cross-cultural study of PWD is an emerging are of interest, especially using a sociocultural model rather than focusing only on biomedical factors, and especially in the developing world. Beliefs about the meaning of disability in a particular culture are one component of a society's general belief system about health and sickness, and they have meaning when considering what form of rehabilitation will be developed in a society. The cultural interpretation of disability depends on how a society attaches value and meaning to a particular type of disability. The interventionist, client, and family may each have a different perspective. Although there is intercultural and intracultural variation, three major categories of social beliefs seem to exist cross-culturally and tend to predict how well an individual will fare in a particular community. These are causality, valued and disvalued attributes, and anticipated role.

Causality

Causality refers to the cultural explanations for why a disability occurs. Few societies have only one explanation, and there may be different explanations for different disabilities. The range of variation in the beliefs concerning cause are considerable. Also, people often "hedge their bets," incorporating the notion of multicausality for one diagnosis. Typically, an informant might preface remarks with "I don't know, but maybe . . ." or "I believe such and such, but my mother (or husband, neighbor, etc.) thinks such and such . . ." "Natural" or "supernatural" possibilities exist.

People from the Euro-American cultures typically ascribe disability to natural causes such as disease (viruses, bacteria), environmental agents (accidents, toxins), or genetic disorders. Natural causation is also an explanation used in other cultures, but some explanations are more "scientifically sound" than others. For example, in Jamaica, a scientifically sound natural explanation could be, "fits damage the brain" or "the doctor say long time it take to born . . . The afterbirth is coming before . . . I had lots of clots . . . ." But some naturalistic belief systems are not supported by scientific reality. Again from Jamaica, "Like how I have the children fast and the food me eat . . . Me had a problem with me big daughter . . . sent her to buy shoes and she run away with a guy and she never come back until long after the baby born. I was very worried." In this case, the diagnosis was Down syndrome (Leavitt, 1992).

In many Asian cultures, naturalistic explanations often focus on the suspected failure of the mother to follow prescribed healthy practices during pregnancy and the postnatal period. For example, Chan (1998) reports a mother being blamed for her son's epilepsy because she ate lamb, a forbidden food, during pregnancy. Excessive "cold wind" and shellfish have also been held responsible for disability.

In contrast to these beliefs are those in which people believe in a supernatural cause for the disability. These explanations, however, must be viewed with caution. It is quite possible that informants underreport their belief in supernatural causes, or alternatively, one can believe in the supernatural but not associate it with one's personal situation.

The following supernatural explanations are more examples from rural Jamaica (Leavitt, 1992). The "duppy," meaning ghost or spirit, is frequently blamed for things that go wrong or are evil. Duppies can be visible and invisible, and they can work through people, animals, birds, and plants. Duppies live and play around the silk cotton tree and are especially fond of the night. They are thought to be unpredictable, sometimes helpful and sometimes harmful.

The duppy . . . well, because babies are small, people who pass off like to play with them. That's what cause the life of my last baby . . . When you leave baby alone, the duppies play with him. The duppies want to give assistance.

When me seven months, I saw a duppy and was frightened. Also, the house family lived in was over a graveyard.

I believe in normal sickness with some addition of evil. The devil throw some sensation on her at the school.

The Kumina Queen (a religious leader), who is the "adoptive mother" of a retarded boy says,

It's a kind of spiritual order . . . the mother leave him at night and when she coming back for it nobody there to look about the baby. Spirit come and fingle it [plays with it or caring for it] . . . me give the child sugar and water and the spirit no like that . . . the father says spirit feed him—him sick and vomit up some green things [the child vomits up the bad spirit food].

In many cultures, religious beliefs are highly associated with a supernatural belief system. For example, a common belief is that the birth of a child with an anomaly is evidence of divine displeasure and punishment due to such things as parental sin or breaking of a taboo. Not infrequently, supernatural belief systems are associated with witchcraft, spirits, or ancestors who are punishing the PWD or, if a child, the parents because of their "inappropriate" behavior. Divine intervention is presumed in the Old Testament, when PWD were not allowed to approach the alter, and in the New Testament, when Christ, upon restoring sight to a blind man, is reported to have said "go and sin no more." The Buddhist and Hindu religions also suggest the theory of retribution whereby a sin in a past life is responsible for a present situation (Groce, 1999; Leavitt, 1992). Alternatively, as reported in Mexico, God can selectively choose parents who will be particularly kind and protective for "special" children (Madiros, 1989). In Botswana, the birth of a child with a disability can be seen as either God's trust in the parents' ability or as a punishment for a past transgression (Ingsted, 1999).

Some examples from Jamaica (Leavitt, 1992) having to do with God's role in a child's disability are the following:

I just believe God make him and he make everyone of us to his own likeness.

Well, maybe he [God] would [have caused the child's disability], he know that I can cope. Because I don't think he going to give you more than what you can manage.

Sickness is not our fault. God gave it to us. We have faith in God.

In contrast, a few people specifically stated that they did not believe God had any connection to their child's problems:

I don't believe that God make him sick like that. Me say is me the problem come from since me was young.

I don't believe God ever give you anything that is bad. If you are sick it's just maybe a natural thing.

God don't make anyone sick. Sickness is from the devil.

For people of Hispanic origin, people may also become sick (i.e., be punished) if they have sinned or violated a taboo, thereby causing the wrath of God or other source of wickedness. The belief in the evil eye is not uncommon. Generally, the concept implies that an evil spell has been put on another, which causes the victim to fall ill. The motive is usually envy. Other folk beliefs include the notion that a pregnant woman must be careful using a sharp object or the child may be born with a cleft palate, and if she is knitting clothes for the child, she cannot wind the yarn into balls, or the child will be born with the cord wrapped around the neck. Alternatively, an imbalance of elements, or humors, may be responsible for the disability. There needs to be a balance of "hot" and "cold." These mutually complementary forces are required for one to be in harmony with nature (Zuniga, 1998).

People of Asian origin may also believe in supernatural causes (divine punishment) and the need to have harmony by balancing hot and cold forces of nature. In the highly acclaimed and very readable book *The Spirit Catches You and You Fall Down*, Anne Fadiman (1997) describes the cultural conflict between a Hmong family whose daughter Lia has a seizure disorder, and her American doctors. The Hmong people are an extremely traditional group from Laos, many of whom have unwillingly immigrated to the United States as a result of the Vietnam War. The Hmong see illness as a spiritual matter linked to everything in the universe, whereas the medical community in the United States denotes a division between the body and spirit. The Hmong call Lia's illness *quag dab peg*—the spirit catches you and you fall down—that is, the soul is taken and you cannot get well until the soul is returned.

Native Americans often consider multiple causal factors as responsible for disability. Supernatural causes may relate to spirit loss, spirit intrusion, spells, or witchcraft. Naturalistic causes may involve the notion of imbalance or disharmony, secondary to breaking a cultural taboo, acculturation, or an accident (Joe & Malach, 1998).

Valued and Disvalued Attributes

Valued and disvalued attributes also play a role in determining a cultural belief system regarding disability. If the society values physical strength and beauty (as defined by that particular culture), then individuals who do not display these attributes will be considered less likable, less worthy, and more disabled. If the society favors intellectual capability, then being physically limited by a wheelchair might be seen as less significant. In most communities, being disabled makes one stand out from the group. In Native American communities, being different and calling attention to oneself is particularly stressful.

Related to the notion of disvalued attributes is that of stigma. Although there is not complete consensus, most often PWD are considered to have an observable deviation from the norm. Associated with deviance is stigma; typically a PWD is branded with stigmata, that is, "marks" or "blemishes." The stigmata are used to assign a negative value to the deviant person (Goffman, 1963). The construction of individual and societal models of stigmatization of PWD seems intimately connected to beliefs concerning causation of disabilities, typically those that are supernatural in origin. As Goffman states, "A disability is often considered evidence of God's displeasure of one's own or one's family's past behavior . . . a stigmatized individual is presumed to be not quite human, and often a sign of danger" (Goffman, 1963, p. 5).

Although there is evidence that attitudes toward PWD are becoming more positive, there is little theoretical research trying to link cultural variables with attitudes toward PWD. One such relatively recent study, "Attitudes Towards Disabilities in a Multicultural Society" (Westbrook et al., 1993), investigates the differences in the attitudes of six cultural groups in Australia with regard to twenty diagnoses. Overall, PWD were accepted most by the German community, followed by the Anglo, Italian, Chinese, Greek, and Arabic groups. It is interesting that the results did not show significant differences with regard to the concept of stigma hierarchy: in all communities, people with asthma, diabetes, heart disease, and arthritis were the most accepted, and people with AIDS, mental retardation, psychiatric illness, and cerebral palsy, the least accepted.

In another study, Leavitt (1992) investigated families with disabled children in a poor, rural area of Jamaica. A majority of the interviewees did not believe that their child was stigmatized. In fact, most noted that their family and neighbors seemed to be quite fond of the child in question. When a subject reported hearing negative comments, it was generally believed to be an isolated incident. The informant typically added, "I don't pay them attention." It is of interest to note that when a child was not taken outside the house in a manner similar to that for other children, caretakers specifically stated that the reason was because doing so posed a physical burden for them. In other words, the child was too heavy to be carried. (Only three children in the study population had a wheelchair.) Some other reasons were that the child has no shoes, the child holds the caretaker back, the child is teased by others, or the child is "rude" (i.e., naughty). Nevertheless, it is likely that stigma may have been a factor in some of the households. Although stigma was not present in most instances at the family and local community level, children with disabilities are not being prepared to fully integrate into Jamaican society. They are rarely able to attend school, and they are not prepared for any future vocation.

Likewise, being labeled as deviant is associated with the notion of contagion. There is fear that a disability might be "caught" or that one could become "contaminated." Some Native American parents discourage their children from having any contact with PWD or even touching assistive technology; and in Kenya, a hut for a PWD might be built far away from those of others, and the person's belongings cannot be touched (Groce 1999).

Anticipated Role

The role that people can play as an adult and how much they can contribute to the household income is the third category to consider. Some may find work outside the home, but more typically a PWD may contribute by watching children, doing housework, or doing farm work. Some may be assigned tasks that others do not want. For example, Groce (1999) cites a study done in Ecuador where rural families who were introduced to iodized salt for the purpose of eliminating iodine deficiency syndrome (mild mental retardation and hearing loss) were concerned that there would be no one to collect firewood, draw water, or herd animals. The material conditions of a community are bound to affect belief systems and decisions regarding disability and adult roles, especially in poor communities.

In sum, there can be a wide range of variation with regard to beliefs about the cause of disability within the larger community or within a family unit. An understanding of the belief system can contribute to the clinician's overall understanding of the client, his or her family, and the sociocultural context in which they live. This understanding will impact the design of the rehabilitation program and the ways in which the therapist might approach the client. For example, if a family believes that the PWD has a disvalued attribute or has no future productive role as an adult, the focus of an intervention might first be on trying to educate the family about what virtues the patient has, what can be realistically accomplished (as opposed to solely focusing on their limitations), and how the person may contribute to the family and society.

Cultural Response to the Presence of Disability at the Individual Level

An individual with a disability is likely to seek some form of intervention in an attempt to "cure" or minimize the effect of having a disability. Beliefs might impact the patient's decision regarding what medicines to use and foods to eat, or what exercises to do. Behaviors vary substantially between and among cultures and can be quite different from those held by the Euro-American. Depending on the individual's sociocultural background, services may be provided for by a "Western" style health professional, "traditional"/indigenous healer, or lay person/family member. Examples of traditional healers include, but are not limited to, curanderos (Mexican-American), espiritistas (Puerto Rican), santerios (Cuban), vodoo priests (Haitian), diviners (Southeast Asian American), singers (Native American), and the more generalized herbalists, astrologers, and more. Each has his or her own repertoire of skills and rituals. In reality, the practical issues of availability, cost, and severity of episode account for the choice of practitioner.

Leavitt (1992) described health behaviors associated with children with disabilities in rural Jamaica. The African heritage is reflected in much of the current Jamaican culture and folk medical belief systems. In particular, the Jamaicans' belief in African forms of witchcraft and animism is relevant to their behavioral response to the presence of disability. *Obeah*, or the practice of witchcraft, is "essentially a magical means whereby an individual may obtain his personal desires, eradicate ill health, procure good fortune in life and business . . . , evince retribution or revenge upon his or her enemies, and generally manipulate the spiritual forces . . . to obtain his will" (Morrish, 1982, p. 41). The *obeah* man or woman keeps his or her "things" in his or her *obi* place. These "things" are composed of such materials as blood, feathers, parrots' beak, grave dirt, rum, and egg shells, and his or her "bush" is a concoction of medicinal herbs. The *obeah* may sometimes cause a problem by "putting" the spirit sickness on a person, or the *obeah* may "work it off." Reportedly, many people visit an *obeah*, even though it is forbidden by law. Strongly linked with the practice of *obeah* is the belief in "duppies."

Jamaican folk medicine practices can be as simple as the use of a bush tea for a cold, avocado to lower high blood pressure, and pawpaw to get rid of a boil, or as complex as the treatment by an *obeah* man or woman employing many of the previously mentioned materials. Most "bushmen" are not *obeah* men or women but rather spiritualists who believe that herbs can strengthen the physical body and therefore help to ward off ailments. Often, the spiritualist believes in the necessity of supporting the healing herbs with religious ceremony, charms, fresh air and sunlight, or other foods such as cock soup or roasted animal testes.

Examples of statements concerning the use of indigenous healing practices for the treatment of a child with a disability in rural Jamaica are the following:

I use baths a whole lot of times, in the night, put wash pan of water over here, and put two sticks and cross them—let it stay overnight, and bathe him in the morning.

Me boils coconut oil and mix with olive oil—use it to anoint her legs. They say it help the stiffness.

Catch water from six in the evening and let it sit all night and get night dew. Wake him at five in the morning and sop [beat] him legs in it.

I put milk in the bath, and no talk with anyone until after the bath.

Bathe her in Old Man Beard bush.

Dig a hole to the level of the waist. Bury him in it for one hour, remove him and stand him.

Me use grapefruit juice and brandy to wet his mole [brain]. It helps to keep his brain steady.

Yes, I wouldn't hide you that [going to a mother lady], cause I had to try all that because I see and get the vision and maybe it can be a different inferior spirit come along and hurt her.

The mother lady sent me to the bush doctor shop. Get some kind oil to use on her and bush to boil.

Associated with these healing practices are folk tales. The following are examples regarding babies, shared by a group of women who worked with a pregnant Peace Corps volunteer.

Place an opened pair of scissors or a horseshoe over the bedroom door where the baby sleeps to keep away evil spirits.

Duppies are afraid of red, newborn babies should have a red ribbon tied around their left wrist and wear red clothes to ward off evil spirits.

Do not let menstruating women hold a baby or it will get stomach cramps.

If a pregnant woman has sex with a man other than the baby's father, the baby will be handicapped.

When baby's navel stump falls off, the mother must bury it outside under a young plant to ensure that the baby will grow strong and healthy.

Do not cut a baby's hair before he can talk or he will have problems talking.

Religion appears to be as important a factor in influencing the caretaker's behavior with regard to treatment practices as it was in influencing the caretaker's belief system.

> When the child does not have a duppy sickness the mother takes her to a doctor. But when it is a duppy sickness, "You get a different power to deal with that. Me lay my hand on him and pray . . . I know when they [the duppies] come and run them . . . I rebuke the spirit and he have to go . . . Only I is safe to do it, because me only one who feel the holy ghost. I is a Christian . . . I speak unto God . . . speak in tongues . . . It happens at the moment and I interpret the word. The Lord will keep away the duppies.
>
> God is able to do all things. I leave him in God's hands.
>
> I think God have a different plan for him. I'm praying to see that plan when it come through. I love him [the child] very much—what hope for him I'd like to be around when that hope come through. God will make him better in a way he can help himself.
>
> I know the Lord can heal him . . . I don't know if my faith is strong enough. You need great faith . . . Darvey [the child] no have faith.
>
> I'm a Christian you know, and he weren't like this you know [the child had been functioning at a lower level]. I took him to the Throne of Grace, and I laid on him right here and I prayed on him day and night and I ask God to touch him because he used to run all over the place as though him mad . . . but I entreated him to God and I laid on down on him and I pray and I say God touch him. I kept on asking the Lord to touch him, and I can see for *sure* him better.
>
> The Kumina Queen says, "You have to call to God before you do anything . . . me deal with God direct . . . me no deal with the duppy one [obeah man] . . . me speak seven different languages and speak in tongues . . . I can't make him [the child] talk, God have to give that."

As one might expect, there is a strong tendency for the Jamaican respondents who believe in the possibility of a supernatural cause of the disabling problem to also use traditional healing practices. For this study population, the concept of intracultural diversity is supported by the range of variation of beliefs and behaviors with regard to disability and rehabilitation.

A majority of Hispanic people, but not all, are Roman Catholic, and generally speaking, Hispanics rely heavily on Catholicism to support them during times of stress. Religious beliefs are again closely tied to folk remedies. Therapists are generally familiar with beliefs such as the power of holy water to ward off evil or bringing a sick elder to pray before the image of a saint. At the period of death and dying, the praying of the Rosary and last rites are representative behaviors. Additionally, the "hot cold" paradigm is relevant. For example, blood is "hot" and is associated with strength, virility, and machismo. If one is anemic, one might eat more "hot" foods such as those organ meats that are considered blood products.

For the Hmong, traditional healing practices, including animal sacrifice and special ceremonies involving such tools as a saber, gong, rattle, finger bells, and a "flying horse," are paramount as is the role of the *txiv neeb* (indigenous healing practitioner). These are not only very different practices from those used in the United States, but the Hmong also believe that American doctors remove organs from their patients to eat or sell as food, that they anesthetize patients to allow the patient's soul to escape, and that they cut the "spirit-strings" from patients' wrists, thus disturbing their "life-souls" (Fadiman, 1997). It is easy to imagine how both a traditional people and the Western medical practitioner view the other as strange, ignorant, and stubborn. Conflict can easily arise.

In summary, once again there is a wide range of variation in the individual response to the presence of disability. It is the professional's responsibility to have a full understanding of the rehabilitation practices that the patient is partaking in to avoid conflict and to improve overall communication, as well as to ensure an overall appropriate treatment program. One must consider whether or not alternative practices are efficacious and safe. Clinicians must acknowledge and accept, rather than ridicule, differing belief systems and behaviors associated with disability as long as they are not harmful to a person. (Some folk remedies do include arsenic, lead, or opium, and these can be dangerous.) Ideally, a PWD should be able to "call upon" a wide range of treatment alternatives, depending on one's own personal comfort level with the activity.

Cultural Response to the Presence of Disability at the Societal Level

PWD have always been part of human society. In Iraq, there is evidence of a skeleton of an elderly Neanderthal with a withered arm and blindness in one eye. The grave site, covered with flowers, gives an indication that he was a valued member of society. Ancient art and early legends from Greece, Rome, India, China, and the Americas all show evidence of the existence of PWD and their oftentimes high esteem (Groce, 1999). Conversely, although exceptionally rare, a small number of groups have practiced infanticide, usually by abandoning an infant after birth. Outright killing of older children or adults because of disability is almost unheard of (Scheer & Groce, 1988). Exceptions include reports of killing deformed babies (the Masai tribe), poisoning children who have polio (Ivory Coast), and country-specific holocausts (Nazi Germany) where people without disabilities were killed as well. Nevertheless, through the preindustrialized era, even when they were perceived as misfits, PWD were generally maintained in a life-supporting environment and somewhat integrated into society.

For Euro-American societies, during the industrial era, society began to think of PWD as sick, helpless, and needing to be taken care of. The lack of attention to the sociocultural context of the patient, along with medical advances, led to a biomedical, institutional service model that called for the segregation of PWD. Patients were presumed to be unable to function in their own best interest and were expected to take the "sick role" (i.e., they are freed from normal social roles and responsibilities). In this model, providers are presumed to be the expert and are likely to view the patient as a compilation of body parts and systems with little attention paid to the whole. The intention is benevolence.

Still, in modern times, many of the points just enumerated with regard to the allocation of scarce resources still hold true. In part, their persistence depends on the cultural explanations regarding cause of disability, valued and disvalued attributes, and anticipated role as an adult. For instance, although Euro-American cultures typically ascribe disability to the germ theory, genetic disorders, or accidents, the idea of blame sometimes remains strong. People might immediately ask a mother of a child born with a disability whether she drank, smoked, or used drugs during pregnancy. A man with paraplegia is oftentimes given more sympathy if the disability is a result of fighting for his country as opposed to resulting from a driving accident while he was drunk. It is especially likely that a child or PWD might be considered a disgrace and thus hidden from public view or not given the benefit of limited resources when the disability is thought to be the result of parental sin or God's displeasure. Groce (1999) contends that this need to ascribe causality is related to one's ability to justify demands made on social support networks and community resources.

An example related to attributes is the value associated with gender. In Nepal, there are many more boys reported to have polio than girls. The assumption is that girls do not survive because they are either placed at greater risk by being less well nourished, not being adequately immunized, or not being given allotted resources to facilitate survival or recovery. As for anticipated role, PWD were, and still are in some societies, expected to contribute to the family income by their role as beggars. In some cases, begging is clearly associated with disgrace. Conversely, in a rural Mexican community, Gwaltney (1970) describes elderly persons who became blind as a result of onchocerciasis and beg for a living, as being treated with respect. The blind villagers derive a sense of approved and purposeful participation in the life of their pueblo, and there has been cultural accommodation on the part of the community.

Hanks and Hanks (1948) hypothesized that the degree to which a society is willing or able to bear the costs incurred in caring for PWD depend on several interrelating materialistic and cultural factors. Some of these determinants are the relative socioeconomic status of the society (which includes such factors as the number and type of productive units, the need for labor, the amount of economic surplus, and its mode of distribution); the social structure of the society (including whether or not the society is egalitarian or hierarchical, how it defines achievement, and how it values age and sex); the cultural definition of the meaning of the disability (does the symptom of the disability require magical, religious, medical, legal, or other measures?); and the position of the society in relation to the rest of the world. Although there are significant differences in health status and health care systems, including rehabilitation, among contemporary societies, the differences are most extreme between the "developed," or "industrialized," societies and the so-called developing, or Third World, societies. These differences, although influenced by sociocultural practices, primarily reflect the wide economic gap between the two groups.

Leavitt (1999) adds to this by noting that a major impediment to the process of public policy development regarding individuals with a disability is the fact that general health care and rehabilitation for PWD have historically been a very low priority throughout the world. There are many reasons for this situation. First, the cost-benefit ratio of providing rehabilitation to PWD has always been considered poor compared with other health programs. Second, there has traditionally been an underestimation of the potential achievements that a disabled person can accomplish. Third, there is a history of negative attitudes toward persons who are disabled. In many societies, PWD have been seen historically to be deviant from the norm and have been considered to have a social stigma or "attitude that is deeply discrediting . . . a failing, a shortcoming, a handicap" (Goffman, 1963 p. 3). Fourth, when discrimination limits participation by PWD in various social roles, their plight becomes even more invisible. Fifth, there is an apparent absence of urgency. Rehabilitation is associated with disease and illness that are, for the most part, neither acute, communicable, nor "exciting." The general public will not be at risk, nor will its opposition be mobilized, if rehabilitation services are not given to the populations in need. Sixth, on an individual level, mainstream biomedical practitioners tend to reflect a value orientation that stresses mastery of disease and stresses taking personal credit for recovery. In cases in which an individual has a disability, often very little dramatic curing can occur; in some instances, further loss of function is anticipated. Although a wide array of simple and complex technologies are available, the provision of these services does not ensure dramatic results. Thus, many caregivers find rehabilitation frustrating and often not worthwhile. Last, individuals with disabilities are a disadvantaged minority and, accordingly, have little political influence when lobbying for the opportunity to affect public policy.

Having said the preceding, there is still room for optimism. More recently, a new paradigm has developed based on self-determination, self-representation, and human rights. The United Nations Year *of* Disabled Persons (as opposed to *for*) in 1981 marked a turning point on the international scene with regard to the perception of PWD. Originally, the action plan called for an increase in bigger institutions and more training of professionals. But, as PWD became more involved themselves, a new model emphasizing cooperation and partnership evolved. The theme of the Year became "full participation and equality." The Decade of Disabled Persons (1983–1992) was built on the promotion of equalization of opportunities and rights for PWD (McColl & Bickenbach, 1998). "Undoubtedly, the major achievement of the Decade was the increased public awareness of disability issues among policy makers, planners, politicians, service providers, parents and disabled persons themselves" (Boutris-Gali 1992, p. 4). Antidiscrimination legislation has since been enacted, to varying degrees, throughout the world. In the United States, the Americans with Disabilities Act (1990) declares that PWD have a right to pursue "equality of opportunity, full participation, independent living, and economic self-sufficiency" (McColl & Bickenbach, 1998, p. 159).

The newest paradigm, focusing on a client- or family-centered model, including community based rehabilitation (CBR), independent living, and paying attention to the client and his or her family's sociocultural environment has yet to be embraced by all. The process of change is slow, as evidenced by the many physical, political, societal, and personal obstacles that a lot of PWD face in their everyday lives. Nevertheless, society and the field of rehabilitation are moving in this direction. Do we not all have a responsibility to work toward a more humane societal response to the presence of disability that can benefit the PWD and society as a whole?

Issues Needing Our Attention to Foster the Development of a Culturally Proficient Rehabilitation Professional

Cross-cultural research investigating the attitudes, beliefs, and behaviors relevant to disability and rehabilitation is in an early stage. As the world—and likely one's place of employment—becomes increasingly multicultural, the need for such research will become both pragmatic and morally vital. To be more specific, the rehabilitation clinician uses a range of interview techniques and functional scales to assess patient status and evaluate intervention efficacy. Most of these tests have been standardized for the Euro-American culture and lifestyle; yet in the United States, people of non-Euro-American heritage are at greater risk for disability and have greater secondary complications and mortality rates associated with disability. Merely translating an assessment tool into another language is insufficient. For example, a data analysis of the Denver Developmental Screening Test (DDST), a commonly used pediatric instrument, has indicated that some developmental skills emerge at significantly different ages for Alaska Native children, as compared with the normative group of white, middle-class children in the United States (Kerfeld, Guthrie, & Steward, 1997).

Similarly, Gannoti (1998) found differences between the normative group and a population of children living in Puerto Rico. For this group, using the Pediatric Evaluation Disability Inventory (P.E.D.I.), Gannoti noted several social customs affecting the age at which developmental skills were expected to occur. For example, young children in Puerto Rico, in contrast to Euro-American children in the United States, typically use a bottle at night for up to six or seven years, may not use a fork for fear of injury, wear diapers for public outings to avoid the use of public restrooms, and do not have the opportunity to put on socks or tie their shoes, because they wear Velcro sandals all year. Is the P.E.D.I. appropriate to use to evaluate children's development if the expected developmental age is different for this population? Also, many typically used functional tests do not take into account activities such as eating with chopsticks, eating with hands, or moving in and out of the squat position. These activities may be everyday requirements for people from Asia. Research in this arena will help lead to cultural proficiency, that is, when cross-cultural research is held in high regard, when it is disseminated, and when new approaches are developed in response to need.

As we enter the new millennium, it is also likely that rehabilitation professionals may face increasingly difficult moral dilemmas. Prenatal screening tests to detect a potential genetic abnormality, disease, or disability in a child followed by selective abortion is likely to become more common with advancing medical technologies. What effect will this outcome have on attitudes toward PWD? Will each individual make choices, in part based on their own cultural belief system? According to Adrienne Asch (1999), an advocate for disability and women's rights, the technology is based on the erroneous assumptions about the adverse impact of disability on life. Asch supports the "pro-choice" perspective, but if we are to assume the value of continued differences within the society and family, she "challenges the view of disability that lies behind social endorsement of such testing and the conviction that women will, or should, end their pregnancies if they discover that the fetus has a disabling trait" (Asch, 1999, p. 1650). Asch argues that PWD are often healthy individuals who describe their conditions as givens of their lives. Societal rules and laws, such as the Americans with Disabilities Act, can alter existing discriminatory practices, although there is a long way to go. It should not be assumed that PWD do not have fulfilled and satisfying lives.

Case Study (Leavitt 1992)

Sara is a bright three-year-old girl who has a right hemiplegia. Her right arm assists her left, and she walks with several deviations, although she does not use a brace or an assistive device. She came to the United States two years ago from Jamaica and lives in a two-room home with her parents and four siblings. Both father and mother have part-time jobs.

When asked to describe the history of Sara's illness, Mom said: "She didn't born that way . . . She born, and when she was about eight months, she was walking. She took sick, take her to the doctor, we have been visiting the doctor with her for pretty nearly a month, and she make no change. She just droopy . . . the fever comes on . . . the fever left her, but she still looks weepy and droopy . . . The father carry her to hospital. They say she malnourished . . . Saturday she have fits about two times . . . They put her on the drip . . . she go through it nearly a month. . . . When she come home we have to learn her to walk all over again." Upon further questioning about the perceived cause of the disability, Mom says, "in the first instance when she sick, when she was having the fever, he [the husband] say it was me cause I bathe her late and such . . . I see no problem in that, because I do it with all the others . . . and nothing ever wrong with them." Upon further prodding, Mom admits that the grandma and others ". . . tell me the duppy on him. A lady that die in here, and shortly after she buried, she [Sara] take sick, so they say . . . because she used to go up and down and round the yard . . . I don't know . . ."

Regarding the name of Sara's "problem," mom says, "I don't really call it anything you know . . . but people call her cripple." After some time at home, the mother went to the pediatric clinic, where she learned some exercises. When asked more about exercise, the mother responded: "The father exercise the foot morning and night . . . and he take time and stretch the foot and fingers right out . . . They (the physiotherapist at the hospital) say we have to do it early morning before the food and if she feed or you exercise it after feedin it don't have any use to her because the food goes in the bone already gettin it a little stiffer, so do it early mornin and late evening." When asked about home remedies, Mom says she uses "olive oil . . . they say I must get the olive oil blessed . . ." As for divine intervention, "God will make she [Sara] get better, because she start walking again, . . . she's coming on."

In order to understand Sara and her family better—from their (emic) point of view—and for a clinician and the family to develop appropriate goals and activities, one should do a medical ethnography, that is, one should study the culture of the people involved. Arthur Kleinman (1980) sees the health care system as a special kind of cultural system that includes such elements as patterns of belief about the causes of illness, decisions about how to respond to specific episodes of sickness, and the actions taken in order to effect a change. The beliefs and behaviors exhibited by an individual are influenced by macrosocial and bioenvironmental factors. Specifically, Kleinman has developed the theory of an "explanatory model" (EM) in order to analyze this kind of cultural system. "EM's are the notions about an episode of sickness and its treatment that are employed by all those engaged in the clinical process. The study of patient and family EM's tell us how they make sense of given episodes of illness, and how they choose and evaluate particular treatments" (Kleinman, 1980, p. 105).

To elicit an EM, the rehabilitation professional might ask the following questions to gain the client's (or family's) personal point of view regarding the disability and the role that you will take to facilitate rehabilitation:

Questions

1. What do you call your problem?
2. What do you think caused your problem?
3. What do you think your sickness/disability does to you?
4. What are the chief problems that your illness/disability has caused you?
5. What are the most important results you hope to get from your treatment?
6. What are the consequences that you most fear as a result of your disability?

An understanding of Sara's family's EM should facilitate an improved outcome for Sara and greater satisfaction for the family and therapist.

Summary

It is presumed that there are PWD in every society and that there will be specific medical care and sociocultural systems and explanatory models that account for the beliefs about the disability and the cultural patterns of behaviors having to do with disability diagnosis and treatment. The social construction of disability is undoubtedly related in part to societal attitudes toward disability, the material realities of the environment, and the adaptation mechanisms that are available for any individual and his or her family. Rehabilitation clinicians must believe that the notion of cultural competence is as important as clinical competence. Cultural proficiency acknowledges and incorporates at all levels the importance of culture, the assessment of cross-cultural relations, vigilance toward the dynamics that result from cultural differences, the expansion of cultural knowledge, and the adaptation of services to meet culturally unique needs (Cross, Bazron, Dennnis, & Isaacs, 1989; Lynch & Hanson, 1998). I believe that it is our professional moral imperative to embrace diversity and to develop the most appropriate service models and public policy to enhance the lives of all PWD, no matter what their cultural heritage.

Questions

1. Discuss some of the many reasons people give for having disability (causality).
2. What kind of influence would a client's belief about causality of disability have on his or her participation in their rehabilitation?
3. Relate the dominant cultural values of the United States to the attitudes that are often shown to the disabled.
4. Why is it important to have a full understanding of the patient's belief about disability and the healing practices that the patient may be carrying out?
5. Discuss the reasons that rehabilitation has historically had low-priority status throughout the world.
6. Name some strategies to help raise community awareness about the value of rehabilitation.
7. Discuss some reasons that assessment tools must be culturally appropriate to any given population.
8. What are some benefits of being able to perform prenatal genetic screening?
9. What are some moral and ethical problems that can arise with the ability to perform prenatal genetic screening?
10. Evaluate your own cultural beliefs about people with disabilities. Compare and contrast your own beliefs to those of a different culture.

References

Asch, A. (1999). Prenatal diagnosis and selective abortion: A challenge to practice and policy. *American Journal of Public Health, 89*(11), 1649–1657.

Boutris-Ghali, B. (1992) *Message of the Secretary General: World Programme of Action Opens Way to Full Participation in Society* in *Disabled Persons Bulletin,* No.2, Publication 64. Vienna, Austria: United Nations Center for Social Development and Humanitarian Affairs.

Chan, S. (1998). Families with Asian roots. In E. W. Lynch & M. J. Hanson (Eds.), *Developing cross-cultural competence: A guide for working with children and their families.* pp. 251–344. Baltimore: Paul H. Brookes.

Cross, T. L., Bazron, B. J., Dennis, K. W., & Isaacs, M. R. (1989). *Towards a culturally competent system of care*, vol. 1. National Technical Assistance Center for Children's Mental Health, Georgetown University, Washington, DC.

Fadiman, A. (1997). *The spirit catches you and you fall down.* New York: Farrar, Straus and Giroux.

Gannoti, M. (1998). Ph.D dissertation. *The Validity and Reliability of the Pediatric Evaluation of Disability for Children Living in Puerto Rico.* University of Connecticut, Storrs, CT.

Goffman, E. (1963). *Stigma: Notes on the management of spoiled identity.* Englewood Cliffs, NJ: Prentice Hall.

Groce, N. (1999). Health beliefs and behavior towards individuals with disability cross-culturally. In *Cross-cultural rehabilitation: An international perspective.* R. Leavitt (Ed.). 37–47. London: W. B. Saunders.

Gwaltney, J. (1970). *The thrice shy: Cultural accomodation to blindness and other disasters in a Mexican community.* New York and London: Columbia University Press.

Hanks, J., & Hanks, L. (1948). The physically handicapped in certain non-occidental societies. *Journal of Social Sciences, 4,* 11–20.

Ingstad, B. (1999). *Problems with community mobilization and participation in CBR.* In *cross-cultural rehabilitation: An international perspective.* R. Leavitt (Ed.). London: W. B. Saunders.

Ingstad, B., & Reynolds, S. (Eds.). (1995). *Disability and culture.* Berkeley: University of California Press.

Joe, J., & Malach, R. (1998). Families with Native American roots. In E. W. Lynch & M. J. Hanson (Eds.), *Developing cross-cultural competence. A guide for working with children and their families,* 127–164. Baltimore: Paul H. Brookes.

Kerfield, C., Guthrie, M., & Steward, K. (1997). Evaluation of the Denver II as applied to Alaska native children. *Pediatric Physical Therapy, 9,* 23–31.

Kleinman, A. (1980). *Patients and healers in the context of culture.* Berkeley, CA, and London: University of California Press.

Leavitt, R. (1992). *Disability and rehabilitation in rural Jamaica: An ethnographic study.* Associated University Presses, Inc. Rutherford, N.J.

Leavitt, R. (1999). *Cross-cultural rehabilitation: An international perspective.* London: W. B. Saunders.

Loveland, C. (1999). The concept of culture. In *Cross-cultural rehabilitation: An international perspective,* 15–24. R. Leavitt (Ed.). London: W. B. Saunders.

Lynch, E., & Hanson, M. (1998). *Developing cross-cultural competence: A guide for working with children and their families.* Baltimore: Paul H. Brookes.

Madiros, M. (1989). Conception of childhood disability among Mexican-American parents. *Medical Anthropology, 12,* 55–68.

McColl, M., & Bickenbach, J. (1998). *Introduction to disability.* London: W. B. Saunders.

Morrish, I. (1982). *Obeah, Christ and Rastaman: Jamaica and its religion.* Cambridge: James Clarke and Co.

Scheer, J., Groce, N. (1988). Impairment as a human constant: Cross-cultural and historical perspectives on narration of social issues *44*(1), 23–37.

Westbrook M., Legge, V., & Pennay, M. (1993). *Attitudes Towards Disabilities in a Multicultural Society. Social Science and Medicine, 34*(5), 615–623.

Zuniga, M. (1998). Families with Latino roots. In E. W. Lynch & M. J. Hanson (Eds.), *Developing cross-cultural competence: A guide for working with children and their families*, 209–250. Baltimore: Paul H. Brookes.

14

Poverty in the United States: Making Ends Meet

Shannon Munro Cohen

Key Words

poverty   socioeconomics   health insurance

Objectives

1. Discuss the influence of poverty on the access to rehabilitation services.
2. Identify resources to assist clients in need of financial assistance.
3. Identify how your own social class either promotes or inhibits your access to health care services.

Introduction

The United States is considered one of the richest countries in the world, yet it has a large number of homeless individuals and many more people who live in poverty. Although social class is less distinct in this country, it deserves an introduction in the context of poverty in the United States. This chapter begins with a review of the socioeconomic classes: upper, middle, and lower class. In each class, there are additional distinctions between levels as well. Briefly addressed are problems of urban versus rural poverty; hunger; violence; homelessness; the effect of poverty on women, children, and the elderly; and the needs of immigrants to this country. In addition, recent changes in legislation and the health and rehabilitation needs of this group are outlined.

Socioeconomic Class

Social class is influenced by many variables including income, lifestyle, political power, and behavior. Values and role expectations are similar among members of each social class. The upper level, or the affluent, comprises about 6 percent of residents, with an annual income greater than $100,000. They own businesses or work in highly respected professions. The affluent family is usually well educated, contributes to the community through volunteerism and donations, and influences the politics in this country. With privileges come expectations of altruism and responsibility. The upper class value privacy, education, success and initiative, and competence and control. They believe that hard work brings rewards and are generally thought to possess a sense of limitless possibility.

The lower-upper class comprises well-known people such as famous physicians and athletes who have prestige and earn high incomes. They are viewed differently by the upper-upper class, who have long-established wealth. Upwardly mobile professionals and managers may be included in this group. They share values of competition and the desire for acquisition. However, they believe less strongly in philanthropy.

The upper-middle class consists of college educated, highly paid professionals including physicians, lawyers, dentists, and engineers. They value stability and may have political and social involvement. This class has a strong work ethic. Children earn an allowance, and they work as adolescents. They value initiative and achievement with little concern about financial matters.

The middle class consists of people who have some status related to their education or occupation but who are not wealthy. Their occupations do not involve hard manual labor. Examples of professions associated with the middle class include health care providers and educators. The middle class is involved in community activities and organizations, and develops close ties with neighbors. This group is family oriented and shares many of the values of the upper-middle class such as preventative health care and education.

Blue-collar workers make an important contribution to society. They make up the lower-middle-class working level. This group includes carpenters, farmers, waiters, and others who work at more physically demanding jobs to support their families. Men and women tend to have more traditional roles in this group, with the burden of child-rearing resting primarily with the mother. People in this group may seek out health care only when it affects their work. The lowest-paid members of this group live close to poverty with less formal education.

The last social group are the poor, the focus of this chapter. The poor lack funds to meet basic needs and may possess a sense of powerlessness to change their circumstances. Acute poverty is a result of job loss and/or major illness, with an expected return to the lower-middle class. Individuals and families living in chronic poverty hold little hope of improvement. The poor have the least education, and they work in low-paying jobs, most often without medical insurance or job security.

Frequently poverty is described as a distinct culture within America's overall culture. Individuals become acculturated to a life of poverty, becoming resigned or adapting to their circumstances. Economics influences societal attitudes and behavior toward the poor as well as within this group. Negative images abound in America, "the land of opportunity," where people are expected to be successful and self-supporting.

Poverty brings to mind several images. One image is the swollen belly and the thin legs of a malnourished child from a war-torn or starving nation as seen on television. One may envision the struggle of the single mother with many mouths to feed. Another is the image of the person down on his or her luck, out of work after a series of mishaps. These mishaps may include poor financial decisions and choices, substance abuse, and criminal behavior. Negative images of poverty include the drug addict receiving government aid and the person too "lazy" to find employment.

Regardless of the circumstances, the results are similar. People living in poverty are unable to seek adequate health care. Prescriptions are left unfilled in order to pay for heat and food. Children miss opportunities to reach their highest potential. Thus the cycle of poverty continues.

The current U.S. poverty rate is 12.1%, the lowest rate since 1979 (U.S Census, 2003). This percentage amounts to 34.6 million children and adults in this country. Household incomes are highest for Caucasians followed by Asians and Pacific Islanders, American Indians, Alaska Natives, Hispanics, and African Americans. Poverty rates are highest among American Indians, Alaska Natives, and African Americans at 23%. The U.S. Census Bureau has not differentiated between whites, American Indians, and Alaska Natives until recently, with an estimated poverty rate of 10% that does not differentiate between those mainstreamed versus people living on reservations and native villages.

Rural Poverty

Many Native Americans live far from medical services. The remote location of many Native Americans leads to medical staff recruitment problems and limitation of care to emergency cases (Noren, Kindig, & Sprenger, 1998). Repeatedly, after staff members develop rapport with the people and become more culturally sensitive, they are promoted to more urban administrative positions, leaving a void in rural health care. Funding is also an issue. The federally funded Urban Indian Health Program budget currently meets the needs of one-fourth of the population and equipment, and facilities are outdated. Chronic diseases such as diabetes are on the increase in this group, as well as problems associated with substance abuse.

Urban Poverty

The cities have become a refuge for the poor, as professionals and the working class leave urban areas for residential neighborhoods in the suburbs. Mortality rates in Harlem, New York, for persons between ages 5–65 years old are higher than those in Bangladesh, which has the lowest incomes in the world (Prewitt, 1997). High mortality rates in inner cities are linked to cardiovascular disease, diabetes, pneumonia, influenza, alcohol and drug abuse, and violence. In addition, sexually transmitted disease and communicable diseases such as tuberculosis are increasing in prevalence.

Social Problems and Poverty

Violent crimes are increasing in the United States. Crowding, decreased job opportunities, and economic inequality escalate conflicts in urban areas. For white males, the lifetime risk of being murdered is 1 in 280, and for African American males the risk is 1 in 40 (Fox & Zawitz, 1999; Martinez, 1996). Among 10 to 24-year-olds, homicide is the leading cause of death for African Americans and the second leading cause of death for Hispanics. Those living in low-income communities become desensitized to the violence around them and are unable to afford housing in safer neighborhoods. Fewer than 5% living in violent communities report crime to the police or join together to prevent crime in their community.

Most violence, however, occurs within the family. The American Medical Association (1998) reported that 80% of homeless mothers have experienced family violence and that 70% reported physical, sexual, and/or emotional abuse during childhood. This abuse continues into adulthood by the partner or spouse. The victim of abuse is often prevented from achieving independence through education and employment. For example, efforts to find employment may be sabotaged by spousal abuse the night before an interview.

Children who witness or experience such violence perpetuate abuse. Sons who witness abuse by their fathers have a 1,000% (astonishing) greater chance of battering as adults (Germain, 1995; Kenning, Merchant, & Tomkins, 1991). The financial cost of domestic violence in the United States annually is estimated to be $67 billion in housing for domestic violence victims, social services, health care, and criminal justice (Laurence & Spalter-Roth, 1996).

The picture of homelessness has changed from transient men to single parents with children, mostly families headed by single women around 30 years of age (United States Department of Health and Human Services, 2003). There are an estimated 400,000 homeless families in shelters. Of these shelter inhabitants, 1.1 million are children averaging five years of age (Nunez & Fox, 1999). Family homelessness continues to rise with African Americans making up the majority of homeless families.

Inadequate low-income housing and domestic violence are the main reasons for homelessness. Most of the homeless are single mothers with children fleeing abusive situations. Families rotate through shelters after exhausting their stays with relatives and friends. They avoid the streets for fear of losing their children to foster care. Absence of heat and electricity or shelter overcrowding are the primary reasons children are moved to foster care. Onetime events such as job loss or a house fire are rarely the cause of homelessness.

Adolescent pregnancy and lack of education contribute to homelessness. Over half of the homeless receive less than a high school education because they have a child as a teen. Work inexperience and chronic unemployment are common among the homeless. Lack of a permanent address and the lack of adequate child care and transportation compound the problems.

Homeless individuals are at greater risk for medical and social problems. They present with advanced stages of disease, often requiring aggressive treatment and hospitalization for conditions that could have been prevented. Many chronic illnesses such as coronary heart disease, frequently seen among this population, are worsened by their living conditions. Communicable diseases such as tuberculosis, hepatitis, HIV, and influenza are common. In addition, it is difficult to ascertain whether high rates of mental illness and substance abuse among this population contribute more to homelessness or are a result of homelessness.

Children and the elderly have recently exchanged places in poverty statistics. This change is likely due to the powerful government lobbying of their representatives in the American Association of Retired Persons (AARP). If lobbying were directed at helping women and children, poverty levels would surely fall among this group as well.

Children comprise 16.7%, which amounts to 26 million children, higher than any other age group (Dinan, Fass, & Cauthen, 2004). As many as 5.8 million are living in extreme poverty, which is defined as $6,500 annual income for a family of three. The child poverty rate in the nation's capitol at 45% exceeds that in New York at 24%.

Enrollment of children in Medicaid has fallen despite extension of coverage for those losing welfare benefits. The Balanced Budget Act of 1997 included $20 billion over five years for states to develop health insurance plans for uninsured children. With this funding, Congress enacted the State Child Health Insurance Plan (SCHIP). It has not been widely publicized, with low enrollments reported. Of the 8.5 million uninsured children in this country, one-fourth are eligible for SCHIP, and half are eligible for Medicaid (United States Census, 2002). Food stamp usage for children has fallen due to the new legislation.

In Massachusetts and Virginia, legislators chose to use their federal SCHIP funding to establish the Children's Medical Security Plan (CMSP). This plan covers children under 18 who are uninsured for primary or preventative care. Other states have opted for school-based insurance programs and/or managed care programs.

Children need a stable environment and education in order to grow and flourish. Poor children are often left unattended or in substandard child care while parents struggle to make ends meet. Perinatal complications, substandard nutrition, less cognitive stimulation, lower teacher expectations, and poor academic readiness all contribute to lower school achievement. Homeless families relocate frequently, disrupting schooling and increasing dropout rates. In stark contrast to children in more financially secure homes, 62% of homeless children read below grade level, 28% are behind in math, and 37% have repeated a grade (Nunez, 1996).

As poverty among children has increased, so have the number of children enrolled in special education. Forty percent of adolescent mothers live below the poverty line, thus contributing to lower birth weight and premature births that are directly associated with physical and learning disabilities (Roth, Hendrickson, Schilling and Stowell 1998).

The number of children in special education has risen from 3.7 million in 1976 to 6 million children in 2004. These children receive services through the Individuals with

Disabilities Education Act (IDEA) part B state grants. IDEA funds programs to meet the educational needs of children with disabilities through specialized school programs. Disability is more prevalent among male children, single-parent households, and those living under the poverty level (Newacheck & Halfon, 1998).

Families receiving aid have a high burden of illness. Chronic illness in children was reported by half of families receiving benefits, with an increased risk for health problems such as asthma, injuries, lead poisoning, developmental and behavior problems, physical abuse, and neglect. Living in crowded homeless shelters puts children at increased risk for communicable disease such as chicken pox and upper respiratory infections.

Poor children with asthma often require hospitalization that could be prevented through close monitoring of symptoms, avoidance of secondhand smoke and allergens, assistance with administration of medication, and adequate medical care. Parents working minimum wage jobs do not have the flexibility or sick leave to be with their chronically ill child. Parental nicotine use may outweigh the needs of the child for a healthy environment, higher-quality food, and medicines to prevent illness.

Another issue is the lack of continuity of care with health care providers (often because of inconvenient clinic hours and rotating staff) and the unnecessary use of hospital emergency rooms for sick care (Beal & Stein, 2000). These families have many unmet needs. The emergency room setting does not provide appropriate and needed education, prevention screening, and follow-up care. Developing a long-term relationship with families in an outpatient setting provides opportunities for support and anticipatory guidance to prevent illness and injury.

Injuries, a leading cause of death among youth, are increased with insufficient housing and adult/parental supervision. Children are often kept indoors because of community violence and lack of safe play areas. Witnessing familial and community violence leads to feelings of hopelessness, anxiety, low self-worth and depression, and mirroring destructive behavior. Many adolescents living in public housing do not believe that they will live to adulthood.

Women

For every dollar that a man earns, a woman is paid $.74 (2003, United States Census Bureau, 2000). This figure compares weekly median income. This finding means that men occupy higher-paying positions. The inability to pursue employment in higher-paying jobs results from lack of educational opportunity often due to early childbearing and family obligations. Income discrepancy, combined with the burden of child-rearing and caring for elderly parents, leaves women unable to deal with unexpected crises. Friends and family in like circumstances are often unable to help.

Unlike that for men, women's health care includes reproductive issues and concerns. Many women receive all their preventative health care from their obstetrician. This tendency is especially true for women with low incomes, if they receive any health care at all. Regardless of income, women deserve control over their bodies and need ready access to education and contraception. Killion (1998) found several reasons for poor women's choices regarding childbearing and denounces the misconception that "by having children, the poor create their own poverty."

It is a paradox and an injustice that society expects poor women with the fewest resources to be more "in control" of their reproductive lives than women from other segments of society. (Killion, 1998)

In her 5-year ethnographic study, Killion found that homeless pregnant women had little choice in the timing, place, partner, and circumstances surrounding pregnancy. Lack of access to contraceptives, victimization and economic survival, uncertain fertility due to irregular cycles, desire for intimacy, and "hope for the future" are reasons for pregnancy among the poor. Most women conclude that if they were to wait until they could afford children, they would never have them. Medicaid currently provides coverage for birth control, but the lack of transportation and long waits for obstetric and gynecologic services limit this benefit.

The Elderly

Current poverty rates for the elderly remain stable at 10.4%. The median income for a person over age 65 in 2001 was $25,098 (United States Census, 2003). It is increasingly difficult to obtain reimbursement for medical care and nursing services. Elders are discharged from the hospital sooner with little provision for their care. Family members assume uncompensated care of the elderly with an estimated annual cost of $196 billion (Arno, 1999).

Over 7 million family members and friends provide the elderly with daily assistance. However, of the 1.4 million requiring daily care, 22% have family incomes below the poverty level (Kennedy, 1997). Unpaid middle-aged daughters make up 72% of the caregivers for the elderly, many of whom still have children living at home. Thirty-two percent of these caregivers live with incomes less than 125% of the poverty level themselves (Robinson, 1997). With the recognition of the value of home care, the national budget request in 2001 included $125 million in financial support for caregivers through respite and adult day care.

Problems for the elderly include inadequate nutrition, substandard housing, exorbitant utility payments, and high health care costs. During weather extremes, food may be purchased with money left after paying heating or cooling costs. Over 60,000 lives are lost each year to cold weather through fires and carbon monoxide poisoning from portable heaters, as well as hypothermia, pneumonia, and influenza from inadequate heating compounded by chronic illness (Bollwahn, 1999).

The elderly on "fixed" social security incomes often cannot afford to keep their homes in good repair, and preventable medical problems progress because they lack transportation or funds for prescription medications. Lost to many are the abilities to recognize and implement their skills to adapt in ways such as pooling resources and establishing small group living environments, offering support and shared resources.

Immigrants

Family size, level of education, work experience, and number of years in this country affect poverty for immigrants. This group faces similar problems compounded by language and cultural differences. Many suffer from depression and mental illness after fleeing war-torn countries. Immigrants avoid applying for Medicaid for their children born in the United States, because they fear that they will be viewed as a burden and refused citizenship. They also face hostility from the community since immigrants are perceived as taking jobs away from the native born and may be targets of violence in low-income housing areas.

Language barriers are cited as the greatest obstacle to health care, followed by lack of cultural understanding and transportation for new immigrants. Flores, Abreu, Olivar & Kastner (1998) found that lack of Spanish-speaking staff or interpreters led to poor medical care for Latino children, including misdiagnosis and prescription of inappropriate medication. Cultural differences include the Hispanic expectation that health care providers have a positive respectful attitude. The neutral attitude and casual demeanor of most American health care providers may be viewed negatively by other cultures.

Preventative health care, such as screening for hypertension, papanicolau tests (Pap smear) for cervical cancer, and mammography, is often not available in other countries. Therefore, immigrants do not use these screening methods.

Immigrants often arrive undervaccinated with contagious diseases such as tuberculosis (TB). It is difficult to explain to individuals who test positive for TB that they must take medicine for over six months with potentially dangerous side effects when they themselves feel fine. Asian and Latino populations are more likely to have drug resistant forms of TB and gonorrhea because of incomplete treatment for disease (Flaskerud & Kim, 1999). Hepatitis B, HIV, and other sexually transmitted diseases are common among the poor and homeless.

Welfare Reform

In 1996, the government announced plans to end the welfare program with the goal that families would find employment and become self-supporting. The Personal Responsibility and Work Opportunity and Reconciliation Act of 1996 (PRWORA) has eliminated $55 billion in funds. These federal funds support welfare, food stamps, and disability income support. The act eliminated Aid to Families with Dependent Children (AFDC) and replaced it with a capped, block program, Transitional Aid to Needy Families (TANF). The TANF caseload dropped 59% in 1993 to 2.1% of the population receiving benefits.

The TANF program limits recipients to five years of benefits during their lifetime; 23 states have time limits of less than 5 years. States require parents to work after 2 years of assistance. Single parents must work a minimum of 30 hours a week. Parents with children under 1 year of age are exempt; 12 states offer exemption only for parents with children under age 3 months. Parents of children who are disabled must meet strict Supplemental Security Income (SSI) disability standards to be exempt from the work requirement. Several states require community service of those who cannot find employment. Benefits may be withheld from immigrants for five years after their arrival. Victims of domestic violence may be given a time waiver, but this choice is at each state's discretion.

In addition, the government has enacted several requirements to decrease unmarried and teenage births. In order to receive assistance, unmarried adolescent parents are required to live with a responsible adult. To receive aid, the teen parent must stay in school. This requirement, of course, places the burden of raising the child on middle-aged grandparents. Immediate employment is expected from support recipients in many states. Individuals who have more children while receiving benefits receive no additional funds. Many states base benefits on identifying paternity and "compliance" in obtaining child support.

Young parents have a difficult time because they do not have the job experience and skills to secure adequate employment. Acquiring job-skill assistance and/or education is not a requirement of state funding in the plan; pursuing a high school diploma equivalency or college education does not alter work requirements. States are strongly encouraged to use available funds to develop transportation programs to help the poor seek and maintain employment. Hidden costs such as reliable transportation, work clothing, easy-to-prepare foods, and increased child-care fees are not calculated in the cost to families.

Employment, however, does not guarantee adequate support for families. One parent works in 87% of poor families with children (Dinan, 2004). A family of four supported by full-time employment at minimum wage is 36% below the poverty line (USDHHS, 2003). Transitional services such as food stamps and Medicaid are underutilized because of stringent state rules and confusing eligibility requirements. The Earned Income Tax Credit is seldom used; it assists families of four with incomes of approximately 35,000 by taxing at a lower rate. Individuals who take advantage of this tax break may receive income "disregard" as much as 50% of earnings (Dinan, 2004; Schlosberg & Ferber, 1998).

Hunger

Recent decreases in food stamp enrollment reflect changes in legislation, not individual or family need. An estimated 31 million people in the United States experience food shortage and hunger (Anderson, 2000). Requests for food assistance from volunteer organizations and subsidized school lunches for children continue to increase. The poor experience frustration over technical problems and the limited hours of the food stamp office. Recertification requires salary verification from one's employer as often as every three months. This requirement is a source of embarrassment to workers. Of interest, owning a reliable car worth more than $4,650 disqualifies one from receiving such assistance.

The effects of poor nutrition are long-standing. Undernutrition, in the form of inadequate calories, folate, iron and other nutrients, leads to poor growth and iron deficiency anemia. Iron deficiency anemia affects more than 1 million low-income children with serious implications for future cognitive development (Sherman, 1999). In addition, the risk of lead poisoning increases in children living in older homes, resulting in lasting brain and kidney damage and hearing loss in severe cases.

The food supplement program for women, infants, and children (WIC) helps to fill the nutritional void for pregnant women and their children up to age five. This program also lost much of its funding despite the fact that good nutrition decreases the number of low-birth-weight premature infants, pregnancy complications and hospitalizations, special education needs, and disability payments.

Adults also have poor nutrition and hunger. Parents feed their children first, often skipping meals. In one study of diabetic hypoglycemic (low blood sugar) reactions, many were directly related to inadequate food at home (U.S. Government, 2000). Up to 16% of the elderly population have experienced food shortage with profound implications to their health (Wellman, 1997). The elderly tend to utilize community food banks and church assistance rather than obtaining food stamps. Malnourished elderly patients take twice as long to recover from illness and have longer hospital stays.

Health Care Needs

One of my nursing students recently described her care of a homeless man. He had fallen and broken his hip. He had no money and no one to supervise or assist with his rehabilitation after discharge. The shelters would allow him to stay only at night for a limited number of days. He saved food from his hospital trays and stored it in the bedside table. He appeared worried when the student noticed his drawer full of food. She gently asked him to save only food that would not require refrigeration, as she was concerned about his health. We left the unit disturbed, as he did not qualify for a longer length of stay in a rehabilitation facility and social services had not devised a solution (U.S. Government Printing Office, 2000).

In the United States, 43.6 million people have no health insurance (U.S. Census, 2002). Other options and free services are often unattainable because of lack of transportation, missed work for appointments, child care costs, and language barriers. Generally, health care services provided for the poor are comparable, but the people do not receive the continuity and individualized attention received by those with private insurance. After waiting all day at clinics, patients often receive impersonal, abbreviated visits with "the next available" caregiver.

Additionally, Medicaid is of little benefit if the neighborhood lacks providers who accept government reimbursement. Health care providers may avoid caring for this population because they receive less reimbursement for services and because they experience frustration with those who miss appointments and do not follow recommendations for treatment. Extended hours, support, and information about available resources in the community are essential to meet the needs of this group.

Interpreters and Spanish-speaking health care providers are needed, since Hispanics now outnumber African Americans as the largest minority in the United States. The 38 million Latinos in this country exceed the total population of most Latin American countries (U.S. Census, 2003). Of this group, 24 million are children.

Cultural awareness regarding degree of formality, eye contact, space, and independence and family involvement are all issues that health care providers need to consider and respond to appropriately to when planning and implementing treatment. Asians may prefer to squat when eating and to use chopsticks, which demands unique dexterity and requires considerable flexibility. Culturally specific treatments may be sought before allopathic medical treatment. Many Vietnamese believe that they require less medication because of smaller body size and therefore may not follow directions without considerable discussion, education, reassurance, and support.

Many homeless individuals are unemployable because of substance abuse and/or chronic mental illness. Major depression is reported by 12% of mothers receiving welfare assistance (Manisses, 2000). Addiction and illegal drug use were reported by 21%, with 5% of those on welfare using cocaine (3% using crack). Therefore, it is imperative that health care providers screen for substance abuse, cognitive impairments, and mental illness.

In addition to increased rates of communicable disease and substance abuse among the impoverished, diabetes is a major cause of morbidity and mortality. High rates of insulin dependent diabetes among poor Latinos and African Americans often result in end stage renal disease and other complications. Because of the Western diet and sedentary lifestyle, non-insulin dependent diabetes is a serious risk factor that is increasing among people from the Philippines. The cumulative degenerative effects of diabetes are seen most dramatically among the poor who do not have access to or receive consistent medical care and follow-up, education, and screening.

Hypertension and cardiovascular disease are common across all socioeconomic and racial groups. African Americans and Hispanics are at highest risk. The New England Journal of Medicine (Gornick, 1996) reported substantial effects of poverty and race on mortality. Researchers found that African American males had fewer life-saving procedures such as coronary artery bypass surgery and more debilitating surgeries such as amputations resulting from diabetes than Caucasian males had. Delay in seeking treatment and less preventative care are believed to be the primary causes.

Rehabilitation Programs and Legislation

Veterans are frequently counted among the poor in the United States, and often they do not use services available to them. The Veteran's Administration offers support to veterans with service-related disabilities through the Vocational Rehabilitation and Employment program (VR & E). This program provides veteran's assistance in preparing for, finding, and maintaining employment. Other veterans with more severe disabilities are assisted in living as independently as possible. Vocational rehabilitation is available for veterans for a maximum period of 48 months.

In 1990, the Omnibus Budget Reconciliation Act allowed states to redirect nursing home funds to home health programs that aid the elderly with day-to-day activities such as bathing (referred to as activities of daily living, or ADLs). Ever-changing political agendas have brought proposals to limit funding to the "most severe" cases.

The Rehabilitation Services Administration (RSA) has many services available for the disabled poor. Most of the programs listed here share federal and state government funding:

- Independent living services for older individuals who are visually impaired assist these individuals either to find suitable competitive employment and/or to function at the highest nonemployed level possible. The goal is independent living for participants.
- Independent living programs funded by state grants maximize the abilities and functioning level of individuals with disabilities.
- Supported employment, a states grants program, works to maximize the potential of the most disabled persons through supported employment such as sheltered workshops, job coaching, and adapted environments and tasks.
- Migrant and seasonal farmworker's program offers comprehensive vocational rehabilitation services for migrants or seasonal workers with disabilities.
- Projects with industry program are provided to expand job opportunities and assist with placement and training of individuals with disabilities.

- Client Assistance Program (CAP) advocates for individuals with disability, informs individuals of programs available, and offers legal and administrative assistance to protect the rights of each individual.
- Basic Vocational Rehabilitation Services prepares people with disabilities for careers through individual assessment of abilities, provision of assistive technology, and medical care.
- Rehabilitation Training Program supports the training of rehabilitation providers through educational training grants and payback programs.
- Demonstration and Training Programs provide grants for projects and activities that improve delivery of care to impoverished individuals with disabilities.

Rehabilitation Issues and the Role of Health Care Providers

An occupational therapist tells the following story: "I had a home health referral for a fifty-year old African American female. She had a stroke at age 38 and lived in an older two-story home. She was divorced with four grown children living in her home. Two of her grandchildren also lived with her as well as her sister and the sister's teenage daughter. The woman was unable to leave her home because she could not negotiate the multiple steps and walkways from the front porch to the sidewalk due to her unsteady gait and need for new eyeglasses. The combination of impaired vision and hemiplegia (spasticity of both upper and lower right extremities) made descent impossible. While she could get up the steps because there was a handrail on her left side when going up, she could not descend because she could not grasp that same rail because it was on her affected side. In addition she had visual depth distortions that created paralyzing fear. She spent her days cooking and cleaning for all those who lived in her home. It did not occur to them to install a handrail for her and when it was suggested, they did not have the money to build it. When she had to go to the doctor's office, she struggled out the home's backdoor to a small porch and scooted down six steps to the back yard over uneven terrain. From there she had to be carried by a male relative across the backyard to the car awaiting her in the back alley. I made a referral to the Independent Living Center who, with city and state funding, assured me that they would assess the need and put her on the waiting list for a handrail. Two months went by and no handrail came. My call to the agency received a response of 'We don't have any more money left in this year's budget. Unless she can secure the funds for the railing herself, she'll just have to wait' It is so frustrating." (Levan, 2001)

There are many issues to consider when planning rehabilitation for those living in poverty. Most receive little or, at best, inconsistent health care. They often have no records of health care received. The person who is homeless cannot be contacted for appointments and has no safe place to keep equipment, medications, or supplies. The family living in a battered women's shelter may be placed in danger when a provider tries to contact them. New immigrants may not speak or read English well enough to secure employment or needed resources. And they may fear accessing available health care because of fear of deportation; whether justified or not, the result is most often the same.

Impoverished school-aged children may qualify for free lunches; however, preschool and younger children not in subsidized programs often do not have their total nutritional needs met. Parents reluctantly bring their children to homeless shelters for fear of losing custody of them. Homeless families have no refrigeration for food or liquid antibiotics for their children at a time when good health is critical for development.

Access is a critical component in the poverty equation; transportation is an issue for all age groups. Elders who no longer drive or cannot afford alternative transportation are unable to get to appointments or to care for basic necessities such as groceries. Free services are costly for the poor if there is no affordable transportation.

The role of the health care provider is multifaceted. The provider should begin with a thorough need and cultural assessment listing health care values and beliefs, as well as strengths and weaknesses of the individual and family unit. This assessment includes the family's "issues," such as lack of transportation, needed adaptations, financial resources, and support. Literacy and language assessment are paramount to the use of services and written materials.

The second step is to determine the available community resources—social and support groups such as religious and philanthropic organizations that may assist in obtaining needed adaptive equipment. Collaboration with other disciplines provides key information regarding availability of services and offers additional needed services or referral for teaching parenting skills, providing respite for caregivers, obtaining nutritional support and information, and finding volunteers to teach English as a second language to new immigrants.

Implementation is the next step in the process that includes family members in the plan of care to increase commitment and assistance with changes. The therapist aids the client in developing problem solving skills and in learning new ways to adapt to change. Formulating short- and long-term goals with the individual's perspective of need and input is essential. The provider empowers the individual and family to care for themselves by including practical information and skills such as vocational skills, résumé writing, the way to apply and interview for a job, including dressing appropriately and understanding the importance of being on time. Job coaching and support during early employment and securing necessary adaptive equipment further ensure their success.

Finally, the health care provider evaluates the process, noting the approaches that were successful and making changes as necessary. It is essential that the benefits of these resources and positive outcomes are made known to policy makers and decision makers. Providers can make a tremendous difference in our community through careful consideration of the relevancy of information provided and by giving the tools to meet each person's needs.

Case Study 1

A group of undergraduate students is planning a health promotion project for their community. After weeks of developing rapport with the residents at a homeless shelter, the students determine that there is a need for education regarding wellness promotion; one of many possible interventions. The homeless residents are primarily women with young children. The students plan a health fair to be held at the shelter, offering information on nutrition, dental hygiene, smoking cessation, childhood safety, and self-breast examination.

Question

1. How does one determine the highest priority needs of a community? Of a family? Of an individual?

In the planning stages, the students attempt telephone contact with the shelter manager, who does not return their calls. With faculty assistance, the students set a date for the health fair. They make posters alerting shelter residents to the date of the health fair and discuss their plans and preparations with intended shelter participants. The health care community provides many pamphlets and supplies. The students bring food that they have prepared and a large basket of bath supplies as a door prize. Thirty minutes before the health fair is to begin, the shelter staff take most of the residents on a spontaneous community outing. Five people attend the health fair. The students are very disappointed.

Questions

1. What could the students and faculty have done differently?
2. What are the immediate needs of the homeless?
3. How might one best bridge a socioeconomic gap?

Case Study 2

A single parent with two children describes her life as "just getting by." She has little family or financial support. She has a job that does not give her the flexibility she needs when her children are ill. They are too young to be left alone without adult supervision. Her son may require surgery. The child's physician does not agree to move the date of diagnostic testing just "to suit her schedule." You are working in the doctor's office.

Questions

1. Will you intervene on the parent's behalf?
2. How might you intervene most effectively?

Case Study 3

An elderly man you are caring for tells you that he is noncompliant with his medicine because he cannot afford it.

Questions

1. How do you approach this problem?
2. What might you do to respond to this situation?

You later learn that the same man panhandles to buy alcohol on a daily basis.

Question

1. How might you handle the situation differently given this new information?

Summary

The author has discussed how social class is influenced by lifestyle and power in the United States. It is followed by a description of different economic classes in this country. Those living in poverty are unable to seek adequate health care and are more vulnerable to violence in both rural and urban communities. The author also has described how poverty affects children, women, the elderly, and immigrants throughout the communities in the United States. The chapter concludes by addressing specific issues and offering some guidelines for rehabilitation professionals working with people in poor communities.

Questions

1. After reading the summary of social classes in the United States at the beginning of the chapter, determine your own class. What values do you espouse? How have your values come to be?

2. Review the scenario about the woman with residual deficits from a stroke who had difficulty maneuvering her stairs. List three community service organizations or interest groups in your community that would be most appropriate for this individual and her family.

3. A nine-year-old child with cerebral palsy has outgrown her wheelchair. What agencies in your community can help this child acquire new needed and appropriate equipment?

4. A family has arrived in your community from a war-torn country. They speak no English, and you do not speak their language. List several ways that you can enhance communication with this family. Name two community resources, agencies, and/or individuals you could access to assist new immigrants.

5. A young man with spina bifida has recently been promoted and transferred to a new office. The restroom in the facility is not wheelchair accessible. He must leave the building in his wheelchair to use the bathroom in the restaurant down the street. He is concerned about his job security and about how long the restaurant owner will allow him to use the restroom. He resents having to travel a long distance, especially in bad weather. What aspects of the Americans with Disabilities Act could be brought on behalf of this client?

6. Collaborate with your classmates in compiling a community resource guide including contact information and addresses. Describe the process for obtaining Medicare/Medicaid, food stamps, emergency shelter and clothing, rehabilitation equipment, and free or reduced-cost medical and dental care.

7. If your home was destroyed, what alternative housing might be available for your family, and for how long?

References

American Academy of Medicine. (1998, January). Statement on poverty and violence.

Anderson, G. M. (2000, April 22). Hungry in America: Thirty-one million people in the United States experience either food insecurity or actual hunger. *America, 182*(14), 18.

Arno, P. S., Levine, C., & Memmott, M. M. (1999). The economic value of informal caregiving. *Health Affairs, 18*(12), 182–788.

Beal, A. C., & Stein, R. E. K. (2000). A single source of health care: Does it affect health experiences for inner city children? *Journal of Health Care for the Poor and Underserved 11*(2), 151–162.

Bollwahn, P. E. (1999, June 23). Poverty's misery cascades from budget cuts. *Los Angeles Times Syndicate.*

Centers for Disease Control and Prevention. (2000, April 26). Community indicators of health related quality of life—United States 1993–1997. *Journal of American Medical Association, 283*(16), 2097–2098.

Davis, T. C., Meldrum, H., Tippy, P. K. P., Weiss, B. D., & Williams, M. V. (1996, October 15). How poor literacy leads to poor health care. *Patient Care, 30*(16), 94–99.

Dinan, K, Fass, S., & Cauthen, N. K. (2004). State policy choices: Supports for low income working families. *National Center for Children in Poverty.* [On line]. Available: http://www.nccp.org/pub_swf04.html [7/31/04].

Flaskerud, J. H., & Kim, S. (1999, June). Health problems of Asian and Latino immigrants. *Nursing Clinics of North America, 34*(2), 359–380.

Flores, G., Abreu, M., Olivar, M. A., & Kastner, B. (1998, November). Access barriers to health care for Latino children. *Archives of Pediatric and Adolescent Medicine*, 1119–34.

Fox, J. A., & Zawitz, M. W. (1999). Homicide trends in the United States. [On line]. Available: http://www.ojp.usdoj.gov/bjs/homicide/homtmd.htm [12/22/00].

Gardner, J. W. (1987). *Excellence: Can we be equal and excellent too?* Norton Publishing. New York, N.Y.

Germain, C. P. (1995). The children of the shelter for battered women. In P. L. Munhall (Ed.), *Women's experience:* vol. 2. New York: National League of Nursing Press.

Gibran, K. (1923). On children. *The prophet.* New York: Knopf.

Gornick, M. E., Eggers, P. W., Reilly, T. W., Mentnech, R. M., Fitterman, L. K., Kucken, L., & Vladeck, B. C. (1996, September 12). Effects of race and income on mortality and use of services among Medicare beneficiaries. *The New England Journal of Medicine 335*(11), 791–799.

Kennedy, J. (1997, July–September). Personal assistance benefits and federal health care reform: Who is eligible on the basis of ADL assistance criteria? *The Journal of Rehabilitation 63*(3), 40–46.

Kenning, M., Merchant, A., & Tomkins, A. (1991). Research on the effects of witnessing parental battering: Clinical and legal policy implications. In Steinman, M. (Ed.), *Women battering: Policy responses.* Cincinnati, Ohio: Anderson Publishing.

Killion, C. M. (1998, July/ August). Poverty and procreation among women: An anthropologic study with implications for health care providers. *Journal of Nurse Midwifery 43*(4), 273–788.

Laurence, L., & Spalter-Roth, R. (1996, May*). Measuring the costs of domestic violence against women and the cost effectiveness of interventions: An initial assessment and proposals for further research.* Washington, DC: Institute for Women's Policy Research.

Levan, N. (2001). Unpublished interview.

Manisses Communications. (2000, September 4). Study confirms treatment needs of welfare recipients. *Alcoholism and Drug Abuse Weekly 12*(34), 5.

Martinez, R. (1996, May). Latinos and lethal violence: The impact of poverty and inequality. *Social Problems 43*(2), 131–152.

McLoyd, V. C. (1998, February). Socioeconomic disadvantage and child development. *American Psychologist 53*(2), 185–204.

Meyers, M. K., Lukemeyer, A., & Smeeding, T. (1998, June). The cost of caring: Childhood disability and poor families. *Social Science Review 72*(2), 209–225.

National Center for the Dissemination of Disability Research (NCDDR). (1999, April). *Disability, diversity, and dissemination: Cultural and other considerations that can influence effectiveness within the rehabilitation system.* United States Department of Education. Washington, DC.

Newacheck, P. W., & Halfon, N. (1998). Prevalence and impact of disabling chronic conditions in childhood. *American Journal of Public Health 88*, 610–617.

Newacheck, P. W., Pearl, M., & Hughes, D. C. (1998, November 25). The role of Medicaid in ensuring children's access to care: Policy perspectives. *Journal of American Medical Association 280*(20), 1789–93.

Noren, J., Kindig, D., & Sprenger, A. (1998, January–February). Challenges to Native American health care. *Public Health Reports 113*(1), 22–42.

Northam, S. (1996, October). Access to health promotion, protection, and disease prevention among impoverished individuals. *Public Health Nursing 13*(5), 353–364.

Nunez, R. (1996). *The new poverty: Homeless families in America.* New York: Insight Books/Plenum Press.

Nunez, R., & Fox, C. (1999, Summer). A snapshot of homelessness across America. *Political Science Quarterly 114*(2), 289–307.

Prewitt, E. (1997, March 15). Inner city health care. *Annals of Internal Medicine 126*(6), 485–490.

Raphael, J. (1996, April). Prisoners of abuse: Domestic violence and welfare receipt. In C. T. Kenney & K. R. Brown, *Report from the front lines: The impact of violence on poor women.* New York: NOW Legal Defense and Education Fund.

Roberts, H. (1997, April 12). Socioeconomic determinants of health: Children, inequalities, and health. *British Medical Journal 314*, 1122–1125.

Robinson, K. M. (1997, September–October). Family caregiving: Who provides the care, and at what cost? *Nursing Economics 15*(5), 243–247.

Rosenbach, M. L., Irvin, C., & Coulam, R. F. (1999, June). Access for low-income children: Is health insurance enough? *Pediatrics 103*(6), 1167–1186.

Roth, J., Hendrickson, J., Schilling, M., & Stowell, D. W. (1998, September). The risk of teen mothers having low birth weight babies: Implications of recent medical research for school health personnel. *Journal of School Health 68*(7), 271–275.

Schlosberg, C. L. Ferber, J. D. (1998, January). Access to Medicaid since the personal responsibility and work opportunity reconcilliation act. *National Center on Poverty Law.*

Sherman, A. (1999, Winter). Children's poverty in America. *Forum for Applied Research and Public Policy 14*(4), 68.

Sherman, P. (1998, October). Health care for homeless children: A clinician's perspective. *Healing Hands 2*(6).

Shiono, P. H., Rauh, V. A., Park, M., Lederman, S. A., & Zuskar, D. (1997, May). Ethnic differences in birthweight: The role of lifestyle and other factors. *American Journal of Public Health 87*(5), 787–793.

Smith, G. D., Neaton, J. D., Wentworth, D., Stamler, R., & Stamler, J. (1998, March 28). Mortality differences between black and white men in the USA: Contribution of income and other risk factors among men screened for the Multiple Risk Factor Intervention Trial. *The Lancet 351*(9107), 934–936.

United States Census Bureau (2003). Current health insurance coverage, poverty statistics, 5th report to Congress. [On line]. Available: http://www.census.gov/hhes.

United States Department of Health and Human Services (2003). Annual update of HHS poverty guidelines. Washington, DC.

United States Department of Health and Human Services, Administration for Children and Families (2003). Welfare: Temporary assistance for needy families (TANF). [On line]. Available: http://www.acf.dhhs.gov/programs.

United States Government Printing Office (2000, October 20). Self-reported concern about food security—eight states, 1996–1998. *Morbidity and Mortality Weekly Report*, 933–937.

Wellman, N. S., Weddle, D. O., Kranz, S., Brain, C. T. (1997, October). Elder insecurities: Poverty, hunger, and malnutrition. *Journal of the American Dietetic Association 97*(10), 120–123.

Appendix

Groups in Poverty Without Health Insurance for the Entire Year (U.S. Census Bureau, 2003)

Below poverty line	30.4%
Male	33.3%
Female	28.1%
Caucasian	14.2%
African American	20.2%
Asian and Pacific Islander	18%
Hispanic	32.4%
Under 18 years of age	20.1%
18–24 years of age	43.9%
25–34 years of age	48.6%
35–44 years of age	46%
45–64 years of age	33.1%
65 years and older	1.9%
Native born	25.6%
Foreign born	55.3%
Work full time	47.4%
Work part time	44.4%
Did not work	38.1%

43.6 million people in the United States without insurance (15.2% population).

Barriers to Health Care (Northam, 1996)

Money is required before being seen.	38%
Costs too much.	36%
Do not have insurance.	26%
There is no way to get there.	15%
Personnel do not speak my language.	13%
Did not know where to go.	12%
Waited too long to get an appointment.	10%
Staff are rude.	7%
Lose pay from work.	7%
Have no confidence in staff.	7%
There is no child care.	6%
Hours are inconvenient.	6%
Waited too long in the office.	3%

15

Gender and Culture

Margaret Drake

Key Words

gender roles	male	cross-cultural studies
female	culture	

Objectives

1. Indentify how the culture you live in influences gender roles.
2. Discuss gender roles within Maslow's hierarchy of needs.
3. Examine your own beliefs about gender roles, and compare and contrast them with those from another culture.

Introduction

Gender is considered to be both biological and learned. The biological aspect has to do with genetics, as well as primary and secondary sex characteristics. Primary sex characteristics are the obvious ones of penis and vagina. The secondary sex characteristics are the ones that appear at puberty when the sexual hormones begin to activate, such as facial and underarm hair or the voice changes that are so obvious in males. The learned part of gender includes the individual's gender identity and gender role. Most modern health researchers include both aspects in their description of gender. Gender identity has to do with how one identifies oneself as male, female, or androgynous. Gender role is what one thinks of when presenting oneself to the public, such as a family member role (Chetwynd & Hartnett, 1978; Loue, 1999). Culture has been defined in previous chapters.

Within a culture, gender roles can vary widely (Glanville, 2003). Through history and throughout the world, there have been individuals who have challenged the dominant culture's vision of gender. A few of these challengers were Hildegard of Bingen, the eleventh-century abbess and scientist; Anna Morandi Manzolini, the eighteenth-century Italian anatomist; Harriet Tubman, a conductor on the Underground Railroad for fleeing slaves in the United States; George Washington Carver, the African American teacher and botanist; Madam Curie, the French discoverer of radium; and Mohandas Ghandi, the peacemaker and leader of India. However, these women and men have not been representative of the prevalent attitudes and stereotypes in their milieu (Campbell, 1997; Caspar & Hine,1996; Cieslak-Golonka & Morten, 2000; Ghandi, 1948).

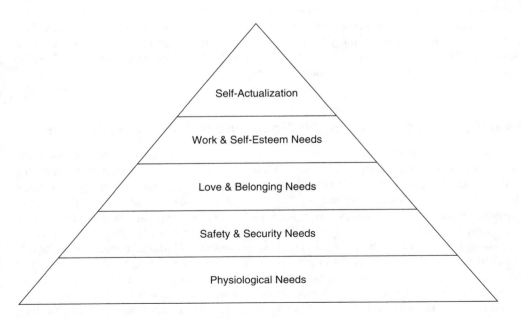

FIGURE 13.1 Maslow's Hierarchy of Human Needs

Because it would be impossible to list all the different ways in which cultures think about gender, a developmental approach is used to describe experiences and issues that affect both sexes and that are common to many cultures. Abraham Maslow's Hierarchy of Human Needs (1968) is used as a framework upon which to hang the stories for each stage of life in a genderized world. This hierarchy says that if one has not filled one's physiological needs such as for fluids and food, one will be unable to attend to one's safety and security issues such as shelter. If one does not feel safe, Maslow averred that the person would not be able to feel loving and belonging in relationships. Furthermore, if the individual were unable to belong and feel love, success and self-esteem would be out of one's reach. Unless all these needs were filled, self-actualization, such as spiritual ideas and artistic expression, would be impossible.

Examples will be given from different cultures that can illuminate the issues in many cultures. It is common in Western culture to present "developmental theory" within the context of Caucasian heterosexual males, thus ignoring half of the worlds' developmental experience. In this chapter, the stories will use the developmental progression through stages to share experiences of both genders in many cultures. Sometimes the stories will be of females, sometimes of males (Erikson, 1963; Groce 2001; Horsley, 1996; Maslow, 1968; McGoldrick, 1998; Neufeldt, 2001).

Infancy

Infancy is usually defined as birth to two years (Kaluger & Kaluger, 1984). It is during this time that infants begin to realize how they will be treated during their life. Little girls will be cuddled and petted. Little boys will be thrown in the air and treated more roughly. This behavior seems to happen in many cultures. It is difficult to delineate between each of Maslow's (1968) different levels. Sometimes one level of the hierarchy seems to flow up into the next level. This tendency becomes apparent in the discussion of infancy.

Physiological Needs—Air, Water, Food, and Human Reproduction

Infanticide has more commonly been practiced in sex selection by allowing female babies to die. This method of population control has usually been practiced by societies such as the ancient Greeks, in which women's value was little. Both Greek and Roman fathers could legally end their baby's life for any reason. For the past several centuries, the birth of males has usually surpassed that of females, but male babies were more prone to die before reaching their first birthday. Consequently, by allowing girl babies to die, the ratio of male to female was more even according to theory. Girls were seen as a liability because they would need a dowry when they married. The mothers of the infants were often forced by the father or the father's family to leave their female child in a place where hopefully a kind stranger would find the child, such as by a pathway. Some abandoned female infants in Greece were expected to be found and made into slave prostitutes. However, historians believe that wild animals often ate them. Some believed that infanticide was the most common crime in Europe until the nineteenth century. The debate continues today about infanticide, eugenics, and handicapped infants (Horan & Delahoyde, 1982; Keuls, 1985; Pernick, 1996).

Safety and Security

Infanticide obviously involves the safety and security of the infant; however, there are other issues for girl and boy infants. Cradleboards used by many native and peasant people provide a measure of security for infants. The stability of being held tightly on a flat surface is thought to increase an infant's feeling of safety. Mothers are able to stand the child up against a tree or fence while they work. Even though it is an ancient practice, many modern tribal women still continue to use this method of carrying infants and providing safety. In Iran, babies are often not named immediately after birth. A girl infant may be allowed to remain on the cradleboard all day not being changed, so that she remains wet. Boys, on the other hand, have their tiny penis threaded into a tube that drains to the outside of the swaddling used for the cradleboard. Amulets and azure beads to keep off the "evil eye" are attached to the board (Friedl, 1997).

"Girl Baby" was left on her cradleboard against a stone wall near the irrigation channel that ran about a quarter mile from the family compound where her mother went to wash clothes. Girl Baby was the third girl born to this 18-year-old mother and 28-year-old father. The Iranian family very much wanted a boy. The couple and their three girls lived with the husband's parent in a village. Both the mother-in-law and the husband were angry with this third girl, whom they wished were a boy. Consequently, the young mother was not as eager and attentive to the child as she had been to the two previous girls. She sometimes delayed breast-feeding. This Girl Baby did not show some of the developmental responses that her older sisters had shown. This lack of engagement further discouraged the young mother from interaction with Girl Baby. Although the mother felt that her baby was safe and secure, the child actually suffered from being immobile. Therapists are rare in the village, but the nurse at the public health clinic was able to intervene and encourage the mother to interact more with Girl Baby.

Love and Belonging

Harlow (1971) showed how important a soft, lifelike mother was for infant monkeys when he made a wire-covered surrogate with padding cloth. Responses to this figure were compared with that of a wire monkey, which was not soft. He concluded that babies need to have a realistic adult caretaker in order to develop emotionally. If the baby does not have a realistic mother surrogate, development will probably be impaired. This problem has become increasingly apparent as U.S. families have adopted infants from Russia, China, and Romania.

Maili was two years old when she was adopted by a Caucasian couple from Kansas City, Kansas. Her new parents were well-educated professionals who were prepared to deal with issues that they had learned to expect from adoptees from China. They knew that many such female infants were neglected in orphanages because of lack of resources, staff training, and available personnel. However, their adoption agent had assured them that Maili, their prospective daughter, was from one of the better orphanages and that she did not appear to have those problems. Maili was six months old when the agent viewed her in the orphanage. The actual adoption process took one-and-a-half years. Her new parents flew to China to get her. They became aware during the next few weeks that she had some delays in development. Because the new adopted mother of Maili was a physical therapist, she immediately started Maili in an enrichment program.

Success and Personal Esteem

Since babies have not mastered their muscles well enough to be able to manipulate most objects, the way in which an infant feels successful is to engage others in interpersonal activity. The child babbles with delight when another person approaches. The child responds to the high-pitched vocalizations that humans instinctively make when interacting with babies (Kaluger & Kaluger, 1984).

Jared, an African-American 10-month-old, had to stay in the hospital for many months after he was diagnosed with leukemia. Because he was such a friendly infant, the nurses and therapist who worked with him all developed an attachment to him. They interacted with him at every opportunity. Jared's teen mother was unable to get to the hospital oftener than once per week, since she was enrolled in a high school two hours away in her hometown. She took the bus on weekends to see her infant son. She became jealous when she saw the close relationship that the staff seemed to have with her baby. The occupational therapist who worked every third weekend was able to figure out that the mother was jealous when she interviewed her for the patient assessment. The OT persuaded the young mother to make both audiotapes and videotapes of her talking to Jared in the high voice commonly used by mothers. Although it was not a perfect solution, it assisted the young mother to see herself as taking some action to improve her own relationship with her baby.

Self-Actualization

Probably laughter exemplifies best the self-actualization of infancy. This expression of pure pleasure is as close to spirituality as a baby can get. Babies laugh at funny faces and sudden movements. The occupational therapist played "funny face" games with Jared and sometimes tickled him. If Jared were too ill to play, the occupational therapist would get the music therapist to come and sing nursery songs and lullabies while holding him (Cousins, 1989).

Childhood

Childhood is often divided into three stages; however, space does not allow doing so in this instance. For the purposes of this chapter, childhood refers to the ages of two to approximately eleven years or the onset of puberty. When there is a cross-cultural marriage, childraising issues often cause strain. Assisting families to be aware of their own ethnic issues is a place to start. The therapist may be most helpful in becoming the *culture broker* (Erikson, 1963; Horsley, 1996).

Physiological Needs

The customs of many cultures include nursing children into their third and fourth year. Female children are nursed for a shorter length of time in several Middle Eastern countries. In Iran, if a male child is judged weak, it is thought that he will be strengthened if he is nursed with the milk from the mother of a baby girl. Some mothers claim that their male infants survived because of the "girl milk" that the mothers begged from other female relatives who were mothers of baby girls.

Ahmed was afflicted with what Western medicine would have called *colic*, or "wind in the stomach." His mother went around to all her female relatives with female babies and begged them to nurse Ahmed for small lengths of time. The mother firmly believed that Ahmed's survival had to do with "girl milk." This custom is thought to be part of the idea that females enhance the lives of males throughout all their lives, even in early childhood. (Drake, 1982; Friedl, 1997; Sebai, 1981)

Safety and Security

Although both sexes are vulnerable to sexual predators, females are at much greater risk. Throughout history, women have been considered "the spoils of war." In the last half-century, in civil wars over the world, female children have suffered from sexual assault and rape by conquerors. African, East-European, and Asian female children have all suffered from such actions by their invaders and occupiers (Goodwin, 1997a; Goodwin, 1997b; Upchurch & Kusunoki, 2004).

One such case was Trawrly, a Rwandan Tutsi girl of 6 years who was gang-raped by Hutu soldiers during the 1994 genocide. She and her pregnant mother were fleeing when they were caught, and the child was assaulted before her mother's eyes. In the refugee camp where they were subsequently sheltered, the child showed all the symptoms of *post-traumatic stress disorder.* Trawrly demonstrated repetitive reenactment of parts of the flight and the rape. She did not respond to U.N. caregivers in the refugee camp who attempted to interact with her. She frequently awoke others in her tent when she screamed during bad dreams. A psychologist who was sent to assist, offered the child crayons. She drew a picture of her pregnant mother standing by a tree with herself on the ground and three soldiers with guns pointing at her. This picture opened the floodgates of tears and initiated discussion of the rape.

Love and Belonging

Clitoridectomy is a practice in many cultures in Africa and the Middle East in which the female clitoris is excised, usually before puberty. This practice is considered a right of passage for the girl in some tribes. The clitoris is thought to be greatly involved in the enjoyment of coitus. Consequently, removing it will keep the young woman from experiencing too much pleasure from sex, thus curbing her wish to stray from her husband. She will keep her love for her husband because there is no temptation to have sex with anyone else, thus preserving her "belonging" in her husband's family (Daly, 1978). Clitoridectomy is a controversial issue, because some believe that it is a cultural practice that defies intervention by Western reformers. It is not felt to be a gender issue, since the surgery is most frequently performed by other women, not by males. However, others feel that it should be considered a sufficient threat to girls so that they should be allowed to have political asylum in Western countries (Purnell & Paulanka, 2003). It was an issue discussed at the 1996 Women's conference in Beijing, China. Generally, women of the world think the practice is detrimental and should be stopped.

Ashai, a 10-year-old girl from Sudan, was taken to the local hospital for surgery to excise her clitoris after a celebration with the women of her family. There had been food and jokes about womanhood and manhood mixed with much hilarity. Her grandmother and mother accompanied her into the surgery. She was praised for being so brave upon becoming a woman. She had not yet begun to menstruate as most women in her family had by this age. A woman surgeon anesthetized her and did the excision with her grandmother and mother present. When Ashai awoke in the hospital recovery room, her female relatives were there to welcome her into the world of womanhood. Despite the pubic pain, Ashai felt proud to have advanced to the status of marriageable woman.

Another kind of belonging is exemplified in African American cultures. African American family boundaries are often more blurred than in some other cultures. Children are often sent to relatives to be raised if the situation for the birth parents makes child-rearing difficult. This arrangement may cause confusion for therapists when they try to identify family relationships (Horsley, 1996).

Andrew was the son of unmarried high-school-age parents. His mother, Tanisha, planned to finish high school and go on to college. Her family wanted to support Tanisha in this endeavor. Her maternal aunt offered to raise Andrew while Tanisha completed her education. During a screening for IDEA (Individuals with Disabilities Education Act) in preschool at age three, Andrew was identified as having difficulty with age-appropriate motor skills. Because his mother was in her first year at college, his great aunt with whom he lived came to his first IEP (Individual Education Plan) meeting. His maternal grandmother came to the second meeting. At the third meeting both his maternal and his paternal grandmothers attended. The therapist was sometimes confused about whom she should address in describing Andrew's program. She decided to give copies to both grandmothers and to send a third copy to the absent great aunt with whom Andrew lived.

Success and Personal Esteem

In the modern world, success frequently means capability to interact in the world of technology. The American Association of University Women has consistently studied the deficits that girls experience as they proceed through the educational system. The following studies have been published in the 1990s: *Shortchanging Girls; Girls in the Middle; Voices of a Generation: Teenage Girls on Sex, School and Self; Separated by Sex: A Critical Look at Single-Sex Education for Girls;* and *Gender Gaps: Where Schools Still Fail Our Children.* The theme throughout these studies is that girls do well in language but that they begin to lose their educational edge as they approach puberty and are exposed to the belief that boys like "dumb" girls rather than "smart" girls. Success for prepubescent and pubescent girls is often having the attention of male peers.

Mary, a European American 10-year-old, had been the class *star* in her early elementary grades. The suburban Denver, Colorado, school had provided her many positive responses for her intellectual achievements. When she entered fourth grade, several of the girls in her class were already menstruating. Sexuality became the most frequent topic of the girls' conversation. As Mary saw her classmates begin to receive more attention for their physicality than she did for her intellectuality, she subtly changed her behavior. At the same time, her parents divorced, and Mary and her younger sister missed their father, who moved to Chicago. In the infrequent visits with her father, Mary became more and more distant from him, avoiding his affection. Her breast development and menstruation were delayed, and she began to doubt herself, because she no longer felt like a *star*. Her working mother sent Mary and her sister to an "after-school" program in the same suburban school that they attended all day. A young adult recreation worker recognized Mary's situation and began to give her special attention for participation in pretrack activities. Soon Mary was leading the pack of girl-friends in sports. She got enough reinforcement from these girls that she postponed her need for attention from boys. (Stepp, 2000)

Girls from some Middle Eastern countries such as Saudi Arabia have their self-esteem built around following Islamic rules and customs of dress. Girls start early in emulating grown women, covering their hair and faces with clothes. However, prepubescent girls are not required to conform to adult women's dress requirements.

An Egyptian eight-year-old girl, Sadika, whose parents were employed in Riyadh, Saudi Arabia, had her self-esteem eroded when she went into a bookstore on the main boulevard with her father. She was clothed in a long dress as were all little girls in Saudi Arabia, but the dress had short sleeves. Only postpubescent females are required to cover their arms. Nonetheless, the *mutawah,* a religious policeman, followed Sadika and her father into the bookstore. He tapped Sadika's bare arms with his staff and verbally threatened her father with arrest if he ever saw Sadika in public with bare arms. (Drake, 1982)

Self-Actualization

Over the last few decades, it has been verified that physical activity often provides the same feelings as do spiritual experiences. Mary, the girl from Denver, became so skillful at running and jumping that she realized that running became as effective as prayer for her when she felt that she needed a change of pace in her emotional life. She was not yet sophisticated enough to call the experience spiritual, but it did indeed function in that way for her. When she was running, she felt truly alive in the way described as self-actualization (Dossey, Keegan, Kolkmeier, & Guzzetta, 1989).

For many children, the stimulation of the mind is self-actualization. In the case of Sadika, the threat to her father and herself by the *mutawah* interfered with the self-actualization she would have experienced through buying and reading books, because the *mutawah* ordered them out of the bookstore.

Adolescence

Adolescence means the period following activation of previously latent sex hormones. Because of the physical changes in both males and females that this causes, almost every culture has ways of marking these developments, such as the Jewish Bar Mitzvah for boys and the Bah Mitzvah for girls. In many cultures, this change means new gender role requirements. The terms *girlhood* and *boyhood* in the English language span the time of infancy through the teen years. However, there are different descriptions of girlhood and boyhood throughout the world. Often small children have mimicked their older siblings and so are well prepared for the new requirements of this transitional stage between childhood and adulthood. Females who enter puberty at an early age are more prone to body dissatisfaction and consequent depression than their age mates (Inness, 1998; Seeman 1995).

Physiological Needs

Maslow considered reproduction to be part of human physiological needs. African and African American females have often seen procreation as an important duty. Because their men were so vulnerable to persecution and death, reproduction seemed a compensation for this threat. Some writers rationalize polygamy in Africa as a method of assuring children in a society where infant and child mortality is high. This attitude is often still subtly in effect. Churches and governments may discourage having a child out of wedlock, but the culture itself does not. Women of the paternal side of the family often maintain a connection with the mother and the child despite the absence of marriage (Glanville, 2003; McGoldrick, Anderson, & Walsh, 1991).

Latisha was the third child of an unwed mother in the United States South. She was raised in the religious home of her grandfather, grandmother, and single mother. Along with her brothers, Latisha attended a Missionary Baptist Church and Sunday School from infancy. At age fourteen, she became pregnant despite careful supervision by her mother and grandparents. The father of her child was a neighbor boy whom the family liked. Latisha did not tell her mother, but her mother realized when she was six months pregnant that her enlarged waist was symptomatic. Her mother asked her whether she was pregnant. Although her mother was dismayed at this development, she realized that Latisha was reenacting her own life of unwed motherhood. The grandparents were also disappointed but saw their role as being supportive of Latisha no matter what. Latisha was not pressed to marry the father of the child. Abortion was not even discussed as an option. Her high school had a program for pregnant teens. After a premature birth, Latisha returned to school. When the baby was released from the neonatal unit, the infant was enrolled into the day care for children of students at the high school. People in the church took both baby and mother into their hearts and gave support as needed. Messages from the predominant culture were negative, but within her own church and school community, Latisha felt supported.

Safety and Security

In teenage years, the younger a girl is, if she is forced into sexual activity, the more likely she is to have sexually transmitted diseases (STDs) (Upchurch & Kusunoki, 2004). However, boys have different teen problems related to STDs. Mozambique Prime Minister Pascoul Mocumba stated that in tribal language in Mozambique, the name of AIDS means "women's disease." Consequently, males do not consider it a threat because the terminology describing the illness makes males think that they are not vulnerable. This is a severe safety problem in a country where AIDS occurs in 16% of the population and HIV infection in 25% of the population (Mocumba, 2000).

Midogo, 17, was raised in an extended polygamous family in Beira, Mozambique. Because he was raised in the city, many of the village values of his Sena tribal grandparents had been diluted. He grew up living and playing with dozens of cousins in several family compounds within the city. Some members of his parent's generation had intermarried with members of other tribes. Like his male cousins, the lure of Western technology and economics overlaid his traditional family culture. However, they still used their tribal Sena language, rather than the more universal Portuguese, for most conversation and communication. Midogo discussed "woman's disease" with his cousins and brothers, never dreaming that he could catch it. However, on a rare trip to the beach, he met a female tourist from another city. They began a sexual relationship. Seven months after the girl went back to her home, Midogo began to cough and have symptoms of pneumonia. He discussed his cough with the health worker at the local clinic, who told him he had HIV. He did not believe the diagnosis because it was "a woman's disease." Shortly thereafter, he became betrothed to a cousin. During the betrothal time, he infected her. Before they could wed, Midogo's disease killed him.

African American males aged 15 to 19 are vulnerable to both murder and suicide. They are ten times more often victims of shooting than European American males. Suicides among 15- to 19-year-old African American males have increased over 100% during the past decade (Kliman, 1998; Mitchell, 2000).

Kareem was one such young man. He was a high school athlete and had named himself Kareem after the famous basketball player, Abdul Kareem Jabaar. His rural Alabama family still worked their 160-acre farm. The small nearby town had remnants of the plantation culture left from previous centuries. Because the schools had been integrated, the European American town fathers and mothers had used the economics of real estate to maintain segregation. When Kareem advanced from middle school to high school, his mother, who was a schoolteacher in the community, appealed to the school board to allow Kareem to go to the school that had *advanced placement* classes to prepare him for college. Most of the students in that school were white. During his first two years in high school, he became friends with several of his white classmates, both boys and girls. Kareem became aware of hostile looks from some of the other white students and some coldness from formerly encouraging teachers. His difficult situation appeared to him to have no solution. He began to think about how he could avoid this racial problem. He didn't want to bring trouble to his family, nor did he want to reject his new friends. Like many other Southern males, he had his own gun, which he kept in his closet. One afternoon his mother arrived home early and opened his bedroom door to find Kareem with his head resting on the muzzle of the gun. This was her first indication that he was suicidal. She persuaded him to avoid causing such grief to his family and to enter a psychiatric unit for treatment.

Love and Belonging

It is often repeated in the African American culture, "raise your daughters but love your sons." This saying gives the message that females need to be taught strength to deal with the dominant racist culture but that boys need to have their self-esteem built. When translated, this message says that boys should be spoiled. They are expected to be at higher risk of physical harm, so they are forgiven behavior that would not be tolerated in African American females (Boyd-Franklin & Franklin, 1998).

His grandmother gave Michael, an African American 16-year-old, a car soon after he passed the driving license test. He frequently parked his car in the driveway of his home in a middle-class neighborhood that had residents of diverse ethnic origins. Michael's radio was usually so loud that the neighbors could hear the music inside their air-conditioned houses. When Michael failed to respond to several requests to lower the volume of the music, neighbors called the police. The third time police came, they issued Michael a citation, which cost $200. His grandmother paid the fine after Michael persuaded her that he was a victim of prejudice. The love shown by his grandmother was unconditional.

Success and Personal Esteem

The self-esteem of teenage girls has been a subject of intensive study for the last decade. Teenage girls have been so sexualized that it appears to girls through media such at TV and magazines that problems can be solved only by sexual means. In order to be the sexual object that can attract partners, girls are led to feel that they must use make-up, creams, and soaps that will make them acceptable. In other words, they must become consumers of commercial products in order to be acceptable (American Association of University Women, 1998; Haag, 1998, 1999; Lemish, 1998).

Sandy, a 16-year-old European American girl from Northern California, was encouraged by her psychologist mother and physician father to be assertive. When she was prepubescent, she had plenty of friends of both sexes. However, as she grew into womanhood as a teen, she found that her assertiveness and competence in math and computers made her "geeky" and not a desirable female friend for either boys or girls of her own age. Through the relationship she built with her male math teacher, she was able to develop some healthy self-respect for her math skills. It was only as she approached college that she was able to fully appreciate herself, because previously the public culture had not supported her academic accomplishments.

Self-Actualization

Sandy found that she was able to meet with other girls who enjoyed math in a computer *chatroom* for girls, NUMBER ONE FEMALES. She spent hours discussing feelings about herself with other girls from across the world. Her feeling of connection to like-minded young women gave her a feeling akin to a religious experience such as she had felt in summer camp when she was in the fifth grade.

Young Adulthood

Physiological Needs

Asian Americans are more often victims of the hepatitis B virus (HBV) than whites in the United States. This virus is 16% more common among Asian Americans than among all other Americans. It is attributed to a lack of immunization. One outcome of this infection is that Chinese American males have a much higher rate of hepatocellular carcinoma (Loue, 1999).

Mei-Ling, a 24-year-old Taiwanese woman was married three weeks before she and her new husband left Taiwan to attend graduate school in Seattle. She had had some periods when she felt ill in the year between graduating from National Taiwan University and her wedding. Finally, she was diagnosed with the hepatitis B virus in time to have treatment before the wedding. During the four years in Seattle, she and her husband returned to Taiwan each summer. After completion of doctoral studies, the couple returned to Taiwan with plans to finally start their family. Mei-Ling had another episode of hepatitis symptoms, which further delayed and complicated their plans. Her doctor asked her to postpone pregnancy until her symptoms were diminished. Meanwhile, Mei-Ling felt her *biological clock ticking.* Eventually she was able to conceive and bear a healthy baby. This event is commonly part of this stage of life for a woman and this level in the Hierarchy of Human Needs.

Safety and Security

In the United States, somewhere a woman is beaten every 18 seconds, on the average. Physical abuse is the most frequent cause of injury to women (Kramer, Lorenzon, & Mueller, 2004; U.S. Department of Justice, 1994).

Karen, a white Midwestern kindergarten teacher, came to her doctor with many complaints, which he diagnosed as psychosomatic. It seemed that she was trying to get the doctor to prescribe medication. During the initial evaluation, the doctor learned that her husband had lost his job as a cable repairman. The doctor asked how the unemployment was affecting the couple. She said that at first, her husband had begun to spend a great deal of time at home watching TV rather than out looking for work. Then he began to call her on her cell phone in the classroom to ask what she was doing. A few weeks later, he began to show up at her classroom as the children were leaving. The rural community where they lived was tolerant of many kinds of behavior such as this. However, recently he had begun to start drinking and be quite drunk by the time she came home. He had ordered her to stop calling her sister. The doctor, recognizing the symptoms of a batterer, asked if the husband had ever hit her. Karen burst into tears and recounted that only last evening he had questioned her about why it took her so long to do the grocery shopping. He had twisted her arm painfully behind her back and struck her in the back. The doctor examined her back and discovered a painful bruise. At this point, the doctor asked her to have her husband make an appointment to see him. Karen's story is typical of the abuse cycle in many different economic and ethnic groups in the United States (Bobes & Rothman, 2003).

Love and Belonging

In Hispanic families, it is still a common practice for men to ask the father-in-law-to-be for his daughter's hand in marriage. The culture is very definite about virginity and the category of "good women" versus "bad women." Good women are virgins when they marry. This requirement is sometimes difficult in the modern United States in which it is not uncommon for 13- and 14-year-olds to be sexually active (Horsley, 1996; Stavans, 1996).

Rosa, a Hispanic woman in California, had been living with her *Anglo* fiancé Alex, several years before marriage. Her sisters had all followed the cultural ritual of having their fiancés ask for their hands in marriage, but not Rosa. This behavior had alienated her from her large family so that when she was in a car accident that caused a head injury with the need for extended rehabilitation, it was necessary to coach her fiancé into rebuilding the relationships so that her family could be supportive for her. Rosa's father had declared that he hated Alex for taking Rosa's virginity so that she was no longer a *mujere buena,* or good woman. The therapist suggested to Alex that he approach Rosa's mother rather than her father. This was a successful approach, and Rosa's family gradually reaccepted her.

When a man of European American culture marries, he often enlists his wife in maintaining his close relationship with his mother. A Mexican man, on the other hand, usually does not expect his wife to participate in maintaining this close relationship. He is able to maintain the relationship on his own (Falicov, 1998).

Raul was a 27-year-old Mexican-American man who married a high school classmate shortly after they graduated. He was the second of two boys. Every Sunday, he spent the afternoon with his mother while his wife went to her own mother's house. The couple had three children in three years. Raul would always take the boys with him to his mother's home. When his mother had a stroke and was in a rehabilitation center, Raul changed shifts at his food packaging job, to be at his mother's bedside while his older brother stayed with her at the other times of day. The therapist was puzzled about why she never saw Raul's wife. When the therapist asked Raul about the whereabouts of his wife, he was surprised that the treatment team expected his wife to visit her mother-in-law.

Success and Personal Esteem

Women who have schizophrenia appear to benefit more than men do from psychosocial treatment. Males appear to respond better to neuroleptic drugs. Theories about this difference have both biological and social explanations (Seeman, 1995).

Jessica was a thirty-five-year-old European American woman recently diagnosed with schizophrenia. Although her medications were adjusted every three months, still they did not seem to be optimal. A slot opened at a Community Mental Health Center (CMHC) in a program for the chronically mentally ill. The program involved an occupational therapy activity group, a recreation group, and a psychosocial group coconducted by a licensed counselor and the occupational therapist. The occupational therapist, recreation therapist, and the counselor collaborated with each other and with Jessica to remind her whenever her paranoia seemed unreasonable and her behavior inappropriate for the situation. After three months of such an approach, Jessica showed marked improvement in her socialization, grooming, and ability to initiate activities. Meanwhile, twenty-eight-year-old European American Bob, at the same CMHC, started to attend the psychosocial program, but his lack of improvement, as perceived by Bob, soon made him drop out. However, he always attended his regularly scheduled psychiatrist visits at the CMHC and reported much improvement from his medication, Prolixin.

Self-Actualization

For Mei-Ling, Karen, Rosa, and Raul, attendance at religious services offered hope and inner calm. Mei-Ling took her baby and went to visit the grave of her grandparents in the southern part of the island of Taiwan, to pray and burn incense. This Chinese custom gave her great peace. Karen had been raised in the Methodist Church, whereas her husband had been raised as a Catholic. During counseling, they decided to attend the Lutheran Church. Joint worship strengthened their commitment to solving their differences. Rosa, a Catholic, and her Baptist boyfriend found a source of support from attending a couples support group conducted by the staff of the Catholic hospital where Rosa received her treatment. The support group had a strong element of religion. Attending worship together, in a group, was encouraged. Raul was with his mother while the chaplain prayed with them. The mother expressed her gratitude for his presence. Each of these individuals and couples found self-actualization through religious participation.

Middle Adulthood

Middle adulthood can include people from ages 30 to 50 years. It is during this time that most women begin to develop premenopausal symptoms such as increased menstrual flow, skipped menstrual cycles, and decreased skin elasticity. Menopausal symptoms include cessation of menstruation, vaginal and urinary tract changes, hot flashes, night sweats, and occasionally mood swings. Cultures provide support for menopausal women in different ways. In the Arab culture, for example, when a woman becomes menopausal, she becomes an honorary man, consequently being allowed to do things she was unable to do as a younger woman, such as speak up more to the males in her family (Drake, 1982).

Physiological Needs

African American women are more likely than Caucasian women to suppress anger about the ways in which they are treated in the health care system. Consequently, some researchers attribute their generally higher blood pressure to this reaction (Krieger, 1990), which means that their physiological state will be affected on a regular basis. Over a lifetime of such increased pressure, African American women have an increased risk of stroke and heart attack (Glanville, 2003).

Antoinette was a 45-year-old female businesswoman. Her childhood was spent in a small, rural African American community in the U.S. South. She had attended a traditional African American state university. When she graduated from college, she took a job with a communications company. This was her first thorough immersion in the European American culture and daily exposure to the presence of many white people. It greatly increased the tension in her life as she attempted to understand her new situation. She married a college classmate. During her first pregnancy, she discovered that her blood pressure was labile, frequently rising to frightening heights. Her African American obstetrician discussed her risk for high blood pressure. Following the birth of this first child, one strategy she chose was to join her husband in his courier business rather than subject herself to the constant tension of working with only European Americans.

Safety and Security

Despite development of equity in most areas of family life in the developed world, distinct role expectations still exist no matter what the ethnic group. Males grow up having the expectation that they will be in control of their family household. Females grow up expecting to be the family caregiver and nurturer. "Men were expected to control their families, and women were expected to take care of the needs of all the family members" (McGoldrick p. 13).

As Irwin, a Jewish American man, began to physically degenerate because of his Parkinson's Disease, he came to understand that he was no longer in control of his household. First, he found it necessary to be classified as disabled in order to receive some income as well as no longer being able to drive the car. He could no longer light the candles at the Friday evening worship service. Moreover, he felt unsafe in leaving his home without a family member. These areas of diminishing function reinforced to Irwin that he was no longer in control. He became more irritable with his family as his role changed, whereas his wife became even more nurturing than she had been before as her role expanded.

Love and Belonging

A woman's relationship with her eldest son is used to increase her influence over her husband in a number of cultures, particularly the Chinese and Arabic cultures. If the eldest son is emotionally bound to the mother, she can rely upon that relationship to secure her a place of importance in the family. Consequently, a young man's loyalty may be to his mother rather than to his wife, thus causing the younger woman to experience loneliness and to feel rejected in her husband's family.

Fareeda, an Egyptian homemaker who had immigrated to Ontario, Canada, with her engineer husband and their five children, continually told her eldest son, twelve-year-old Sadik, that he was her security in this new continent. She told him that he must always take care of her no matter what happened. After five years in their new home, the father wanted to divorce Fareeda; however, she prevailed upon Sadik, now 17 years old, to persuade his father not to divorce her. Sadik took it as his mission to persuade his father not to abandon his mother. He cajoled and threatened until the older man agreed not to leave Fareeda.

Success and Personal Esteem

Hispanic males often refrain from alcoholic beverages for some time and then go on a binge. Drinking is such an integral part of festivals and celebrations that it is particularly difficult for Hispanic males to remain abstinent (Gonzales, 1996; Loue, 1999).

In a California rehabilitation center for substance abusers, the *Anglo* female occupational therapist planned a holiday party with the Hispanic patients. As the planning committee of six male patients and the OT sat together, the male patients began to joke about drinking and to recount stories of past alcoholic exploits during the holidays. The occupational therapist had difficulty getting the group to focus on what needed to be planned, because the men were so busy remembering and joking about alcohol. The therapist initiated a discussion of how important drinking was to Hispanic celebrations. The men readily agreed that no celebration was complete without drinking until they passed out. The OT brainstormed with the men about what could be substituted for alcohol to give a feeling of celebration. Some ideas suggested were to use many candles on the dining table, to make a piñata, and to make *menudo,* a special Mexican soup. The OT asked the men to consider whether these suggestions would sufficiently substitute for alcohol.

Women are particularly vulnerable to depression at the times when their hormones are changing, such as at menopause or during the premenstrual phase of their cycle. Reproductive hormones affect neurotransmitters associated with mood (Seeman, 1995).

Roberta, a 36-year-old Minnesotan, came from a mixed European background. Her grandparents on one side were Irish, and on the other side, Norwegian. Roberta had married immediately after high school. She and her Scandinavian American husband had two children who were teenagers before Roberta realized that her periodic bad moods were related to her menstrual cycle. She had had two episodes in which she had been hospitalized after becoming suicidal. After Roberta had tried antidepressants, her physician put her on birth-control pills to help even out her mood swings related to hormones. This treatment, along with joining a church-related women's group, helped Roberta maintain a tolerable level of emotional cycling.

Self-Actualization

The action by the Southern Baptist Convention, May 2000, to deny further ordinations to women clerics demonstrates the continuing difficulty that many denominations have with women as religious leaders. Religious leadership is considered by many women to be the penultimate way of self-actualization. Midlife is often the time in which women come to the decision to use their leadership skills to influence others' spiritual paths. In many denominations, this road to self-actualization still excludes them.

Alyce Sue, a white Southern Baptist woman who had planned for the ministry since her two children reached their teens and needed her less, became clinically depressed when the Southern Baptist Convention publicized their ruling. She was initially hospitalized when she expressed suicidal thoughts to women in her Bible study group. The women decided to tell her husband, who was a businessman and church member, about the suicidal thoughts Alyce Sue had expressed. He took the initiative to have her hospitalized. This spiritual crisis was treated through outpatient visits with the female chaplain and the female social worker. The chaplain was able to model for Alyce Sue a different way of utilizing her skills.

Older Adulthood

"Older" is an entirely subjective term. Some individuals define themselves as old at age 30, and others at age 75. For the purposes of this chapter, "older" means approximately 50 years to 75 years. It is a time when people retire from regular paid employment or home-making and still may have fairly good health.

In 1900 the life expectancy was 49 years of age. By the year 2000, most American citizens expect to live to their late 70s. As people have begun to live longer, U.S. society has come to accept that there is another stage in which people are older but healthy and that they do not consider themselves elderly (Apple, 1990).

Physiological Needs

Since most women at this time of life no longer have reproductive capability, birth-control is no longer an issue. With the diminishing of reproductive hormones, some women have diminished sex drive. For males at this life phase, sex drive may also diminish; however, new drugs such as Viagra appear to allow men to extend their time of youthful virility.

Joe, who is 54, and Cindy, who is 45, both European Americans, married each other after divorcing their first spouses. They had met at a Baptist Church Divorce Recovery workshop. Joe felt strongly that it was important for him, as a newly married man, that he should be able to have sexual relations with Cindy at least once per day during their honeymoon. Cindy, mother of two grown children, on the other hand was still concerned about getting pregnant and began taking birth-control pills again. One of the issues that came up for discussion during their prenuptial counseling with other couples was that insurance would pay for Joe's Viagra but that it would not pay for Cindy's birth-control pills. This issue made for a lively discussion between the men and women in the group.

Safety and Security

For older persons who experience the natural results of aging, such as hair color change and diminished muscle mass, the fear of being vulnerable to attack is often present. Some think that gray hair is an invitation to predators. Although most often it is older women who color their hair to maintain a youthful appearance because of the emphasis on youth in Western culture, some older males color their hair to prevent attack from thieves (Peach, 1998).

Love and Belonging

Asian women hide their own emotions. They try to be polite and to please people in authority, such as the husband and the father. This feeling is so strong that even after a trusting alliance with the therapist has been established, these women often cannot keep promises that they make. It is not uncommon for it to take one year or more for them to feel free enough to discuss their most difficult family problems (Kim, 1998).

Kim Lee, a 65-year-old female Korean immigrant to the United States, was in the rehabilitation center subsequent to having had a burn on her right arm and hand during cooking. She always told the occupational therapist and physical therapist that she was feeling fine and doing better even when she was obviously in pain. She returned to the outpatient clinic for treatments for one-and-a-half years. It was nearly at the end of her treatments before she could share with her Japanese American occupational therapist that she was still in great pain and that she was embarrassed about her arm's disfiguration and about her inability to assist in the care of her grandchildren. It took her another week to decide to share that her husband sometimes derided her for her accident and the resulting problems.

Success and Personal Esteem

At this stage of life, success is often achieved through grandchildren, volunteer work, and hobbies. Many men in particular have a difficult time adjusting to retirement because they have totally immersed themselves in work, with their life having been scheduled by their employment. Without the requirement of a work schedule, retired men frequently feel less valuable unless they have anticipated this situation. Retirement planning workshops attempt to prepare those considering retirement for this event. Women, on the other hand, have less difficulty because they have learned to be involved in a number of overlapping tasks at the same time. This involvement prepares them for the time of life when demands are fewer and schedules less rigid.

Jordan, aged 65, and Etta, aged 62, both European Americans, were anticipating simultaneous retirement from their jobs as an engineer and as an elementary music teacher. They had coordinated their retirements to start on the same day so that they could rent a motor home and make a trip around the North American continent. When the actual day came for Jordan to stay home and start his "golden years," he felt a deep sense of despair and stayed in bed until 11 A.M. This pattern continued for several weeks. Etta had to call Jordan's brother on the West Coast to get him to call Jordan and cajole him into preparing for the continental trip during which they expected to visit the brother.

Self-Actualization

Older black women are often assigned the job of transmitting their cultural values and instilling religious ideas. Black women spend more time in church than black men do (McGoldrick, Anderson, & Walsh, 1991).

Jonetta, a 67-year-old African American, had retired from her job as a technician in the University Hospital because of diabetic and kidney problems. These problems caused her to spend a great deal of time in doctors' offices and clinics. However, weekends were completely devoted to her African Methodist Episcopal Church. She cooked food for the church to take to the local soup kitchen and she led the women's prayer breakfast committee. On Sunday, Jonetta arrived at church an hour before Sunday school. She made sure that her five grandchildren came to Sunday school and that they were quiet during the worship service, which often lasted until 1:30 P.M. Oftentimes Jonetta was called upon to lead hymns and to testify about how religion fulfilled her life. These experiences compensated her for the many discomforts of her illnesses.

Philanthropy is often a privilege of this stage of life. Middle-class people often have accumulated enough money to be able to give to their favorite charities. Even if they do not have money to give at this time, people at this stage often make out their will. It is not uncommon for people making their wills to include endowments to institutions. Some researchers have found that there are differences in the motivations for giving by men and by women. Men often give to preserve an institution they have known all their lives. Women, on the other hand, frequently write wills to give money to institutions that want to change the world for the better. Women have more often faced the threat of poverty and "baglady-dom." Some people who study philanthropy think that this experience affects giving patterns (Matthews, 1997).

The Wise Elderly

Although the United States has a culture that in many ways worships youth, the culture of many other countries reveres the elderly and the wisdom that they have acquired from living a long life. If a person lives until 60 to 70 years of age, that person has seen so many changes that he or she knows how to adapt to different circumstances. This valuable knowledge can inspire those around them.

Physiological Needs

As people age, their metabolism changes. Many factors are involved, for example, decreased activity level, decreased liver blood flow, higher protein requirements, and diminished thirst. Elderly females are more likely to be living alone and thus to be more vulnerable to malnutrition because of decreased metabolic activity. Because there is no other person to be concerned about, they may skip meals. In congregate eating situations such as in assisted living facilities, balanced meals are more likely to be prepared (Lewis, 1990).

Edith was an 80-year-old retired European American schoolteacher and a writer of children's books. She owned her own condominium in a mid-sized city. Edith had a rich social life; however, retirement decreased the times that she ate together with others. Gradually, over the years, she developed malnutrition despite her financial capability to buy what she needed. Eventually, her poor nutrition and decreased metabolism took its toll, and she was unable to fight off a systemic infection. She was therefore hospitalized, followed by placement in a skilled nursing facility from which she never emerged.

Often one of the daughters in a large Hispanic family will tacitly be designated as the caretaker of the parents. Such daughters will remain single and will sacrifice for the sake of the elderly parents and the family (McGoldrick, Anderson, & Walsh, 1991).

Josephina, a 47-year-old spinster and the youngest daughter of Carlos, aged 79, and Maria, aged 75, had never married. She had remained in the parental home. Every time she had attempted to find an apartment and move away, all her four brothers and three sisters had prevailed upon her to live at home. They had used reasons such as "single women living alone are targets for unscrupulous men." At age 40 when she met a man through a church singles group, again her siblings persuaded her to give up the relationship in the interest of caring for her parents. Carlos and Maria had not had to do the persuading because their other children did it for them. Josephina did not appear to be embittered about this sacrifice. Carlos and Maria did not think she had made a sacrifice; rather, they thought that she loved them as a good daughter should. Josephina agreed with them.

Safety and Security

Females in the United States seek medical care more frequently than men do, because women have more physical complaints. Women have a greater variety of cancers to which they are vulnerable; ovarian, breast, uterine, and cervical. It seems as if their bodies appear to betray them more often. Nonetheless, they live longer than men (Loue, 1999).

Love and Belonging

In many places in the world, as in the island of Tonga, great respect is shown to elders both while living and at death. Elders are perceived as the wealth of the group. When there is a death in a Tongan family, the women sit together and drink kava, the national drink in Tonga, and they mourn the dead person.

Tupou, a Tongan man, and his wife, a California Caucasian woman, were visiting his people on his Pacific island homeland. His mother-in-law died in California while the couple was in Tonga. All the women of the Tongan island community held a *fi bong bong,* or memorial service, for the California woman whom they had never met (Horsley, 1996).

Success and Personal Esteem

Elderly Chinese women were raised to respect all their elders and to know that when they became elderly, then their turn to receive such respect would come. Now, however, they may live in a youth-centered culture such as that in the United States. They are unable to command the respect that they gave to elders all their life and thus feel extremely cheated (McGoldrick, Anderson, & Walsh, 1991).

Case Study

Mrs. Lo, age 75, came to the rehabilitation center following her stroke. Because her family members were all in medical professions, they recognized the symptoms and quickly got her to the hospital. Having grown up in Hong Kong, Mrs. Lo, as a new bride, knew that her main task was to be obedient and respectful to her mother-in-law. After her husband died, in 1996, she immigrated to Vancouver, British Columbia, where her son had a medical practice. Mrs. Lo's Canadian English daughter-in-law was also a physician and spent most of her days working in a community health clinic. Mrs. Lo's daughter-in-law hired a young immigrant woman from Hong Kong to care for her two children while she was at work. When the daughter-in-law returned home in the evening, she ate the dinner cooked by a servant and then went into her home office and worked. Mrs. Lo felt abandoned and disrespected by her daughter-in-law's behavior. When she attempted to discuss her feelings with her son, whom she expected to support her complaint, he instead defended his wife.

Questions

1. Why do you think that Mrs. Lo felt disrespected?
2. What strategies can you think of to help the family resolve this situation?

Self-Actualization

Many elderly find religious practices important to their acceptance of the approaching end of their lives. Despite Mrs. Lo's participation in the Anglican support group, she maintained her Taoist/Buddhist religious practices. She regularly tended the family altar in the living room of the condominium, dusting the altar, lighting the candles, placing flowers and fruit, and burning incense. These rituals gave Mrs. Lo feelings of peace and connection with her family roots in Southern China.

Gender and Immigration

Immigration is a common occurrence in modern society because of the ease of travel. In past centuries, many more men immigrated than women. This trend is beginning to change. Consequently, there are some new issues related to gender and immigration.

Because food is central to all cultures, immigrant women who generally have been in charge of food preparation in their home country easily find work in the North American continent, starting restaurants and cooking for others. Cooking the food of their homeland offers a kind of emotional connection to the past while providing a livelihood. This activity assists in linking their new world with their old world (Walsh, 1998).

U.S. servicemen have brought back to America many "war brides," a euphemism for an immigrant wife. It is not uncommon for a European American husband to threaten his immigrant wife with deportation if she does not obey him. In addition, part of the threat is that the children will stay with the husband, thus depriving the woman of her children. In reality, a husband of an immigrant woman has no such power. Rehabilitation professionals can reassure an immigrant wife (Kim, 1998).

Women are raised in most cultures to be adaptive in their relations with others. Males, on the other hand, are educated to be in control and often become more rigid when confronted with new uncontrollable situations. This reaction causes them difficulties as new immigrants when they would benefit by being more flexible.

Mario, an Italian husband, had difficulty learning English after immigrating with his wife, who was a test cook for a food magazine. Because he was unable to find a job as a result of his poor English skills, he attempted to compensate by becoming more controlling at home. As his wife gained more power, Mario tried to compensate by making more rules at home about when she should arrive from work, when she could visit with her sister who lived in the same city, and the like. He became physically abusive and was arrested when a neighbor reported a domestic disturbance. His male therapist in jail provided therapeutic activities in which Mario was compelled to release control (McGoldrick, Anderson, & Walsh, 1991).

Irish immigrant women often do better with a female therapist because their family structure often had a female in authority. Irish men are often seen as less strong than the mother. Metaphors and parables often work better than direct confrontation with Irish clients (McGoldrick, Anderson, & Walsh, 1991).

When immigrants find it necessary to hide part of their traditional life's practices and rituals from health professionals, doing so causes them to feel extremely isolated. It is important for health professionals to be sensitive to these issues and thus to avoid causing the immigrant patient to feel personal rejection (Mirkin, 1998).

Summary

Male and female roles differ in almost every culture. After race, gender is the next most important thing that people notice about other people when meeting them (Glanville, 2003). Those working with rehabilitation patients must consider the importance of gender in achieving success in patient recovery.

Questions

1. What are men taught regarding their primary responsibilities toward their children, and how do you imagine that women's teaching on this topic is different?
2. What do you think is the rationale for the insurance company to pay for Joe's Viagra and not to pay for Cindy's birth-control pills?
3. Which of the vignettes in this chapter on gender has a rationale for behavior that would be most difficult for you to accept? Why?
4. Examine how the gender roles of the adults in your life as you were growing up have influenced your own gender roles.

5. Discuss the ways in which patients' beliefs about appropriate gender roles may influence their health outcomes (either positively or negatively).

6. Discuss the ways in which parents promote gender-specific roles in young children.

7. What are some approaches to help patients discuss difficult issues?

8. Do you think that the United States shows respect to elders? Why, or why not?

9. How would you plan a health education campaign to educate men who believe that AIDS affects only women?

10. How do you think that the number of males and females in your chosen profession affects the way the profession is perceived by the general public?

References

American Association of University Women (1998). *Gender gaps: Where schools still fail our children.* Washington, DC: American Association of University Women Educational Foundation.

Apple, R. D. (Ed.). (1990). *Women, health, and medicine in America.* New Brunswick, NJ: Rutgers University Press.

Bobes, T., & Rothman, B. (2003) *Doing couple therapy: Integrating theory with practice.* New York: W.W. Norton & Company.

Boyd-Franklin, N., & Franklin, A. J. (1998). African-American couples in therapy. In M. Mc-Goldrick (Ed.), *Revisioning family therapy: Race, culture, and gender in clinical practice* (pp. 268–281). New York: The Guilford Press.

Campbell, C. T. (1997). *Civil rights chronicle: Letters from the south.* Jackson: University Press of Mississippi.

Caspar, D. B., & Hine, D. C. (1996). *Black women and slavery in the Americas: More than chattel.* Indianapolis: Indiana University Press.

Chetwynd, J., & Hartnett, O. (1978). *The sex role system: Psychological and sociological perspectives.* London: Routledge & Kegan Paul.

Cieslak-Golonka, M., & Morten, B. (2000). The women scientists of Bologna. *American Scientist 88,* 68–73.

Cousins, N. (1989). *Head first: The biology of hope.* New York: E. P. Dutton.

Daly, M. (1978). *Gyn/Ecology.* Boston: Beacon Press.

Dossey, B. M., Keegan, L., Kolkmeier, L. G., & Guzzetta, C. E. (1989). *Holistic health promotion: A guide for practice.* Rockville, MD: Aspen Publishers, Inc.

Drake, M. (1982). *A california woman sees behind the veil.* Unpublished manuscript.

Erikson, E. (1963). *Childhood and society* (2nd ed.). New York: W. W. Norton.

Falicov, C. J. (1998). The cultural meaning of family triangles. In M. McGoldrick (Ed.), *Revisioning family therapy: Race, culture, and gender in clinical practice* (pp. 37–40). New York: The Guilford Press.

Friedl, E. (1997). *Children of Deh Koh: Young life in an Iranian village.* Syracuse: Syracuse University Press.

Gandhi. M. K. (1948). *Gandhi's autobiography: The story of my experiments with truth.* Washington, DC: Public Affairs.

Glanville, C. L. (2003). People of African-American heritage. In L. D. Purnell & B. J. Paulanka (Eds.), *Transcultural health care: A culturally competent approach* (2nd ed.). (pp.40–53). Philadelphia: F. A. Davis Company.

Gonzales, R. (1996). *Muy macho.* New York: Anchor Books.

Goodwin, J. (Spring1997a). A nation of widows. *On the Issues. 6/2,* 28–32, 56–58.

Goodwin, J. (Fall 1997b). Rwanda: Justice denied. *On The Issues. 6/4,* 26–33.

Groce, E. G. (2001). Health beliefs and behaviors towards individuals with disability cross-culturally. In R. L. Leavitt (Ed.), *Cross cultural rehabilitation: An international perspective.* (pp. 37–47). London: W. B. Saunders.

Haag, P. (1998). Single-sex education in grades K-12: What does the research tell us? In American Association of University Women Educational Foundation, *Separated by Sex: A Critical Look at Single-Sex Education for Girls* (pp.13–38). Washington, DC: American Association of University Women Educational Foundation.

Haag, P. (Ed.). (1999). *Voices of a generation: Teenage girls on sex, school and self.* Washington, DC: American Association of University Women Educational Foundation.

Harlow, H. F. (1971). *Learning to love.* San Francisco: Albion.

Horan, D. J., & Delahoyde, M. (1982). *Infanticide and the handicapped newborn.* Provo, UT: Brigham Young University Press.

Horsley, G. C. (1996). *In-Laws: A guide to extended-family therapy.* New York: John Wiley & Sons, Inc.

Inness, S. A. (1998). *Millennium girls: Today's girls around the world.* Oxford: Rowman & Littlefield Publishers, Inc.

Kaluger, G., & Kaluger, M. F. (1984). *Human development: The span of life.* St. Louis: Times Mirror/Mosby.

Keuls, E. C. (1985). *The reign of the phallus: Sexual politics in ancient Athens.* New York: Harper & Row, Publishers.

Kim, B. C. (1998). Marriage of Asian women and American men: The impact of gender and culture. In M. McGoldrick (Ed.), *Revisioning family therapy: Race, culture, and gender in clinical practice* (pp. 309–319). New York: The Guilford Press.

Kliman, J. (1998). Social class as a relationship: Implications for family therapy. In M. McGoldrick (Ed.), *Revisioning family therapy: Race, culture, and gender in clinical practice* (pp. 50–61). New York: The Guilford Press.

Kramer, A., Lorenzon, D., & Mueller, G. (2004). Prevalence of intimate partner violence and health implications for women using emergency departments and primary care clinics. *Women's Health Issues, 14,* 19–29.

Krieger, N. (1990). Racial and gender discrimination: Risk factors for high blood pressure? *Social Science and Medicine, 30,* 1273–1281.

Lemish, D. (1998). Spice Girl's talk: A case study in the development of gender identity. In S. A. Inness (Ed.), *Millennium girls: Today's girls around the world* (pp. 145–167). Oxford: Rowman & Littlefield Publishers, Inc.

Lewis, C. B. (1990) *Aging: The health care challenge* (2nd ed.). Philadelphia: F. A. Davis Company, Publishers.

Loue, S. (1999) *Gender, ethnicity, and health research*. New York: Kluwer Academic/Plenum Publishers.

Maslow, A. (1968). *Toward a psychology of being* (rev. ed.) New York: Van Nostrand.

Matthews, A. (1997). *Bright college years: Inside the American campus today*. New York: Simon & Schuster.

McGoldrick, M. (1998). *Re-visioning family therapy: Race, culture, and gender in clinical practice*. New York: The Guilford Press.

McGoldrick, M., Anderson, C. M., & Walsh, F. (1991). *Women in families: A framework for family therapy*. New York: W. W. Norton & Company, Inc.

Mirkin, M. P. (1998). The impact of multiple contexts on recent immigrant families. In M. McGoldrick (Ed.), *Revisioning family therapy: Race, culture, and gender in clinical practice* (pp. 370–383). New York: The Guilford Press.

Mitchell, J. (July 8, 2000). Suicides among black male teens on the rise. *The Clarion-Ledger*, Jackson, Mississippi.

Mocumba, P. (April 12, 2000). Interview with Charlie Rose at 11:00 P.M. on National Public Television.

Neufeldt, A. H. (2001) "Appearances" of disability, discrimination and the transformation of rehabilitation services practices. In R. L. Leavitt (Ed.), *Cross cultural rehabilitation: An international perspective* (pp. 25–36). London: W. B. Saunders.

Peach, L. J. (Ed.). (1998). *Women in culture: A women's studies anthology*. Oxford: Blackwell Publishers Ltd.

Pernick, M. S. (1996). *The black stork: Eugenics and the death of "defective" babies in American medicine and motion pictures since 1915*. New York: Oxford University Press.

Purnell, L. D., & Paulanka, B. J. (2003). *Transcultural health care: A culturally competent approach*. Philadelphia: F. A. Davis Company.

Sebai, Z. A. (1981). *The health of the family in a changing Arabia: A case study of primary health care*. Riyadh, Saudi Arabia: Tihama Publications.

Seeman, M. V. (1995). *Gender and psychopathology*. Washington, DC: American Psychiatric Press, Inc.

Stavans, I. (1996). The Latin phallus. In R. Gonzales (Ed.), *Muy macho: Latino men confront their manhood* (pp.143–164). New York: Anchor Books.

Stepp, L. S. (June 20, 2000). Distant dads spell trouble for daughters. *The Clarion-Ledger*, Jackson, Mississippi.

Strehlow, W., & Hertzka, G. (1988). *Hildegard of Bingen's medicine*. Santa Fe, NM: Bear & Co.

Upchurch, D. M, & Kusunoki, Y. (2004). Associations between forced sex, sexual and protective practices, and sexually transmitted diseases among a national sample of adolescent girls. *Women's Health Issues, 14,* 75–84.

U.S. Department of Justice. (1994). *Violence against women: A national crime victimization survey report.* Washington, DC.

Walsh, F. (1998). Beliefs, spirituality, and transcendence. In M. McGoldrick (Ed.), *Revisioning family therapy: Race, culture, and gender in clinical practice* (pp. 62–77). New York: The Guilford Press.

16

Age as Culture in Rehabilitation

Tana L. Hadlock and Jeffrey L. Crabtree

Key Words

cohort theory

ethics

continuity theory

age

rehabilitation

Objectives

1. Appreciate and understand the construct of age, or age groups, as subcultures apart from ethnic or gender diversity factors.
2. Understand the considerations necessary for a rehabilitation professional in providing effective and ethical services for persons who are members of different age-culture groups.
3. Identify and understand typical assumptions that rehabilitation providers may have about aging.
4. Identify and understand cohort theory and ethical concerns peculiar to rehabilitation practice with older recipients.
5. Identify and explain continuity theory as a way of explaining the life and treatment goals of older persons who seek our services.

Introduction

This chapter proposes a construct of age, or age groups, as subcultures in themselves and as apart from ethnic, racial or gender diversity factors, and also explores the considerations necessary for a rehabilitation professional in providing effective and ethical services for persons who are members of different age-culture groups. The chapter will explore assumptions about rehabilitation providers and mainstream, Western recipients as members of particular age-cohort "cultures"; will examine cohort theory and ethical concerns peculiar to rehabilitation practice with older recipients; and will discuss continuity theory as a way of explaining the life and treatment goals of older persons who seek our services.

In this chapter, we assume that most rehabilitation providers are in their twenties to forties and that most of the individuals who receive rehabilitation services are older than the practitioners. In addition, we assume that people of different generations are likely to misunderstand, and occasionally to mistrust, each other. Also, we assume that different age groups function as different subcultures even within ethnic and other cultural groups and that they are likely to hold different beliefs and values (including those about health, illness, and disability), which are at least partly determined by their experiences during their early decades of life. Finally, we assume that this misunderstanding and mistrust is the source of communication problems, ethical dilemmas, and practice problems.

Certainly not all rehabilitation practitioners are in their twenties or thirties. In addition, not all rehabilitation practitioners misunderstand older adults. However, for the purpose of this chapter and in order to highlight the need for cultural competence in rehabilitation, we will explore these potential differences from the perspective of a large variance of ages between providers and those receiving services. Because it would be impossible, within the limits of this chapter, to examine the impact of generational subcultures within all the major cultural-ethnic groups currently viable worldwide, or even within the United States, we will confine our examination of the issue to Western, Euro-American cultural groups of persons of different ages.

Why examine the potential problems that arise from misunderstandings among diverse age groups in the rehabilitation setting? Since cultural beliefs influence how people view their roles and responsibilities and also influence their decisions about health care (Bonder, 2001, pp. 18–19), age-related misunderstandings between rehabilitation providers and their clients can lead to miscommunication and an array of conflicts over issues of informed consent, individual autonomy, the role of the family, end-of-life issues, and the most appropriate rehabilitation goals for a given consumer. A competent rehabilitation practitioner must consider an important central question: What are this client's or patient's likely expectations for his or her rehabilitation, and more important, how do I maximize my chances of relating to him or her in a culturally effective way when providing my services?

Throughout this book the authors have described a number of different cultural groups within American society and have discussed how cultural distinctions may affect an individual's beliefs, values, and behaviors regarding health, disability, and rehabilitation. Although everyone recognizes that ethnicity, country-of-origin, and other inherent characteristics can be categorized as "cultures" that have distinct values, mores, and rituals, it is somewhat uncommon to consider age itself as a characteristic that defines groups as cultures. If we think about age difference at all as a factor that influences beliefs and behavior, we are likely to categorize the human family into *age-grade* groupings. Ember and Ember (as cited in Helman, 2000, p. 5) define age-grade as "a category of persons who happen to fall within a particular culturally defined age range (such as child, adult or elder)." Sociologists throughout the past century have studied and articulated an awareness that age-grade divisions function as cultures within the larger body of human groups. Helman (2000) noted that "both children and the elderly can be said to have their own cultures, or rather sub-cultures; their own unique view of the world, and ways of behaving within it. Although each is always imbedded within the wider culture, they also have certain distinct characteristics of their own" (p. 6). Psychosocial dimensions of age-grade "define quite precisely how people within an age-grade should behave, and how other people should behave toward them" (p. 5). Age-grade groups not only behave in different ways but they also think differently and hold different values, as every parent and every teenager are much aware.

However, for the rehabilitation practitioner providing services to patients including children and elders, it is no longer sufficient to understand that "elders" and "children" constitute, for practical purposes, two subcultures different from their own "adult" age-grade culture. For the first time in history, humans live in a world wherein the traditional division of human beings into three age-grades is no longer sufficient. During the course of the past two centuries, Western culture (and more recently, most of the remaining cultures of the world) have added two age-grades to their understanding of the "ages of man": adolescents and those of middle age. These two periods of human life were not generally considered distinctive life periods before the early nineteenth century, when some writers began to refer to "youth," a vaguely defined period between childhood and the full responsibilities and gravity of adulthood. The turn of the twenty-first century presents us with the reality that old age also cannot any longer be considered a single life period. Longevity continues to increase worldwide because of improvements in diet, preventive health care, and disease treatment, and we continue to define old age as beginning around 60 or 65 years. We now find, therefore, that the category of "old age" includes individuals ranging from their sixties through their hundreds, encompassing more than five decades. According to the Huffington Center on Aging at Baylor College of Medicine (Houston, Texas), there are currently 76,000 Americans aged one hundred years or older, and the U.S. Census Bureau estimates that figure will grow to be 129,000 by 2010 (Krach & Velkoff, 1990). In the United States, at least, "old age" now comprises three distinct generations. It should be noted that Helman did not distinguish age-grades into more discrete categories than child-adult-elderly and that he was writing about humans in general. Therefore, his tri-level concept of age distinctions cannot be generalized to other cultural groups. It is likely that some cultures distinguish more age-grades than others. American health care providers have become familiar with the categories of pediatric versus adolescent medicine and commonly conceive of elderly persons in subgroups that typically include categories such as "young-old" and "old-old" (Bonder, 2001, p. 11).

Morgan saliently points out the vagueness inherent in an age-grade hierarchy of only three levels:

> Unfortunately, studies of aging over the past few decades have paid little attention to the concept of generational cohorts. Instead, we talk about "the older generation" as if turning 60 or 65 somehow wipes out any differences between the experiences of one generation and the next. Yet, will the elderly of 2025—who grew up in an age of affluence, fought in Vietnam, and spent midlife in an era of "downsizing"—really be the same as today's elderly—who grew up in the Great Depression, fought in World War II, and retired in a time of relative security? (Morgan, 1998a, p. 7)

In the course of providing rehabilitation services for these older adults, many rehabilitation practitioners discover that a patient of 60 has quite different expectations about his or her disability, therapy, and progress than does a patient of 95, and that these differences cannot entirely be explained by differences in physical and cognitive condition.

Mrs. Gagne, a 64-year-old woman, is referred to the physical therapy department for evaluation and treatment following a total hip replacement necessitated by a severe fracture sustained in a fall. Prior to interviewing the patient, the physical therapist suspects, on the basis of the patient's age, gender, and diagnosis, that she has some degree of osteoporosis, that she is deconditioned, and that the goals of treatment will include patient education in hip precautions, recovery of general ambulation, and reconditioning to allow the patient to return to her usual homemaking and activities of daily living. During the interview, however, the physical therapist discovers that the patient is a university professor who works 50 to 55 hours a week, engages regularly in tai chi, weight-lifting, and long-distance cycling for exercise, and that she broke her hip falling from a rock cliff during a wilderness hike. Her bone densitometry was negative for osteoporosis.

Rehabilitation professionals who provide services for older adults are about to experience a significant change in the context of their practice with the "arrival" of a huge new population of consumers. The oldest of the Baby Boomers, born between 1945 and 1960, are about to turn 60, and over the next 20 years, 78 million of them will enter the stage of life defined as "elderly" (Lancaster & Stillman, 2002; Mitchell, 2000; Smith & Clurman, 1997). These older consumers will not necessarily have the same values, beliefs, behaviors, and expectations about their health, health care providers, and disabilities as had earlier generations.

Generational Cohort Theory

Rehabilitation practitioners can comprehend the issue unearthed by Morgan by using a sociological theory of generational cohorts when interacting with their older consumers. Mannheim, in an essay originally written in 1927 (published in 1952), and Rider, in 1965, have given us classic works in this theory. However, more recent and popular exploration of the issue is widely available in the business literature, where generational differences have had great impact both on marketing and on the management of employees and consumer relations (Lancaster & Stillman, 2002; Mitchell, 2000; Smith & Clurman, 1997). William Strauss and Neil Howe have also written several books for the popular press in the past decade, emphasizing the sociopolitical implications of generational differences. Current health care literature, however, generally classifies all "elders" as a chronologically homogeneous group, although significant attention is given to ethnic and other cultural group distinctions. According to Rider, "A cohort may be defined as the aggregate of individuals (within some population definition) who experienced the same event within the same time interval" (1965, p. 845). Generational cohorts are usually defined by their year of birth. The writers cited in the previous paragraph have described and defined a sequence of generational cohorts whose life experiences and resulting values and "collective personality" have affected many aspects of public life through the twentieth century in America. The authors differ somewhat in their choices of the range of birth years of each cohort and in the names they assign to these cohorts. Table 16.1 represents a summary of these authors' works.

Readers of this book will rarely encounter a consumer of the Lost Generation, those who fought in World War I, suffered the disillusionment and losses of that devastating conflict, and frenetically danced and drank their way through the recover-and-forget period of the Roaring Twenties. Generation X and the Millennials may concern the reader as fellow employees, and the works cited in the previous paragraph explore in depth the possible difficulties in and results of integrating these younger workers into the workforce that is currently dominated by Baby Boomers. However, the focus of this book is on relationships between professional caregivers and the recipients of their services. The caseload of the

TABLE 16.1   Generations of the Twentieth Century

Birth Cycle	Generation	Age Range (in 2003)
1880–1900	The Lost Generation	100 years +
1901–1926	The GI Generation	77–99 years
1927–1945	The Swing (or Silent) Generation	58–76 years
1945–1960 (or 1964)	Baby Boomers	40–57 years
1961/65–1980	Generation X	23–39 years
1981–	Millennial Generation	3–22 years

rehabilitation professional will sometimes include members of all of the six generations listed in Table 16-1. With the exception of practitioners in the public schools, however, the majority of the rehabilitation professional's practice is with people whose aging process and its associated conditions lead them to seek intervention with their debilitation and their orthopedic, neurological, arthritic, and chronic disease conditions. The so-called elderly make up a significant proportion of rehabilitation practice. The Silent and the GI Generations (those persons currently in their sixties, seventies, eighties, and nineties) are the cohorts currently making up the majority of this population. Soon 78 million Baby Boomers will begin to join them (Mitchell, 2000).

Cohort Values

No general description of the values, expectations, and beliefs of a given cultural group can be applied to any individual representative of that cultural group without careful examination of the individual. All African-Americans do not hold the same cultural values and beliefs. All American gay men do not share the same expectations. Even in a group as specific as Cuban-American Roman Catholic females, the interviewer will find significant variations of values. Just so, a description of the cultural distinctions of generational cohorts must, of necessity, be a gross generalization. Therefore the following descriptions must be taken as guidelines only.

The GI and the Silent Generations

The GI Generation and the Silent Generation (sometimes called the "Matures") shared some common societal experiences in their formative years that contributed to the development of a number of shared cohort characteristics. Economic times were hard for both these groups, constrained by the deprivations of both the Great Depression and the rationing of World War II. They learned that success and even survival depended on their own hard work as well as the collaborative efforts of families, communities, and of squadrons, brigades, and armies. They held joint-ownership with all their generation of the goals and victories of World War II and the booming economy and political simplicity of the postwar years. They learned that "we're all in this together" and that "working together, we can get out of it." These cohorts are characterized by loyalty to their group and to authorities, governmental and expert. They value frugality, patience, hard work, and the achievement of common goals through cooperation and delaying personal gratification (Lancaster & Stillman, 2002; Mitchell, 2000; Smith & Clurman, 1997). The members of these cohorts have looked forward to leisure and retirement as a reward for their many years of effort. After the war, many took advantage of the GI Bill to achieve an education and higher-paying jobs in order to pursue a better standard of living and better opportunities for their children. In addition, they learned early that wellness meant avoiding disease, and doing that meant relying on medical experts. They also learned young that the world was not always a safe place, although they grew up largely in either urban or rural environments where neighborliness was essential. Satisfaction, they realized, wasn't something that they necessarily deserved but was something that they might achieve if they worked hard enough, long enough, and cooperatively enough. Financially, they have become the most comfortable group of elders in America's history through hard work and frugality and the benefits of both federal entitlements and decades of steady employment with retirement and health care benefits in abundance (Mitchell, 2000).

Baby Boomers

Baby Boomers, in contrast, benefited from the hard work and gains achieved by their GI parents. Growing up primarily in the suburbs, in a time of a huge middle class, they were blessed with the highest collective level of education and the highest national standard of living in American history (Mitchell, 2000). Most attended college, had allowances and cars in their teens, and adopted their parents' message that with enough persistence and know-how, anything was possible. As children, teenagers, and young adults, they understood that the family was focused on *their* future and *their* success (Mitchell, 2000). Although they knew the distant, constant threats of the Cold War, their immediate suburban environment was quite safe, and they had little fear of sudden, catastrophic disease and death. They felt free to question the authority of their elders and of the government, and the war in Vietnam offered them plenty to be skeptical of. They "tuned in, turned on and dropped out," focusing on self-examination, self-development, and frequently self-indulgence (Lancaster & Stillman, 2002). The good things of life were plentiful and would apparently always be plentiful in the long economic upturn (Smith & Clurman, 1997). Baby Boomers learned to value individual self-expression, individual achievement, and individual autonomy. They also learned to expect a well-functioning, largely disease-free body that modern medical science was supposed to keep functioning for them as long as they wanted.

Between 1979 and 1987, however, the comfortable world of the Baby Boom Generation began to come apart. The inglorious end of the Vietnam conflict taught them that success was not, in fact, inevitable. Renewed Cold War tensions, new troubles in the Middle East, the worsening of the energy crisis, the exposure of widespread cheating in the Stock Market that resulted in widespread unemployment, high energy prices, and the "Reagan recession" revealed that the "good life" they expected might not always be there (Smith & Clurman, 1997). Crime rates skyrocketed. Even medical science betrayed them: the increased longevity that doctors delivered did not come with an attached guarantee of lower disability rates to gladden those extra Golden Years. Differences in generational values may often create ethical dilemmas in the rehabilitative environment, as the professional provider tries to interpret and negotiate the value and expectation factors leading to families' decisions.

Hilde and James Nelson (1998) provide an enlightening snapshot of a typical conflict between the values and expectations of Baby Boomers and their parents, in describing the reactions of a fragile woman in her late seventies and her daughter. The older woman, confronted with requests by the health care team to make decisions about her health care and rehabilitation, continually defers to her Baby Boomer daughter. A product of the GI/Silent generation era, she appears to value consensus and the needs of the entire family as critical factors in making decisions about her own needs. The younger woman, whose value system was developed in the 1950s and 1960s, is unwilling to accept the decision-making role, believing that her mother, as the patient, is the only person with the "right" to decide her fate.

Generation X

Generation X is demographically a small cohort of 45 million Americans sandwiched between two large cohorts; preceding them are 78 million Baby Boomers and following them are about 76 million Millennials (Mitchell, 2000). Most grew up as "latchkey children," since their parents' generation invented the two-paycheck family, the "power breakfast," and the long working week of an intensely competitive economic environment. Generation X children discovered early their own independence and their mutual interdependence on their peer group. They tend to be resourceful and to look for needed information and advice from their peers and to reject "authoritative" sources (Lancaster & Stillman, 2002). They have grown up well aware that the "good life" their parents strived and sacrificed for may not be available to them. They have seen that the Baby Boomers' strategies for success and getting ahead aren't necessarily successful. Generation X-ers are generally skeptical, pragmatic, and technologically sophisticated, and they are comfortable with uncertainty and change. They collaborate primarily with their age-peers and tend to be more committed to enduring personal relationships than were their parents, but they generally distrust institutions and don't expect to develop permanent connections to workplace, community, or setting. They don't "live to work," as so many of the Baby Boom generation did; rather, they view work as a means to quality of life and are not willing to work the long hours and sacrifice family and personal time to the job (Lancaster & Stillman, 2002; Mitchell, 2000; Smith & Clurman, 1997). To predict this cohort's response to aging and health changes would be premature, but it is likely that their values regarding independence, self-direction, and disability will differ from that of their parents. They may also be expected, as a group, to be more tolerant of individual differences, diversity, and pluralism, and therefore may be relatively unaffected by the stigma of disability that all previous generations have had to confront. The role of adult Generation X children in the long-term care and rehabilitation decisions about their Baby Boomer parents is uncertain, but it is expected that there will be value conflicts to resolve.

Overarching Considerations About Aging as Culture

On the basis of cohort theory, there may exist several subcultures of aging among older adults seen in rehabilitation settings in the United States. Despite differences among these groups, however, there are several constructs we will explore that suggest that older adults of different cohorts also share many beliefs, needs, desires, types of experiences, and social dynamics. These common elements need to be explored in order for rehabilitation practitioners to offer culturally proficient services to older adults. These theoretical considerations include the ethics of autonomy vs. paternalism in providing services to older persons; that as people age they perform and think in characteristic ways that offer continuity in the aging process; and that this continuity offers a common strategy for coping with changes not only in the aging process, but in the process with coping with changes due to chronic illness and other disabling conditions.

Ethical Considerations Across Age Cultures

The reader is referred to Chapter 4 for a full discussion of ethical principles, collectivism versus individualism, and their application to cultural diversity in general. However, a brief digression is necessary here to explore the particular ethical considerations that arise when the culture represented by the patient/client is age. The dominant Western cultural value of individual autonomy is often unexpectedly called into question in this circumstance. Rehabilitation providers who would rarely hesitate to accept the care decisions and rehabilitative goals of a young adult with an amputation or multiple sclerosis often find themselves reacting with unusual paternalism when confronted by an elderly client who disagrees with the provider's recommendations. A study done by C. A. Kane (as cited in Kane & Levin, 1998) disclosed that professional caregivers generally stated a belief that older adults "should be free to act against advice of a professional . . . regarding risk-taking," but they also believed that this autonomy should be qualified: "when it does not jeopardize their own safety or that of others." This apparently self-contradictory value held by health care providers, Kane and Levin summarize as "Professionals endorsed informed risk-taking, but apparently only when it was risk-free!" (p. 77).

A recent Australian study by Russell, Fitzgerald, Williamson, Manor, and Whybrow (2002) revealed that occupational therapists working with frail elders variously define *independence* of clients as either the client's physical self-reliance, particularly in basic and instrumental ADL, or as autonomy and independent decision-making, or as both. This variation is also reflected in U.S. occupational therapy literature. One of the occupational therapist respondents in the Russell et al. study (2002) describes a conflict between herself and nursing staff over the definition of "independence" in relation to a client whom the OTR wanted to discharge from the nursing facility but whom the nursing staff did not. The OTR felt that the patient could be independent in the home with "home help three times a day with meals and personal care" (p. 374) (a level of assistance provided in New South

Wales's health care system that Americans may envy). The nurses, however, felt that the client was not "independent" because she could not bathe and dress herself and manage her own ADL, and therefore she could not appropriately return to her own home.

Russell et al. (2002) also noted that although occupational therapists verbalize client autonomy as the highest value and the priority goal of intervention, that goal can be overruled by what Russell terms "the safety clause." That is, if in the opinion of the therapist the client was not likely to be safe exercising autonomy, the therapist felt an obligation either to persuade the client to adopt the opinion of the therapist or to fall back on professional authority to prevent the client from exercising his or her choice. Safety trumps independence regardless of how independence is defined. Some therapists also were reluctant to help the client exercise autonomy if they disapproved of the client's choices.

Rehabilitation practitioners must be on their guard against the potential influence of ageism on such clinical decision making. Traditional, less-industrialized cultures tend to accord more respect and higher status to elders, especially in nonliterate cultures dependent on oral tradition for their history, cultural mores, and wisdom. Modern industrialized cultures tend to view the elderly with reduced respect, at least in part because of the perceived importance of cognitive skill within these societies. As elders are perceived to suffer from decreased cognitive competence, they may therefore be perceived as being of lesser value and even as an irritation or a burden. Non-Western cultures often have a higher tolerance of reduced cognitive capacities usually associated with old age. However, changes in many of these non-Western societies, including increasing life-span (and changes in family/work structures that result in more women moving toward work outside the family home), are resulting in changes in social attitudes toward elders. Non-Western, traditional societies vary considerably in the amount and the quality of care, and overall respect, afforded older adults (Helman, 2000, pp. 7–8).

Russell et al. (2002) do not address the issue of whether older adults have, at some poorly defined milestone of life, lost part of their "right" to take risks compared with younger adults. Very few Americans would argue that young adults should be constrained, in their own best interests, from driving cars, playing football, or bungee jumping because of the high risk of injury deriving from these activities. But many rehabilitation professionals assume their right to persuade, recommend, or even coerce elderly clients, often with the active assistance of the client's children or other family members, into accepting a reduced level of autonomy or increased restrictions of living environment because of the "safety clause," even when there is no question of the client's having reduced cognitive capacity to realistically assess the degree of risk he or she is wishing to assume.

Persons of the GI and Silent generations, having developed a greater orientation to the welfare of the family or group, have usually been persuadable, even if reluctant, to accept such limitations in the interest of "not worrying their family" or "not being a burden." But it remains to be seen whether Baby Boomers, conditioned to value individuality and autonomy above all other ideals, and also accustomed to enjoy, especially in their recreational lives, high-risk activities that often appall their elders, will so compliantly accept similar restrictions. Is it possible that the average elderly Baby Boomer, confronted with a suggestion that he or she leave his or her home for a more restrictive environment to "avoid worrying the children" or to "prevent you from falling and hurting yourself," may feel perfectly willing to cause the children worry or burden, as long as the person is able to continue to live life "my way"?

Continuity of Aging

Notwithstanding the cultural distinctions between different generations of rehabilitation providers and recipients, with all the difficult negotiations and unpredictability that are likely to result, the concept of *continuity* can help to inform the rehabilitation provider's exploration of the values, needs, and expectations of clients of differing ages. Atchley (1999), in his Ohio Longitudinal Study of Aging and Adaptation (OLSAA) study, identified a number of factors in aging individuals' lives that seem to be consistent during the normal aging process. These include mental orientations called *internal continuity*, social arrangements called *external continuity*, and patterns of activity. These factors appear to provide older adults guidance during the aging process and appear to be central to the individual's development. Atchley sees these orientations and social arrangements as long-term patterns of thought and behavior that are resources for, and form the basis of, strategies for coping with change throughout later years.

It is important to note that the notion of continuity is not based on the sameness of the details of daily life. Rather, continuity is defined inclusively as a trend, as a general consistency, or as a pattern over time. For example, although an aging couple, because of poor health, might have to move from a large six-bedroom home to a small duplex in a retirement center, they view living in their own home as a strong source of continuity in their lives. In another example, a person's level of activity, or the vigor with which a person engages in physical activities, may decline, yet the person sees his or her pattern of activity as an important thread in his or her life and as a source of adaptation to aging.

Although this continuity theory needs more research to confirm its usefulness across cultures and ethnic groups, we assume that most rehabilitation clients have a history of these personal thoughts and behaviors that have helped them adapt to all sorts of social, functional, and health-related changes in their lives and that these orientations and social arrangements will be important resources for both clients and rehabilitation practitioners in the rehabilitation process.

In the following section, we identify the personal orientations and social arrangements that Atchley found to offer the strongest continuity across the later years of the subjects of his longitudinal study. In addition, we explore likely rehabilitation implications of those personal orientations and social arrangements, both in terms of how continuity supports normal aging and how discontinuity leads to problems in aging.

Adaptive Capacity

Atchley (1989; 1999) found three characteristics of aging individuals' lives that showed strong levels of continuity. As mentioned before, he organized these characteristics as internal continuity, external continuity, and patterns of activity. The person's internal continuity is individually defined according to the person's remembered structure of ideas about personal agency, experiences, skills, emotional resilience, personal goals, and the like. These characteristics form models of who and what a person is and help people adapt to the countless changes that occur in aging. Atchley found that self-confidence, emotional resilience, and personal goals seemed particularly important in normal aging. He characterized self-confidence as the belief in the ability to achieve goals—the ability to be assertive toward people in general and to authority figures in particular. He considered emotional resilience to be the "perceived capacity to deal with the emotions that can arise from the ups and downs of life" (p. 41). Finally, he said, "people enact their self-reflective values through their structure of personal goals" (p. 44).

External continuity is made up of general social arrangements that provide continuity in the lives of his subjects. According to Atchley (1999), people have one of two types of social arrangements they use to meet their needs: one that assumes they have control over the future, and the other that assumes they are at the mercy of spiritual, economic, social, and other forces. Individuals who assume that they have some control over their future tend to choose from a set of positive values they have chosen for themselves. They construct the most positive lifestyles possible given their personal, social, or cultural limitations. Those who see themselves at the mercy of outside forces tend to make the best of whatever comes their way. Atchley said that those who adopt this latter approach become motivated "to preserve [this view] because it becomes their customary way of adapting" (1999, p. 53).

Regardless of whether aging adults assume that they have control over the future or that they are at the mercy of various forces, Atchley's research found three general social arrangements that provided continuity in the lives of his subjects: first, living arrangements, household composition, and marital status; second, income adequacy (having the income required to support a customary lifestyle); and third, modes of transportation.

In addition, Atchley identified that patterns of activities tended to be continuous over the aging person's life. He found that the majority of the respondents of his study, 55%, engaged in diverse activity patterns that included "socializing, hobbies, organizational participation, physical activities and solitary pursuits" (p. 75). When changes in activity did occur, they tended to be in the frequency of doing the activities rather than in the diversity of the activities. A very small percentage of those studied actually discontinued a favored activity. He noted that among the participants of his study, few took up activities that they had not done before; however, a significant number in his study showed increases in engagement in civic and social organizations.

Continuity theory has three important implications for rehabilitation practitioners. First, continuity theory serves to remind the practitioner that probably the vast majority of older adults have learned over the years how to age successfully. The normal aging process seems to include the development of attitudes and beliefs, social structures, and activity patterns that, although they are unique to each individual, offer the majority of older adults effective ways of coping and adjusting to normal changes in the aging process.

Second, to the extent that older rehabilitation clients have threads of continuity in their lives, the rehabilitation practitioner will want to take a thorough history of his or her clients to understand how they have coped and adjusted to changes in the past. What practitioners learn from their careful history will offer clues to how a client will cope and adjust to the specific challenges that he or she faces in therapy.

Third, older adults are likely to bring to the rehabilitation setting long-term patterns of thought and behavior, social structures, and patterns of activity that have served them well in the past and potentially will serve them well in adjusting to significant functional changes in the future. The individual's level of self-confidence, emotional resilience, and sense of personal agency offer the rehabilitation practitioner cues about how the older rehabilitation client will cope and adjust to changes brought on by serious disabling problems. As Atchley put it, the vast majority of respondents in his study sought "to protect and preserve their customary way of life, not out of fear or defensiveness or rigidity but because their customary way of life was a rich source of potential life satisfaction for them" (p. 153).

Summary

In this chapter, we have proposed a concept of generational cohorts as "cultural" groups whose differing generational experiences, values, and beliefs require consideration by rehabilitation practitioners when planning interventions. We have described typical profiles of the several cohorts that the practitioner is likely to encounter frequently in practice, with the caveat that no individual consumer can be expected to think and act in stereotypical patterns based on his or her cohort, any more than he or she might be expected to do so on the basis of ethnicity or gender preference. We have suggested that individuals strive to maintain continuity throughout their life span despite external and internal changes, and that the practitioner should use continuity theory as a tool for collaborating with the consumer on intervention.

Questions

1. Review Table 16.1. To what generation do you belong? Examine your personal values; how do they resemble, as well as differ from, your generation's values?

2. To what generation do your parents (grandparents) belong? How do you think that your parents' or grandparents' values both resemble and differ from the values of their generation?

3. Briefly outline your beliefs about your health, illness, and death. Then outline your beliefs about the health, illness, and death of someone 75 years old. What are the sources of these beliefs (your culture, religion, professional studies, the popular media, and the like)?

4. Identify several major political, social, or economic world events shared by you and your age cohort that you think will be pivotal in determining the "profile" of your generation.

5. Review the example of Mrs. Gagne presented in a box earlier in the chapter. Collaborate with your classmates to identify what expectations this woman might have regarding her plan of intervention and its outcome, and then determine which of her expectations might be based on generational values. What is likely to be the influence of *internal* and *external continuity* for this woman's rehabilitative course?

6. Imagine that you are in your seventies and are experiencing declining health and physical abilities. You have been referred to rehabilitation services for intervention for a recently acquired disability. What threads of continuity will you most want to communicate to the practitioners as of primary importance in planning your evaluation and treatment?

7. With your classmates, divide into small groups or "debate teams," and then argue both for and against the "safety clause."

Case Study

Remember Mrs. Gagne, a 64-year-old woman referred to physical therapy because of a severe fracture sustained in a fall? Let's fast forward twenty years. This historically active and healthy woman, now 84 years old, lives alone in a retirement center. Her nearest living relative is a niece who lives four hours away by automobile. Mrs. Gagne has fallen twice in the last two months, once causing contusions on her chin and cheek. She often does not have dinner in the center's dining room. When the staff ask her about missing dinner, Mrs. Gagne offers vague excuses about being busy. The niece has spoken with the retirement center management about her concerns regarding her aunt's poor memory and falls.

You have been asked to consult with the retirement center to make suggestions about placement for Mrs. Gagne. There are two nursing homes and a home health agency in the community. Also, the retirement center has an assisted living wing.

Question

1. Considering what you know about Mrs. Gagne's history and taking into consideration what you have read about continuity theory, what kinds of information, in addition to assessing her functional and cognitive abilities, would you want to know about Mrs. Gagne before making a recommendation about placement?

References

Atchley, R. C. (1989). A continuity theory of normal aging. *Gerontologist, 29*(2), 183–190.

Atchley, R. C. (1999). *Continuity and adaptation in aging.* Baltimore: Johns Hopkins University Press.

Bonder, B. (2001). Growing old in the United States. In B. Bonder and M. Wagner (Eds.), *Functional performance in older adults* (2nd ed.). Philadelphia, PA: F. A. Davis.

Helman, C. G. (2000). *Culture, health and illness.* Oxford: Butterworth-Heinemann.

Kane, R. A., & Levin, C. A. (1998). Who's safe who's sorry? The duty to protect the safety of clients in home- and community-based care. *Generations: In-Depth Views of Issues in Aging, 22*(3), 76–81.

Krach, C. A. & Velkoff, V. A. (1990). Centenarians in the United States: Current population reports—special studies. United States Census Bureau. Retrieved January 26, 2005 from http://www.census.gov/pro/99pubs/p23–199.Pdf.

Lancaster, L., & Stillman, D. (2002). *When generations collide: Who they are. Why they clash. How to solve the generational puzzle at work.* New York: HarperCollins.

Mannheim, K. (1952). The problem of generations. In P. Kecskemeti (Ed.), *Essays on the sociology of knowledge.* New York: Oxford University Press. (Original work written 1927).

Mitchell, S. (2000). *American generations: Who they are. How they live. What they think* (3rd ed.). Ithaca, NY: New Strategist Publications.

Morgan, D. L. (1998a). Facts and figures about the baby boom. *Generations: In-depth Views of Issues in Aging 22*(1), 10–15.

Morgan, D. L. (1998b). Introduction: The aging of the baby boom. *Generations: In-depth Views of Issues in Aging 22*(1), 5–9.

Nelson, H. L., & Nelson, J. L. (1998). Care at home: Virtue in multigenerational households. *Generations: In-depth Views of Issues in Aging, 22*(3), 52–57.

Rider, N. B. (1965). The cohort as a concept in the study of social change. *American Sociological Review, 30*, 843–861.

Russell, C., Fitzgerald, M., Williamson, P., Manor, D., & Whybrow, S. (2002). Independence as a practice issue in occupational therapy: The safety clause. *American Journal of Occupational Therapy, 56*, 369–379.

Smith J. W., & Clurman, A. (1997). *Rocking the ages: The Yankelovich report on generational marketing.* New York: HarperCollins.

Strauss, W., & Howe, N. (1991). *Generations.* New York: William Morrow.

Tornstam, L. (2000). Transcendence in later life. *Generations: In-depth Views of Issues in Aging, 23*(4), 10–14.

17

Understanding Sexual Minorities

Suzann Robins

Key Words

gay

lesbian

bisexual

transgender

orientation

gender conviction

gender identity

homophobia

Objectives

1. Define some of the terminology related to sexual minorities.
2. Provide some useful guidelines for rehabilitation professionals working with this population.
3. Identify some problems that gays and lesbians are experiencing in this society.

Introduction

People who deviate from sexual norms and mores have existed throughout recorded history in most cultures. In recent years, some lesbians and gay men have been more vocal and therefore more visible. Because of this willingness to be seen and heard somewhat forced by the AIDS epidemic, this population has come to the attention of medical professionals as a distinct group. This greater degree of willingness to be visible doesn't mean to imply, in any way, that anyone can tell at a glance who is a member of a sexual minority and who is not. Many people, including health care professionals, remain prejudiced toward anyone who does not fit within a predetermined, narrow "normal" range. Unless people who provide rehabilitation learn tolerance and acceptance toward lesbian, gay, bisexual, transgender, and intersexed people, any attempts toward improved health and wholeness in this area will be thwarted.

Despite recent positive steps toward support, many lesbians, gay men, bisexuals, and transgender people (LGBT) remain invisible to most other people. Their lives retain an air of mystery and difference, as well as defiance in some cases. The majority of the heterosexual population tends to disregard sexual minorities and often permits spoken or implied intolerance toward them. In addition, in an attempt to be considered "normal," sexual minorities often remain silent, tolerating these comments in order to protect themselves. This silence allows discrimination to continue. This chapter is an attempt to suggest some concrete ways to eliminate barriers to acceptance and provide a path toward wholeness when this group of people seeks any level of rehabilitation service. Although some gay and lesbian literature has an angry, frustrated tone because of the prejudice and discrimination that sexual minorities have experienced or witnessed, this author is delighted to acknowledge the possibility for change in the future.

Defining Terms

In a rehabilitation setting, it is very important that nothing be taken for granted. The way people look, act, and how they present themselves must become part of the initial interview. Although not all things are noted on the chart when taking a history, an attentive rehabilitation professional needs to be observant of the person sitting before him or her. To do this well, it is important to become aware of personal judgments and prejudices about people in order to go beyond individual interpretations of normalcy.

Rehabilitation programs need to include education and assessment of *sexual orientation*. This term refers to one's primary psychological, emotional, erotic, and social attraction to the opposite gender, the same gender, or both. The current breakdown of orientation includes heterosexual, homosexual, and bisexual. *Bisexuality* refers to an attraction to both the same sex and the opposite sex partners. The term *queer*, referring to any sexual minority, is being reclaimed by the younger generation. *Orientation* is the accepted term, rather than *sexual preference*, according to current Parents, Family and Friends of Lesbians and Gays (PFLAG) literature. All people also have a *sexual identity*, which is the inner sense of knowing one's self with sexual desires and habits; and it is different from ge*nder identity*. Orientation refers to one's primary erotic, psychological, emotional, and social attraction to the opposite gender, the same gender, or both. The current, commonly acknowledged, breakdown of orientation includes: heterosexual, homosexual, bisexual. Carol Queen (1997) suggests we add: pansexual and PoMosexual. She is referring to the post-modern era where we are beginning to acknowledge that neither gender nor orientation is a binary dichotomy. None of us are totally male or female, masculine or feminine, gay or straight, but rather, like all human traits, both gender and orientation are found on a continuum. To be more inclusive, the term *queer*, referring to any sexual minority, is being reclaimed by the younger generation. In addition, sometimes the letter Q is added to *LGBTIQ* to make room for *QUESTIONING*.

Have you ever looked at a tall, large woman with very short hair and immediately assumed that she was a lesbian? Or decided that a short, slight man with long, beautiful hair and small hands was gay? Men and women come in a full range of sizes, as well as skin colors and personality traits. We cannot make assumptions that are based on appearance. Nor should we assume that most women of a particular age are married or that a man living alone is an eligible bachelor. People explore a full range of relationship styles, but even in today's so-called free society, in many cultures any deviation from the heterosexual, monogamous norm remains unacceptable. Therefore, rehabilitation professionals need to consider sexuality as part of overall wellness.

Homophobia refers to the societal assumption and accepted norm that being heterosexual is superior to being homosexual. It expresses the institutional and societal reinforcement of heterosexuality as the privileged and powerful norm, as well as the fear and hatred directed toward gay men, lesbians, and bisexuals. On the other hand, *heterosexism* has become institutionalized in a way that sanctions the discrimination and the denial of the basic human rights for any sexual minority, but this must not be the case when providing rehabilitation. A heterosexist attitude (or orientation) is the assumption that everyone is heterosexual, and it disregards a core component of personal identity, as well as the values, motivations, and preferences of sexual minorities. Because of this generalized assumption, gay, lesbian, bisexual, transgender, and any queer people who don't subscribe to heterosexual monogamous norms, are rarely free to reveal their orientation without suffering significant negative reactions in many situations. Heterosexual people regularly talk about their sexual orientation in ways both explicit (mentioning boyfriends, girlfriends, or spouses) and implicit (such as wearing wedding rings or displaying family photos). Sexual minorities don't have this freedom. Consequently, some of the LGBTI population may adopt an attitude of *Heteronegativism* toward hetersexuals (White, 1999).

According to the Sex Information and Education Council of the United States (SIECUS, 1993), no single scientific theory about what causes sexual orientation has been fully substantiated. Although studies of the association between sexual orientation and genetic, hormonal, and environmental factors are inconclusive, there are many indications that sexuality is deeply ingrained at a very young age. Sexual orientation and *gender identity* are no longer viewed as a result of conscious individual preference or choice; instead, they are formed by a complicated network of social, cultural, biological, economic, and political factors, which includes making a choice for self-acceptance.

In the past, any form of homosexuality was considered a mental disorder or illness. In 1973, the American Psychiatric Association eliminated homosexuality from its list of mental disorders, proclaiming that "homosexuality is no more a sign of mental illness than heterosexuality is a sign of mental health." However, this declaration did not result in the elimination of homophobia. When the fourth Diagnostic and Statistical Manual of Mental Disorders (DSM-IV-TR) was published, gay advocates viewed it as a significant breakthrough, without recognizing that a new "mental illness" had appeared called Gender Identity Disorder (GID) (Boenke, 1999).

The transgender population is even more complex than the gay, lesbian, or bisexual. *Transgender* is an umbrella term for the full spectrum of people whose gender identity and/or expression differ from conventional expectations of masculinity or femininity. In other words, transgender people transgress cultural norms (Goodrum, 2000). Many people have formed opinions about this group on the basis of exposure to the "drag queens" viewed in popular culture movies or television shows. Although the man performing as a flamboyant woman may or may not be part of this group, he or she is by no means representative of the whole. The person may simply be an entertainer or may like the feeling of women's clothing, a preference referred to as being a *cross-dresser* or *transvestite*, a term currently applied to people who cross-dress to achieve sexual arousal. On the other hand, *transsexuals* are people whose gender identity differs from their biological sex (Crooks, 2005). *Intersexed* people, formerly called *hermaphrodites*, are born with chromosomal anomalies or ambiguous genitalia, and will be discussed later in this chapter.

For most people there is no conflict between their gender and their physical sexuality however, many, but not all, transsexual people grow up questioning their identity, which they feel is the opposite from their physical body (Xavier, 2000). In order to understand any sexual minority, or for that matter, any individual, it is important to understand *gender identity*, *biological sex*, and *gender roles*.

Gender identity refers to a person's self-awareness of being male or female. By the age of 3 or 4, this identity is well established; and by the age of 7, the child is able to reason and make choices that are based on the child's awareness of his or her gender identity. *Biological sex* is based on one's genitals and reproductive organs present at birth. Chromosomal composition and the presence of hormones in the individual's body determine both gender and sexuality. *Gender roles* refer to the expectations that a particular culture has regarding how individuals appear, behave, and interact with one another as males and females. These expectations vary dramatically from culture to culture and even among particular groups within the same culture.

In simple terms, the *transsexual* is a person who has a gender identity that is opposite to his or her biological or birth sex. Therefore, a male to female transsexual (MtF), though born with male sexual characteristics, identifies internally as female. Conversely, a female to male transsexual (FtM), though born with female sexual characteristics, identifies internally as male. In some Native American cultures, these people are called *two spirits*. Advances in medical procedures have allowed people to have *sex reassignment*, formally referred to as a *sex-change operation*. The process of sexual reassignment is rare, difficult, and expensive, and although not all transgendered individuals choose surgical modification, those who do often find the process an intense, empowering, positive experience.

North American data indicate that boys are much more likely than girls to be referred for assessment and/or treatment of gender-identity disorders (Cohen-Kettenis et al., 2003). Transgender includes preoperative, postoperative, and nonoperative individuals. Women and men from any of these groups may present in public in any stage of "passing" in their identified gender. Ease in being able to visually appear to the public eye as the opposite gender is related to how easily the individual's physical characteristics conform to societal norms of what is male or female. For example, we have an expectation that men will be taller and women smaller. Many individuals blur those traditional ideas of what it means to look male or female. A biological woman may choose to dress as a man without binding the chest in order to hide breasts. Or a biological male may choose to dress and talk as a woman but may retain a full beard and body hair. On the other hand, a woman might have a great deal of facial hair, even resulting in a beard or mustache, yet will choose not to remove it. This choice does not mean that the woman desires to be a man. Conversely, a man may be completely hairless, but in every other sense truly masculine. Regardless of the outward appearance, one needs to approach each and every individual with openness and acceptance. If you are uncertain which pronoun to use, it is best to ask, "How do you want me to refer to you?" or "How do you identify?" Once you know, try to be consistent. If you slip up, and use the wrong pronoun, simply make the correction. Most trans people will appreciate your efforts.

Several theories have been discussed as to how these various sexual minorities develop. These are, however, only theories—clinical researchers and behavioral scientists are still exploring the intricate ways in which human personality develops and is influenced by biology and environment (Boenke, 1999). Current leading theory holds that transsexualism is the result of purely genetic or biological influences. One such theory that has gained rather widespread acceptance among many researchers and medical professionals is that hormones that influence the development of the fetus in the uterus may affect the development of the body so that it is masculinized, as in the case of MtFs, but that the hormones do not affect the brain, which then continues to develop as female. This process would work conversely in the case of FtMs, so that the body is feminized but the brain develops as male. Thus, the infant is born with the sexual characteristics of one gender but with a brain that has developed as the other gender in construction and processes.

Transsexualism was named Gender Identity Disorder (GID) in the *Diagnostic and Statistical Manual*, 4th edition (DSM-IV-TR), which is used by the psychiatric profession for the diagnosis of clients and for insurance billing purposes. It has been used to justify various forms of therapy in order to change children's perceived sexual orientation and/or gender nonconformity. According to the classification scheme, a person must meet four distinct criteria to be diagnosed as having a gender identity disorder, not merely a desire for any perceived cultural advantages of being the other sex. These include:

1. a strong and persistent cross-gender identification
2. persistent discomfort and a sense of inappropriateness in the gender role
3. disturbance that is not concurrent with a physical intersex condition
4. disturbance that causes clinically significant distress or impairment in social, occupational or other important areas of functioning. (Crooks, 2005)

Although controversial, the designation GID is sometimes important because it allows those who want to physically change their sex access to counseling, hormones, and reassignment surgery; however, currently there is little medical insurance money available for such services (Boenke, 1999). In spite of the lack of medical coverage, some transexuals present themselves to occupational and/or speech therapists to receive help in learning new behaviors.

Even though the term *disorder* is currently used in association with this condition, it is important to understand that transsexualism is not a mental illness or defect, and not everyone fits the diagnosis criteria the DSM-IV lists for GID. Rather, it is a medical condition in which an incongruity exists between a person's biological sex and his or her gender identity. Transsexualism is a conscious choice that a person makes; however, a person may deny or hide the condition for many years because of the dominant insistence in most cultures that only two genders exist and they must be consistent with one's biological sex. There is an ongoing debate in the transgender community about finding a way to balance the need for a diagnosis with the acknowledgment that people are acting on natural feelings and are not "sick" (Boenke, 1999).

The Washington Transgender Needs Assessment Survey conducted by Jessica Xavier, from September 1999 to January 2000, sought to identify the health, housing needs, and concerns of transgendered residents of the District of Columbia. A total of 252 individuals were surveyed, and the summary of the findings included the following:

- There was a suicidal ideation rate of 35%. Of these, 64% attributed their ideation to their gender issues, and 47% report that they had actually made attempts to kill themselves. This group is 16% of the entire sample.
- Only 58% of the participants were employed in paid positions, and 15% reported losing a job because of discrimination from being transgendered.
- Of the participants, 43% had been victims of crime or violence.
- Of the participants, 47% did not have health insurance, and 39% did not have a doctor to see for routine rehabilitation.

This survey, although relatively small *and not a significantly randomized study*, reinforces the need for rehabilitation professionals to be sensitive and open to the unique concerns of these individuals.

It is important to note that transsexual is the umbrella term for transgender and transsexual. It is also essential to understand that gender identity is not the same as sexual orientation. The transsexual person may identify as heterosexual, gay, lesbian, or bisexual, just as the nontranssexual person may. Sexual orientation is understood in relation to the transsexual person's gender identity, not to the biological sex. For example, an MtF transsexual who is sexually attracted to men usually considers herself to be heterosexual, whereas an MtF transsexual who is attracted to women usually will identify as lesbian. The individual needs to be allowed to define her or his sexual orientation. Comments such as "Well, is she really gay because she used to be a man and is now attracted to men?" are pointless and often mean-spirited rather than a sincere effort toward understanding. In many cases, before and during transition, the person may be solely concerned with his or her own identity rather than to whom to relate sexually.

Other conditions that blur the physical appearance and gender identity of individuals include Klinefelter's Syndrome (XXY chromosomes), congenital adrenal hyperplasia, and androgen insensitivity syndrome. Children born with these conditions have genitalia that do not appear to be completely male or female. Such genitalia are commonly described as ambiguous. Others appear genitally normal at birth but develop mixed secondary sexual characteristics at puberty. In the past, persons with such conditions were referred to as *hermaphrodites;* the preferred term now is *intersex,* which occurs in about 1 out of 2000 births according to Colapinto (2000).

Much controversy surrounds the treatment of the intersexed individual. Previously the standard treatment of infants with ambiguous genitalia has been to surgically modify their genitalia to look as normal as possible and to rear the children as the gender that "matches" their surgically modified genitalia. For example, if the child has an undersized penis, the child may be raised as a female. However, intersexuals are not always the gender that their parents and/or medical professionals determine for them. The Intersex Society of North America (ISNA) argues that *genital abnormality* is more accurately *genital variability* and advocates for a non-intervention, child-centered approach (Crooks, 2005). Because of advances in communication via the Internet, much is being learned about sexual minorities in general resulting from the openness and discussion among the intersexed people about what it means to "be" a man or a woman.

Once again it must be emphasized that all of these classifications need to be individualized and must be observed and treated by the professional with thoughtful and sensitive care.

Taking a Medical History

Rehabilitation professionals need to recognize that homophobia may become internalized, creating a form of self-hatred derived from the prevailing negative stereotypes associated with homosexuality. Therefore, it is necessary to allow persons seeking care to reveal their sexual orientation at their own speed. As mentioned earlier, asking the right questions can facilitate this.

With whom one lives and considers family is an important aspect of overall health. The meanings of *extended family* and *nuclear family* are constantly changing and evolving. Families consist of step-moms and dads, half-brothers and sisters, more than one set of grandparents, various aunts, uncles, nieces and nephews, stepchildren, foster children, as well as spouses/partners and lovers. The way that questions are phrased can help create a comfortable atmosphere. For instance, asking "With whom do you live?" may provide basic information, but following this with "Whom do you consider family?" or "Who are in your support network?" allows one to reveal more. Using the words *lovers* or *partners* instead of *husband* or *wife,* or *boyfriend* or *girlfriend,* is one way to indicate an openness to hear someone in a nontraditional relationship. When rehabilitation professionals encourage open and honest communication, they lead the way to a higher level of functioning within the context of both family and community. Communication must be as clear as possible to provide a truly healing community for all people, no matter the sexual orientation or lifestyle. A thorough health history must include questions about family, as well as a more open question like "Who else would you like us to contact in case of emergency?" Asking "Who should we contact first in case of an emergency?" helps to validate that individual's primary relationship. Once it is established that the person is in a same-sex relationship, be certain to refer to the partner appropriately. In the case of a transsexual person, or even if you are unsure whether someone is a male or a female because of the cut of his or her hair or the way the person is dressed, ask what pronoun he or she uses or prefers. Attention to pronouns is a way to show respect. Heightened awareness and sensitivity to these issues will begin to eliminate unconscious assumptions and judgments. Listening carefully to all answers provides a good way to connect with the person coming for help.

In addition to asking about family, questions about other treatments that have been tried must become part of taking a complete history. Even when previous medical records are obtained, they are most often only from the professional prospective. All health professionals must become more knowledgeable about the various integrative modalities available today. People with alternative lifestyles are often likely to have also experimented with alternative health care options. Sensitivity and openness to the entire range of possibilities in the rehabilitation field is imperative. Herbal remedies, vitamins and mineral supplements, homeopathy, chiropractic, massage, hydrotherapy, and hypnosis are just a few of the many complementary and alternative (CAM) health options that people are using to find relief from chronic ailments, boost their immune systems, overcome depression, or even balance hormonal shifts. Asking these questions provides another opportunity for openness and acceptance.

Professionals can decrease barriers to good care by acknowledging their own beliefs, listening with an open mind, and attempting to be as impartial as humanly possible. Active listening means being more open to hearing another person's truth and being able to respond appropriately. It is important to move past the limitations of our own prejudices.

As a rehabilitation practitioner, consider your reaction when someone tells you that he or she is gay or lesbian, or bisexual or transgendered, and you thought that the person was average-looking. A response like "No, not you" or "I never would have guessed" can be just as insulting as saying nothing at all. On the other hand, to respond to someone you are judging to be out of the average range with "Oh, I knew that" leaves the person wondering Why? and How? since gay men and lesbians often do not consider their sexuality to be obvious. It is better to reply with "I see" or "That's fine" or just to nod and continue with the taking of the history.

On the other hand, when someone reveals that he or she has children, does that automatically mean a person is heterosexual? This is too often the automatic assumption. Although sexual minorities are disturbed by society's attitudes, gay, lesbian, bisexual, and transgender people have the same range of mental and physical health problems as other groups. These problems do not stem from their sexual orientation or result from their being psychologically unbalanced or having some sort of deviant behavior. More often the problems stem from society's hostility, hatred, and fear of the unknown, in a word, *homophobia*. Gay, lesbian, bisexual, and transgender people simply deviate from the norm, and most thrive in an understanding environment. It is not necessary for providers to personally condone alternatives, but it is essential to accept the person who comes in for rehabilitation regardless of sexual orientation, gender identity, race, color, or creed.

The Need for Understanding

Although the rehabilitation specialist is not a psychologist, it is important to understand developmental issues in order to provide care for the whole person. The need for confidentiality between the client and the caregiver does not necessarily lead to a need for secrecy.

The fear of rejection is often at the root of anyone's not talking openly about sexual matters. Being able to talk openly is not only a sign of healthy maturation but also an indication of overall good health. The environment created by the rehabilitation professional can convey sensitivity and inclusiveness for sexual minorities to work through issues of abuse as well as sexual and/or gender identity. Items in the office, such as gay-friendly posters on the walls, nondiscrimination statements, diversified reading materials, videos, and other educational material that is inclusive and supportive, can help facilitate the process of talking about sexual issues.

Memories of childhood abuse, which sometime surface when rehabilitation is needed, can become the basis of a healing opportunity. If this occurs, psychotherapy should be suggested, but a rehabilitation specialist can also provide the sensitivity necessary for someone to sort out gender identity and/or sexual orientation issues. Although there is no proven correlation between gender identity or sexual molestation and adult sexual orientation, sexual abuse in childhood can cause some to question his or her identity and/or preferences, thereby leading to underlying years of confusion. Some parents have a narrow definition of what it means to "act like a girl" or "be a man." If these rules are broken, the child may be unjustly punished and become bewildered about his or her identity. Abusive parents too often view their children as "property" and use the child to satisfy their own sexual needs. Because some lesbians may have been abused by men, and, they therefore may be turned off to male advances, it is not a "cause" of sexual attraction to women. Likewise, young boys who are molested by men are not automatically attracted to or repelled by men as adults. Nor do all gay men have domineering or overbearing mothers and absent fathers. These kinds of stereotypes must be eliminated, and every case of homosexuality must be considered on an individual basis. Sexual orientation is affected by many factors; therefore, it should never be assumed that early childhood problems are the cause of homosexual or transgender issues. Post traumatic stress syndrome and other responses to trauma and abuse need to be kept separate from homosexuality and transgender issues.

Teenage Identity Is Difficult for Everyone

The most invisible, yet one of the most vulnerable, groups of people in any culture are lesbian, gay, bisexual, and transgender youth. Children can be cruel to each other simply because someone has an odd name or appears different, for example, a small boy or a large girl. Appearance does not automatically make someone a sexual minority. Too often, a child who is teased and who has internal conflict about sexual identity develops a very poor self-image and is vulnerable to many problems. Too many children become victims of harassment or violence.

A 1997 study found that one-fifth of females and nearly half of males were harassed, threatened with violence, or physically assaulted in school simply because they were perceived to be lesbian or gay. Often harassment takes the form of name-calling, such as queer, homo, faggot, lezzy, or dyke. According to the Report of the Massachusetts Governor's Commission on Gay and Lesbian Youth (GLSEN, 1993), 53% of students report hearing homophobic comments made by the school staff. High school students report hearing

26 antigay comments on a typical day, and 97% of the time teachers do not intervene. Because of this situation, many teens had not previously identified themselves as gay or lesbian because they feared for their safety. Others are too ashamed to even imagine identifying themselves in this way and therefore have suppressed all sexual feelings. In addition, there are some who have so little exposure to role models that they have no way to relate their feelings to their learned or perceived view of the world.

It is a well-known fact that many self-inflicted teenage injuries result from questions regarding sexuality. In addition, Planned Parenthood records show that some teen pregnancies are also due to discomfort regarding sexual orientation. Boys may try to prove that they are not gay by having sex with as many girls as possible. When a girl is willing to have sex and even wants a baby, the assumption is that surely she is not a lesbian. Therefore, it is important to remember that sexual behavior or expression does not always prove one's long-term orientation, making the problem of sexual identity even more complicated. When questioning a teen about sexual partners, the use of gender-neutral language and open discussion regarding possible activities are ways to build trust. The concept of trust-building will be discussed more in detail later in the chapter.

Confidentiality is particularly important when working with teenagers. In many cases, teens may have never had an opportunity to tell anyone how they feel. Like adults, only when they believe that you can be trusted will they let you know what they are thinking and feeling. They must be certain that what they reveal will not necessarily be noted on their chart or spread around the office, not to mention outside the confines of the rehabilitation setting. There are many ways to communicate sincerity, openness, and willingness to listen. If you have those qualities, they will be apparent, but it is very difficult to create the necessary safety if the ability to accept diversity is not sincere. Teenagers, as well as the older population, many of whom have developed a keen sense of awareness, will be able to detect your sincerity.

An Aging Population

The gay and lesbian segment of the United States population is currently estimated at 1 to 3 million people and projected to increase to 4 to 6 million by 2030 (Toledo & Cahill, 2000). This group forms what is in many cases an invisible population. Some older individuals choose to withhold the knowledge of their sexual orientation from all but a close circle of associates. Others, who are willing to be visible, are overlooked by rehabilitation and social service agencies that are not providing the level of support needed because of a lack of knowledge or of prejudice (Berger, 1986). Rehabilitation professionals are facing an elderly population who have been characterized all their lives as deviant, immoral, and promiscuous, and as authors of their own fate who deserve punishment.

When today's older gays and lesbians were young adults, homosexuality was considered a crime or mental illness and was treated as such. Gay people could be refused employment or fired simply because of their sexuality. During World War II, about 9,000 men and women were dishonorably discharged from the military. Being gay or lesbian was considered shameful, even dangerous—an aspect of one's self to be hidden at all costs from employers, friends, neighbors, and family. As a result, some had difficulty acknowledging their sexual identities even to themselves (Bensing, 1996).

In a society that desexualizes older people in general, the additional influence of homophobia fosters a hostile environment for LGBT seniors. Some health care providers have described feeling "a lack of empathy and difficulty in connecting" with people who are viewed as different (Taerk & Gallop, 1993). In the past, some people may have needed to see homosexuals as "different" in order to avoid thinking about one's own sexuality and vulnerability. As with all homophobia, avoidance of speaking about this aspect of human nature may quell anxiety but may also seriously impair the rehabilitation delivery process. This was especially the case at the height of the AIDS epidemic when the number of AIDS patients over age 60 rose steadily (Wallace et al., 1993). Currently, all populations, including HIV positive people, are living longer because of the availability of better treatments.

Men and women who have chosen to live an alternative lifestyle now face a culture that is more open to diversity. But this change can also cause "identity confusion" for an older individual. A researcher at University College in London, Nigel George, found that many older homosexuals did not feel that they fit anywhere in society (Frean, 2000): "Their sexual identity was often a source of embarrassment or ill-will in certain mainstream services, such as day centers or residential care homes." In a 1994 study of New York State's Area Agencies on Aging, 46% reported that openly gay and lesbian seniors would not be welcome at centers in their area. Homophobia and neglect appear widespread, according to the 2000 National Gay and Lesbian Task Force survey of nursing home social workers. More than half said that their coworkers were intolerant or condemning of homosexuality among residents; most other respondents avoided answering the question. This level of discrimination can be avoided as we educate ourselves about the problems this population faces. These individuals have all of the same health and psychosocial issues that aging heterosexuals have.

The physical process of aging, living on a fixed income, finding meaningful activities after retirement, and losing friends and loved ones will occur regardless of sexual orientation. The stress of these situations, however, may be amplified for sexual minorities who often struggle with estrangement from their own biological families. This difficulty, of course, reduces the network of support. Moreover, in the case of illness or death, the grieving partner is often not acknowledged by the family of the partner. This is one of the reasons many are pushing for the recognition of gay marriage.

In the past, pensions and benefits have not been awarded to domestic partners, gay or straight. This increases the risk of poverty and these stressors may force older sexual minorities into a rehabilitation setting.

Lesbians and gay men who move, or are moved, to an assisted living facility or a nursing home may have to relive the entire coming-out process (McKee, 1999). Suddenly, after living for years or decades among a network of friends and acquaintances who know of their sexual orientation, they may have to undergo the arduous process of deciding how safe it is to come out, and to whom, in a strange, new environment. Rehabilitation workers, in all settings, need to be aware that sexual orientation is still an important part of the lives of aging minorities, regardless of how long they choose to be sexually active (Loulan, 1984;

Van de Ven and Rodden, 1997). An open, accepting, and compassionate atmosphere is just as important when working with older clients as at any other point during the life span.

The Search for Community

When any of us is in need of rehabilitation services, we look for support. We may be feeling insecure; something in our life has gone awry. For someone who has been living in a perpetual state of feeling different, not average, or outside mainstream culture, an injury or illness may make things even worse. Rehabilitation professionals can provide a safe place for a healing dialogue when they provide an open and accepting environment. First and foremost, the rehabilitation specialist must acknowledge and be sensitive to the full spectrum of sexual and gender identity issues. This understanding can then be demonstrated by using nonbiased language and responding in a nonjudgmental way. Language is very important. Take time to ask about partners or lovers (rather than spouse, boyfriend, girlfriend, husband, or wife). Use of the words "gay" and "lesbian" in conversation, rather than the more clinical "homosexual," shows that you are open and friendly. Remember that people come from an assortment of backgrounds and cut across every socioeconomic class and educational level and that they are found in all cultures. Small cues can allow someone to open up and share his or her personal stories.

Although sexuality is just one small part of the entire person, it is an important part. But it is often difficult for sexual minorities to find community because they blend in and are a part of all other communities, crossing all ethnic, economic, and racial lines. There can be no sense of family or even familiarity until one admits, first to one's self and then to others, that he or she is having a sexual orientation and/or gender identity issue.

According to many reports, between the ages of 13 and 16, gay men and lesbians, as well as bisexuals, recognize that they are somehow different. Some realize this when they are even younger. This may cause a sense of isolation which can cause a variety of problems until people find others who understand or who feel the same way, until he or she is able to talk about those feelings. This sense of isolation can cause a variety of problems. It is important to keep in mind that not all lesbian, gay, bisexual, or transgender people recognize or acknowledge these feelings within themselves at some appropriate age. The realization is different for each individual, often occurring gradually, and may even change over time. People are able to self-identify much younger than they did in the past, but we are still in an era of "Don't ask, don't tell."

Hopefully, this will change in the near future. In the meantime we must be sensitive to the diversity of people looking to rehabilitation professionals for assistance. Because most sexual minorities are not obvious, many choose to remain *closeted*, which refers to staying behind "closed doors." The *closet* is a figure of speech used to describe an emotional hiding place where it is not necessary to reveal one's true identity. People do not reveal their sexual orientation for a variety of reasons, often having to do with previous discrimination—real or imagined. Sometimes, in the case of gender identity, the confusion cannot be avoided until there is a full opportunity for *gender conviction* (Applegate, 2005, Ellaborn, 2002). Until this happens, they may not be able to conceal the confusion in appearance, and once they are able to "pass" as the other gender, they may choose not to reveal themselves unless appropriate and absolutely necessary.

Many systems within society perpetuate the discomfort of sexual minorities to be open about themselves. Some family systems disproportionately abuse and disown members who do not conform to preset standards. In many areas, employment and housing discrimination are still allowed. Many churches continue to teach that all sexual behavior other than heterosexual, monogamous marriage is wrong. Therefore, it is especially important for rehabilitation professionals to create an atmosphere of acceptance. Staff, at all levels, need to be sensitive to the issues regarding sexuality and gender identity. Those who interface with the public must become aware of how easily they can offend someone who is being viewed as *different* or *other.* In order to avoid discomfort for either person, a level of awareness and sensitivity toward all people must be attained, because "different" in the case of many sexual minorities is NOT always obvious. Sexual minorities face a constant struggle about how and when to reveal their orientation; therefore, it is necessary for health professionals to address questions regarding confidentiality in order to provide a feeling of safety.

Sensitivity and sincerity evolve over time. Educational classes and in-services on diversity are valuable only when time is allowed to have open discussions with people of varying backgrounds and lifestyles. The best way to learn about people who are different, no matter what the difference, is to spend time with them in order to get past the surface stereotypes. Remember that these stereotypes have also been learned over time; therefore, it takes time on both sides to move beyond the fear of difference. As members of a minority group, lesbian, gay, bisexual, and transgender people are subject to oppression from the majority. They can minimize the feelings of oppression only by staying in the closet or by coming out and showing themselves as valuable members of society.

Each meeting with a rehabilitation professional requires a decision to come out or to stay in the closet that one creates in regard to sexual issues. Being in the closet has been described as being "in a void created by fear on one side and silence on the other" (Bennett, 1982, in Andrews, 1997, p. 168). This fear relates to punishment for being different; the silence reflects the inability of the heterosexual majority to respond to sexual minorities by speaking and acting with admiration or appreciation of that difference. Some LGBTIQ people feel that "silence is preferable to active hostility and rejection" (Anderson, 1997). Moving beyond the fear and silence is the ideal for all people, both straight and gay, to become members of a more accepting and loving society. The constant attention to the presentation of identity is, in itself, a stressor that needs to be taken into account by the entire rehabilitation staff.

Too often, the argument is heard that heterosexuals do not display their sexuality openly, so why do gay people have to "make a big deal out of it?" Marriage and pregnancy are the most public displays of heterosexual affection. Moreover, how often do we see opposite-sex people holding hands, kissing, or fondling in public, on TV, and in movies? In addition, sexual innuendos between men and women sell many products. On the other hand, sexual minorities who hold hands in public are told that this is an unnecessary public display and that a parade or a gathering in a park, as a show of support for one another, is very questionable. It is this level of contradiction and put-down that make the coming-out process difficult.

Stages of Coming Out

It is essential to remember that the coming-out process does not end with any single disclosure. As rehabilitation professionals, we must meet each person wherever they are in their process of self-revelation. What is most important to remember in a health care or in any other setting is that either person can take the lead. But a safe place must be created. Until a person fully accepts who he or she is as part of a sexual minority, health problems may increase. In addition to a higher incidence of drug and alcohol abuse, as well as more physical and verbal assaults, suicide attempts, AIDS, HIV, STDs, and vaginal infections are also more prevalent among sexual minorities (Centers for Disease Control, 1995). Unplanned pregnancies, anxiety disorders, and severe depression, as well as lack of self-worth and dignity, are all possible concerns that may require consulting a rehabilitation professional. Prostitution and/or "survival-sex" can also be a way of coping with confusion and dysphoria. Sex workers may also present themselves in a rehabilitation setting, and they are another group we must not denigrate. As health care professionals, we must remain sensitive and caring in all cases.

Remember that the identity of everyone's sexual being, regardless of orientation, evolves over time. To summarize the development of sexual and gender identity and identification, Cass (1979) and Coleman (1974) have created models for various stages of sexual identification. The first step is *sensitization and awareness* of one's own internal response to any kind of sexual stimulation, including fantasy or simple flirtation. When one realizes that this response is female-to-female, male-to-male, or both, *identity confusion* follows. In time, lesbians, gay men, and bisexuals acknowledge that this response is different from that of most peers. In a 1992 study conducted by Remafedi of 34,706 students in grades 7 to 12, 10.7% described themselves as "unsure" of their sexual orientation. Some try to deny homosexual feelings. Some seek "repair" through religious or psychological counseling. Others try to avoid their own same-sex feelings, which manifest in such ways as limitation of opposite-sex exposure so as not to be found out, or in limiting exposure to information about homosexuality to be certain not to know "too much." Others immerse themselves in overtly heterosexual or gender-appropriate behavior or escape through drugs and alcohol, and even the adoption of homophobic attitudes and actions. Another response to confusion is *redefinition*, which means rationalizing behavior by redefining it along more conventional lines, for example, special cases (I'd do this only with you); ambisexual strategy (I guess I'm just willing to be sexual with anybody); temporary identity (This is only a phase); or situational (It was only experimentation). Not all gay men and lesbians use these coping mechanisms. Some respond to identity confusion by moving into a stage of *acceptance*, which means acknowledgment of these feelings and beginning to seek out sources of information. Once a gay or lesbian person with a healthy attitude is able to recognize and believe that this difference is acceptable, *self-identity* is reestablished and explored. Here the process of coming out gradually begins. Only at this stage can one begin to affirm the adopting and accepting of their homosexuality.

Sexual identity is an integral and essentially a permanent part of all people. Becoming fully conscious of one's sexuality can only follow the acceptance of difference that then leads to a commitment to live an alternative lifestyle. The *commitment stage* is a gradual extension of the identity assumption stage and may occur at any age (Allen & Glicken, 1996). The factor most commonly cited as leading to acceptance, or *identity assumption*, is recognition of the larger gay community. Within this select group, the similarities of the struggling sexual minority are recognized, and integration can begin. Open expression often follows this acceptance.

Regrettably for some, this level of recognition never happens. Some people are never able to reach the stage of internal acceptance because of continued oppression and homophobia from the heterosexual community. Unfortunately, many people who do not fall into a normal range of sexual behavior either believe that they are doomed to an unhappy life in which they will never find love and acceptance, or turn to drugs, alcohol, and other unhealthy behaviors. Contributing factors to this kind of hopelessness include the absence of positive adult gay, lesbian, or bisexual role models, and the lack of realistic information about how a successful life could be possible.

Cultural Complications

Every culture has belief systems that discriminate against deviance. Some ethnic and religious groups are more averse to homosexuality than others. Many tend to believe the myths and stereotypes of their culture, which indicate that any deviation from the sexual norm is unacceptable. When deviance is unthinkable it is also ignored. People displaying homosexual tendencies are often excluded from the group. This view often causes a double layer of self-hatred and conflict for people of color who are also sexual minorities. Both internal and external commitment to a particular lifestyle is necessary to formulate a complete identity. This struggle for integration continues to happen every time a person with any alternative lifestyle, of any nationality, is in a new situation. One must decide again whether this is a "safe" place to reveal the intimate, private details of his or her life. One might cycle back through to the stage of confusion when meeting another person and again facing the dilemma of revealing one's sexuality. For these reasons, coming out is often viewed as a complicated, lifelong process. As a concerned and educated rehabilitation professional, you can help to ease this process for the people who come to you for help.

Moving Beyond Acceptance

Dr. Dorothy Riddle (1987) has developed an Attitudes Towards Differences Scale through her work on diversity. The Riddle Scale addresses people's various responses to differences in general and to sexual minorities in particular. The scale includes four negative and four positive levels of attitudes towards gay men and lesbians. The four negative levels all contain an element of dominance rather than equality. *Repulsion* is the lowest negative attitude toward people who are different, for example, seeing them as strange, sick, crazy, immoral, sinful, or aversive. For many people, placing sexual minorities in this light justifies wanting to change them, or in the extreme, kill them. The second negative attitude is *pity*, which means seeing people who are different as "born that way" and feeling sorry for them. The goal at this stage, would be to help these "poor individuals" become as "normal" as possible. Riddle also considers *tolerance* to be a negative attitude that she describes as the belief that people with a different sexual orientation or gender preference are in a phase of development that "most will grow out of." This view implies that gays and lesbians should be treated as children who need to be protected and tolerated. Dr. Riddle also views *acceptance* as a negative attitude, which implies that one needs to make accommodations for another's differences. Acceptance does not acknowledge that varying identities may be of the same value and importance as any other identity.

According to Dr. Riddle's scale, to have a positive attitude, one must move to a *supportive* position. Here, work is being done to safeguard the legal and civil rights of those who are different. Regardless of one's own comfort with or acceptance of homosexuality, all people need to be treated fairly. Supportive work helps to foster the next attitude, which is one of *admiration*. At this stage, one acknowledges that being different takes strength. From this position, an attitude of *appreciation* can be developed by which diversity is valued and one is willing to confront all insensitive attitudes. This leads to *nurturance*, which views sexual minorities as indispensable in our society. Only then can one act as an advocate for those who are different. Once a great majority of gays and straights together have arrived at this stage of maturity, real change can take place.

Guidelines

The following may help you in your practice as a rehabilitation professional.

- Avoid stereotypes.
- Make no assumptions.
- Use gender-neutral language.
- Become knowledgeable and sensitive to the full spectrum of various sexual minorities.
- Know the names of local counselors and support groups for referral when necessary.
- Develop the habit of referring to same-sex practices when interviewing all clients.
- Do not include people's sexual orientation on a medical chart without obtaining permission to do so.
- Do not question a client merely to satisfy your own curiosity.
- Include pamphlets and pictures of people from a variety of minorities, including same-sex couples, in the waiting area and exam rooms.

Summary

The recurring need to decide how transparent to be is something that becomes part of every gay, lesbian, bisexual, or transgender person's life. To have a healthy life, one must accept the differences within oneself, before revealing that difference to another. To attain healthy communities, we must accept the differences among ourselves. Only full acceptance can eventually lead the way to the support and nurturance of these differences.

We must learn to see each person as much more than a collection of broken parts that needs to be fixed. Taking into consideration the mental and emotional aspect of each person is as important as being aware of the physical problem. For many the spirit, or soul, is also damaged when one must seek professional care. If we are going to be adequate healers and helpers in the rehabilitation field, we must be willing to see the whole person without prejudice and treat each case without discrimination. Every person is a unique individual.

Questions

1. Define gay, lesbian, bisexual, transgender, and interesex.
2. What is sexual orientation?
3. What is the distinction between sexual identity and gender identity?
4. What is Gender Identity Disorder?
5. What are some sociocultural, psychological, and emotional issues facing people with different lifestyles?
6. How should rehabilitation professionals deal effectively with this population? List some specific steps that must be taken in order to deal with individuals of different lifestyles.
7. What are some specific issues facing young people of different lifestyles?
8. What are some specific issues facing adults with different lifestyles?
9. Discuss the stages of "coming out" mentioned in this chapter.
10. You just learned that your brother is gay. How would you deal with this situation? What are some of the issues and obstacles that your brother and your family may be facing while dealing with this situation?

Case Study

John and Allen, men in their late 30s who have been partners for ten years, have had much contact and interaction with the rehabilitation establishment since Allen had an accident cutting wood three years ago. Both Allen and John enjoy working outdoors and living in a rural, rather remote area. After a femur fracture and significant knee damage that occurred from falling twelve feet from a retaining wall, Allen has had two knee replacements, numerous bone and skin infections, and significantly impaired mobility. Both of them report a moderate level of acceptance from the rehabilitation professionals whom they encounter. John stays with Allen as much as possible when he is hospitalized; however, most rehabilitation professionals direct questions and comments to Allen's mother when she is present. More to the positive, the medical team has been supportive of John's spending the night in Allen's hospital room when necessary, and

John is listed as Allen's first contact in case of emergency. Even so, they are careful in their personal interactions.

It should be noted that they are both outspoken and fit into the societal norm of "masculine" men. They also have a good understanding of the structure of the rehabilitation system—John's father is a retired physician, and Allen's sister and her partner are registered nurses. Allen's family is supportive and does not restrict John's access to him in any way. Both Allen and John acknowledge that their experience with rehabilitation workers has been significantly more positive than experiences in stories that they have heard from others.

Questions

1. What is LGBT?
2. Identify some issues that sexual minorities are facing in the United States.
3. As a rehabilitation professional, how would you deal with your own prejudices toward this population?
4. While working with sexual minorities, what specific steps you would take toward effective rehabilitation?
5. Define gender identity, biological sex, and gender roles as discussed in the chapter.

References

Allen, L., & Glicken, A. (1996). Depression and suicide in gay and lesbian adolescents. *Physician Assistant, 20*(4), 44–49.

Andrews, S. (1997). Gynecologic and obstetric care of lesbian and bisexual women, in *Varney's Midwifery*. (3rd ed.). Helen Varney (Ed.). Sudbury, MA: Jones and Bartlett Publishers.

Applegate, K. (2005). Private conversation.

Bensing, K. (1996). Being gay and grey. *The Plain Dealer*, May 26, Cleveland. p. 8F.

Berger, R. (1986). Working with homosexuals of the older population. *Social Casework, 67*, 203–10.

Boenke, M. (1999). Our trans children. PFLAG Transgender Network found at http://www.youth-guard.org/pflag-tnet/booklet.html. (Retrieved February 10, 2005.)

Boenke, M., Sharp, N., & Xavier, J. M. (1999). Transforming families 3rd ed. Walter Trook Publishing. Imperial Beach, CA.

Cass, V. C. (1979). Homosexual identity formation: A theoretical model. *Journal of Homosexuality, 4*, 219–235.

Centers for Disease Control. (2005). http://www.cdc.gov. (Retrieved February 10, 2005.)

Cloud, J. (1997). Out, proud, and very young. *Time, 150*, 83–85.

Cohen-Kettenis, P., Owen, A., Kaijser, V., Bradley, X., & Zucker, K. (2003). Demographic characteristics, social competence, and behavioral problems in children with gender identity disorder: A cross-national, cross-clinic comparitive analysis. *Journal of Abnormal Child Psychology*, 31, 41–53.

Coleman, E. (1981). Developmental stages of the coming out process. *Journal of Homosexuality*, 7, 31–41.

Colapinto, I. (2000) *As nature made him: The boy who was raised as a girl.* Harper Collins, Toronto.

Crooks, R. & Baur, K. (2005). *Our sexuality.* Thompson Wadsworth, p. 64.

Diagnostic and statistical manual of mental disorders: DSM-III. (1980). (3rd ed.). Washington, DC: American Psychiatric Association.

Diagnostic and statistical manual of mental disorders: DSM-IV. (1994). (4th ed.). Washington, DC: American Psychiatric Association.

Frean, A. (2000) . . . but not so glad to be gray. July 15. *The Times of London*, p. 13.

Goodrum J. (2000). *A Transgender Primer* from http://www.ntac.org/tg101.html. (Retrieved February 10, 2005).

Loulan, J. (1984). *Lesbian sex.* San Francisco: Spinsters.

Massachusetts Governor's Commission on Gay & Lesbian Youth http://www.mass.gov/gcgly. (Retrieved February 10, 2005).

McKee, V. (1999). Survey identifies double discrimination for senior lesbians. *Herizons*, *13*(1), 9.

Nelson, J. (1997). Gay, lesbian, and bisexual adolescents: Providing esteem-enhancing care. *The Nurse Practitioner*, February, Vol. 22, (2), 94–105.

Queen, C. (1997). PoMosexual: Challenging Assumptions about Gender and Sexuality. SF, CA. Cleis Press.

Remafedi, G. (1994). Death by Denial: Studies of Suicide. Boston, Alyson Books.

Ross, M. W. (2000). *Sexual health concerns: Interviewing and history taking for health practitioners.* Philadelphia: F. A. Davis.

Sharp, N. (1997). Medical abuse of GLBT youth. [online]. http://www.critpath.org/pflagtalk/gid.htm (Retreived August 25, 1997).

Taerk, G., & Gallop, R. (1993). Recurrent themes of concern in groups for rehabilitation professionals. *AIDS Care*, *5*(2), 215–223.

Toledo, E., & Cahill, S. (2000). [online] www.ngltf.org Homophobia, unequal treatment limit quality of life. (March 26, 2001).

Van de Ven, P., & Rodden, P. (1997). A comparative demographic and sexual profile of homosexually active men. *Journal of Sex Research*, *34*(4), 349–361.

Wallace, J. I., Paauw, D. S., Spauch, D. H. (1993). HIV infection in older patients: When to suspect the unexpected. *Geriatrics*, *48*(6), 61–64, 69–70.

Walsh, A & Crepeau, B. (1997) "My Secret Life" *The American Journal of Occupational Therapy.* July/Aug. 1998 Vol. 52 #7, pp. 563–569.

White, S. & Franzini, L. (1999). Heteronegativism? *Journal of Homosexuality* Vol. 37(1), 65–79.

Witten, T. M. (2001). Ramifications of the anthropological dilemma in studies of healthcare needs involving sex, gender, and sexuality: Healthcare Surveys—A social epidemiological problem. TransScience Research Institute. Http://www.transcience.org. (Retrieved (2/10/05).

Xavier, J. M. (2000). The Washington Transgender Needs Assessment Survey. http://www.glaa.org/archive/2000tgneedsassessment1112.shtml. (Retrieved February 9, 2005).

Index

A

Abortion
  Jewish beliefs about, 214
  prenatal screening and, 287–88
  selective, 287–88
Acceptance, 372
Acceptance of Disability Scale, 121
Acceptance stage, 370
Access to health care
  African American, 115
  poverty and, 305
  racism and, 20–21
Acculturation
  definition of, 10
  disability and, 276
  Pacific Islander, 269
Achondroplasia, 266
Achromatopsia, 266
Adaptive capacity, 352–54
Admiration, 372
Adolescence, 321–24
  cohort theory and, 344
  LBGT identity in, 365–66
Advanced directives, 69
Affect, 111
Affluent, the, 294
Afghanistan, 198–99
African Americans, 103–30
  background on, 105–7
  celebrations of, 111–12
  in clinical research, 25
  communication and, 108–9,
    123–26
  culture transmission among,
    333
  demographics of, 106–7
  disability and, 120–22
  eating habits of, 116–18
  family among, 110–12
  health beliefs/practices of,
    112–15
  health care access and, 115
  health disparity of, 115–16
  health risks among, 21
  HIV care among, 29
  hypertension among, 303
  income of, 106
  love and belonging among, 323

mental illness and, 118–20
number of in U.S., 105
religions of, 107
reproduction and, 321
sexism and, 25–26
space concepts of, 108
time concepts of, 107–8
violence and, 322–23
who they are, 105–6
Age, as culture, 342–56
  autonomy vs. paternalism and,
    350
  cohort theory on, 346–47
  continuity theory and, 352
  generational values and, 347–49
Age-grade groupings, 344–45
Ageism, 20, 23–25, 350–51
Aging, continuity of, 352. *See also*
    Elderly, the
Ahmad, S. Omar, 181–202
AIDS, 322
  ageism and, 24
  Asian Americans and, 154
  discrimination and, 28–29
Aid to Families with Dependent
    Children (AFDC), 300
Alsharif, Naser Z., 181–202
Ambiguous genitalia, 360, 362–63
American Academy of Physical
    Medicine and Rehabilitation
    (AAPMR), 61
American Association of Retired
    Persons (AARP), 297
American Association of University
    Women, 319
American Hospital Association
    (AHA), 60–61
American Medical Association, 296
American Occupational Therapy
    Association (AOTA), 61
American Physical Therapy
    Association (APTA) Guide for
    Professional Conduct, 61
American Psychiatric Association,
    359–60
American Psychological
    Association, 61
American Samoa, 245, 248, 249–50,
    265. *See also* Pacific Islanders

American Speech-Language,
    Hearing Association (ASHA),
    61
Americans with Disabilities Act of
    1990, 19
Androgen insensitivity syndrome,
    362–63
Anger, suppressing, 328
Appreciation, 372
Arab Americans, 181–202
  from Afghanistan, 198–99
  art of, 189–90
  definition of, 182
  demographics of, 183–84
  exercise and, 190–91
  family among, 329
  family and, 188–89
  fasting among, 191–93
  immigration of, 184–88
  from Iraq, 196–97
  Islamic law and, 189–94
  from Kuwait, 194–96
  from Lebanon, 197–98
  rapport with, 193–94
  rehabilitative care of, 182
  religions of, 183–84
  from Saudi Arabia, 199–200
  self-esteem and, 320
  stereotypes of, 182
  time concepts of, 186–88
  vocation and, 191
Art
  Arab American, 189–90
  Native American, 138–39
Asch, Adrienne, 287–88
Asher, Asha, 151–80
Asian Americans, 151–80
  Asian Indians, 159–63
  Chinese, 156–59
  demographics of, 152
  elderly esteemed by,
    335–36
  emotions hidden by, 332
  family among, 329
  Filipinos, 166–69
  generational status and, 152
  health-risk factors of, 152–54,
    174–75
  hepatitis B among, 324–25

Asian Americans, *(con't.)*
  information disclosure and,
    65–66
  Japanese, 163–66
  Koreans, 172–74
  mental illness and, 154–55
  planning treatment for, 302
  Vietnamese, 169–72
Asian Indians, 159–63
Assessment, 287–88
  poverty and, 305
Assimilation
  definition of, 10
  Native American, 134
Atchley, R. C., 352–54
Attitudes Towards Differences
  Scale, 371–72
"Attitudes Towards Disabilities in a
  Multicultural Society," 280
Authority
  perception of, in
    communication, 41
  professional autonomy and,
    67–69
Autonomy, 62
  aging and, 350
  client/patient, 68–70
  European American value of,
    75–76
  professional, 67–69

B

Baby Boomers, 345, 346, 351
  values of, 348–49
Balanced Budget Act of 1997, 297
Bar Mitzvah/Bat Mitzvah, 210
Basic Vocational Rehabilitation
  Services, 304
Bedouins, 197
Belgrave, F. Z., 120
Belonging
  in adolescence, 323
  in childhood, 318–19
  in the elderly, 335
  in infancy, 315–16
  in middle adulthood, 329
  in older adulthood, 332
  in young adulthood, 325–26
Beneficence, 64–65
Benton, Jean, 1–16
Bias. *See also* Discrimination
  covert, 20, 22
Biculturalism, 10

Bilingualism, 44, 47–48
Binge drinking, 329
Biological sex, 360
Birth control, 298–99
Bisexuality, 358
Black cultural ethos (BCE), 111
Black English, 108–9
Blanchard, Shirley, 103–30
Blasquez, Eduardo, 218–41
Blood transfusions, 68–69
Blue-collar workers, 294–95
Body Mass Index (BMI), 153
Bond, Sandra, 37–58
Boykin, A., 111
Breastfeeding, 317
Bronowski, J., 61–62

C

Caida de la mollera, 231
Canavan Disease, 215
Cancer
  Asian Americans and, 153
  Jewish Americans and, 215
Cariños, 228–29
Caroline Islands, 251–52
Carr, K. D., 154–55
Carver, George Washington, 313
Ceausescu, Nicolae, 83
Central America. *See* Centraleños;
  Hispanics
Centraleños, 222. *See also*
  Hispanics
Change, as value, 7
Chanukah, 207–8
Cheng, L. L., 271–72
Chicanos, 220. *See also* Hispanics
Child abuse, 365
Childhood, 317–20
Children
  ageism and, 23–25
  Chinese, 157
  communication competency
    and, 48
  in poverty, 26, 297–98, 304–5
Children's Medical Security Plan
  (CMSP), 297
Chinese Americans, 156–59, 329.
  See also Asian Americans
Christian Science, 10
Chuuk, 251–52
Circumcision, 210
  female, 318

Civil Rights Act of 1964, 115
Client Assistance Program (CAP),
  304
Client/patient autonomy, 68–70
Clitoridectomy, 318
Cohen, Shannon Munro, 74–102,
  293–311
Cohesion, 121
Cohort theory, 343
  generational, 346–47
  values and, 347–49
Collectivism, 62–63
  Arab American, 188–89
  client/patient autonomy and,
    69–70
  paternalism and, 350–51
Coming out, 370–71
Commitment stage of coming out,
  370–71
Communalism, 111
  Native American, 132–33, 137
Communication, 37–58
  African Americans and, 108–9,
    123–26
  age and, 343
  Asian Americans and, 175
  barriers to, 43–49
  competency in, 47–48
  components of, 38–39
  cross-cultural, 95
  cultural influences on, 40–43
  definition of, 38
  disorders, 43–44, 45–47
  form vs. content in, 47
  Hispanic, 226–28
  Jewish American, 205
  LGBT people and, 363–64
  limited English fluency and, 44,
    47–48
  mismatches in, 48–49
  Pacific Islander, 257–59, 263–64,
    270–71
  in the U.S., 95
  verbal vs. nonverbal, 39–40
Community based rehabilitation
  (CBR), 286
Community resources, 305
Complementary and alternative
  (CAM) health options, 364
Confidentiality, 364–65, 366
Conflict, 121
Congenital adrenal hyperplasia,
  362–63
Conservative Judaism, 212–13

Contextual considerations, 144–45
Continuity theory, 343, 352–54
Contraception, 298–99
Conversation initiatiation, 40
Cook, James, 250
Countercultures, 9–10
    definition of, 10
Covert bias, 20, 22
Covert cultural destructiveness, 5
CP (colored people) time, 107–8
Crabtree, Jeffrey L., 1–16, 59–73,
    131–50, 342–56
Cradleboards, 315
Croatians, 79–81, 96
Cross-dressers, 360
Cubanos, 221. *See also* Hispanics
Cultural awareness
    definition of, 3
Cultural blindness, 5
Cultural competence, 1–16
    continuum of responses in, 4–6
    cultural sterotyping vs., 49
    definition of, 5–6
    developing, 49
    institutionalized, 6
    Pacific Islanders and, 244
    in rehabilitation, 4
Cultural destructive behaviors, 5
Cultural diversity, 2
    communication and, 37–58
    continuum of responses to, 4–5
Cultural rules
    in communication, 39–40
Cultural sensitivity, 5
Cultural variables, 39
Culture
    age as, 342–56
    characteristics of, 9–10
    communication and, 40–43
    definition of, 2–3
    gender and, 312–41
    LGBT people and, 371
    transmission of, 333, 336–37
Curie, Marie, 313

D

Dawes Allotment Act of 1887, 134–35
Death
    Jewish Americans and, 211–12
Decade of Disabled persons, 286
Decision making
    ethical, 70

European American values of, 76
    Japanese factors for, 165–66
    Koreans and, 174
    Vietnamese factors in, 171–72
Decision-making models, 70
Degenerative conditions, 43
Demonstration and Training
    Programs, 304
Denver Developmental Screening
    Test, 287
Developmental disabilities, 43
Developmental theory, 314
    childhood in, 317–20
    elderly in, 333–36
    infancy in, 314–17
    middle adulthood in, 327–30
    older adulthood in, 331–33
    young adulthood in, 324–27
Diabetes, 303
    Asian Americans and, 153
    poverty and, 303
*Diagnostic and Statistical
    Manual*, 360, 361
Dilmun civilization, 194
Disability
    acculturation and, 276
    anticipated role and, 280–81
    beliefs about, 95
    causality of, 277–79
    cross-cultural meaning of,
        274–92
    cultural beliefs about, 276–81
    cultural competence and, 287–89
    cultural responses to, 281–84
    European American beliefs
        about, 76
    Jamaican beliefs about, 281–83
    Native American concepts of,
        132–33
    Pacific Islanders and, 258–59,
        260–61, 267
    resource allocation and, 284–86
    societal responses to, 284–86
    subculture based on, 275–76
    valued/disvalued attributes of,
        279–80
Disabled people
    African American, 120–22
    anticipated roles of, 280–81
    assessing, 287–88
    children, 23–24
    communication disorders and,
        43–44
    in the United Kingdom, 93

Discrimination
    ageism, 23–25
    institutional, 19
    overt, 19–20
    perceived, 18–19
    poverty and, 26–27
    real, 18
    rehabilitation and, 17–36
    sexism, 25–26
Disease
    African American beliefs about,
        113–14
    Asian American risk factors for,
        152–54
    Asian Indian concepts of, 163
    Chinese concepts of, 158–59
    European American beliefs
        about, 76
    Filipino concepts of, 169
    German beliefs about, 89
    Greek beliefs about, 85–86
    Hispanic concepts of, 229, 231–32
    Italian beliefs about, 87
    Japanese concepts of, 165
    Japanese risk factors for, 165–66
    Jewish American risk factors
        for, 215
    Jewish beliefs about, 214–15
    Korean risk factors for, 174
    Native American beliefs about,
        139–41
    Pacific Islander concepts of,
        264–69
    Polish beliefs about, 79
    Vietnamese beliefs about, 171
    Vietnamese risk factors for,
        171–72
Distributive justice, 66–67
Divorce
    African American, 110
Doing vs. being, 8
Dominicanos, 221. *See also*
    Hispanics
Drake, Margaret, 312–41
Duppies, 277–78, 281–83
Dworkin, G., 62

E

Earned Income Tax Credit, 301
Egalitarianism, 8
Elderly, the
    access to health care and, 305
    ageism and, 20, 23–25

Elderly, the (*cont't.*)
  Asian Indians and, 162–63
  Chinese, 157–58
  developmental theory on,
    333–36
  discrimination against, 19
  family care of, 66–67
  Filipino, 168
  Hispanic, 226
  Japanese, 165
  Jewish, 214
  Korean, 173–74
  LGBT, 366–68
  life expectancy and, 344–45
  nutrition and, 301–2
  paternalism toward, 350–51
  in poverty, 297, 299
  sexuality and, 24, 331
Emotions
  African Americans and, 122
Empacho, 231
Enculturation
  definition of, 10
Environment (natural)
  control of, 7
  Native American views of,
    134–35, 135–36
Espiritualistas, 232
Ethics, 59–73
  codes of, 60–61
  paternalism and, 350–51
European Americans, 74–102
  Croatian, 79–81
  French, 93–94
  German, 88–89
  Greek, 84–86
  health care values/beliefs
    among, 75–76
  Hungarian, 81–82
  immigration of, 75
  Irish, 89–91
  Italian, 86–87
  personal space among, 77
  Polish, 77–79
  Romanian, 83–84
  societal responses to disability
    of, 284–85
  statistics on, 96–97
  time views of, 76–77
  U.K., 91–93
Exercise
  Arab Americans and, 190–91
  self-actualization and, 320
Experiential considerations, 145

Expressive individualism, 111
Expressiveness, 121
External continuity, 352–54
Eye contact, 41, 233–34

F

Fadiman, Anne, 279
Falkland Islands, 223
Family
  African American, 110–12,
    120–22
  Arab American, 188–89
  Asian Indian, 160–62
  belonging and, 319
  Chinese, 157
  Croatian, 80
  disability and, 286
  extended, 363
  Filipino, 167–68
  French, 94
  German, 88
  Greek, 85
  Hispanic, 226, 325–26
  homelessness, 296–97
  Hungarian, 81–82
  Irish, 90
  Italian, 87
  Japanese, 164–65, 166
  Jewish, 213–14
  Korean, 173
  LGBTs and, 363–64
  Native American, 144
  nuclear, 363
  Pacific Islander, 255–57, 269
  in rehabilitation, 120–22
  role expectations in, 328
  Romanian, 83
  United Kingdom, 92
  Vietnamese, 171
  violence in, 296
Fasting, 68–69
  Arab Americans and, 191–93,
    199–200
Feast of the Sacrifice, 200
Federal Patient Self-Determination
  Act (PSDA) of 1990, 60–61
Federated States of Micronesia,
  251–52, 253–54
Festival of Jinadriyah, 200
Festival of Lights, 207–8
Filipinos, 166–69, 303. *See also*
  Asian Americans
  independence and, 64–65

Fluency disruptions, 46
Food stamps, 301–2
Form vs. content, 47
French people, 93–94, 96
Friendliness
  as U.S. value, 9

G

Gannoti, M., 287
Gender, 312–41
  adolescence and, 321–24
  childhood and, 317–20
  elderly and, 333–36
  immigration and, 336–37
  infancy and, 314–17
  life expectancy and, 335
  middle adulthood and, 327–30
  older adulthood and, 331–33
  young adulthood and, 324–27
Gender conviction, 368–69
Gender identity, 313, 359, 360
Gender Identity Disorder (GID),
  360, 361–62
Gender roles, 360
  Arab American, 188–89
  Asian Indian, 160–61
  definition of, 313
  disability and, 285
  Hispanic, 229
  U.S., 9
Generational cohort theory, 346–47
Generation X, 346, 349
George, Nigel, 367
Germans, 88–89, 96
Gestures, 41
Ghandi, Mohandas, 313
Ghost Dances, 134, 141
Gift giving, 228–29
GI Generation, 347–48, 351
Glucose 6 phosphate
  dehydrogenase (G6PD), 85, 87
Goldsmith, Marcy Coppelman,
  203–17
Gone, J. P., 132–33
Greeks, 84–86, 96

H

Hadlock, Tana L., 342–56
Haftorah, 205
Halacha, 214
Hallowell, Bob, 4–5
Hang loose time, 107–8
Hanks, H., 285

Hanks, J., 285
Harlow, H. F., 315
Harmony, 111
Haskins, Awilda R., 17–36
Hassidim, 212
Hawaii, 248, 249–50. *See also* Pacific Islanders
 education in, 261–62
 health care in, 265–66
Head Start, 261–62
Health care
 barriers to, 308
 Croatian, 80–81
 French, 94
 German, 89
 Greek, 85–86
 Hispanic, 229
 Hungarian, 82
 Irish, 91
 Italian, 87
 Jewish American, 204
 Korean, 174
 in Kuwait, 195–96
 Pacific Island, 264–69
 Polish, 78–79
 poverty and, 302–3
 Romanian, 83–84
 traditional Chinese, 158–59
 traditional Native American, 140–41
 United Kingdom, 92–93
Health care professionals
 age of, 343
 guidelines for working with LGBTs, 372
 negative first contacts with, 22
 poverty and the role of, 304–6
 poverty issues and, 304–6
Health education
 Asian Americans and, 153–54
Hearing problems, 45
Henderson, G., 119
Hepatitis B, 324–25
Hermaphrodites, 360, 362–63
Heteronegativism, 359
Heterosexism, 20, 22–23, 359
Hezel, F. X., 271
Hierarchy of human needs, 313, 314
Hildegard of Bingen, 313
Hispanics, 218–41
 alternative health care and, 232–33
 binge drinking among, 329

cariños and, 228–29
Centraleños, 222
Chicanos, 220
communication among, 225–26, 228–29
Cubanos, 221
cultural differences among, 224–25
demographics of, 222–23
disability and, 283
diversity among, 223–24
Dominicanos, 221
elder care among, 66–67, 334
family among, 66–67, 225, 325–26
food/nutrition of, 230–31
health care provider roles and, 300
health risks among, 21, 231–32
Hispanos, 219–20
HIV care among, 29
hot-cold model of disease and, 230
hypertension among, 303
immigration of, 219–22, 224
intervention techniques with, 233–35
languages of, 225
as largest minority, 302
last names among, 230
machismo and, 229
nonverbal communication and, 233–35
palanca and, 229
Puerto Riqueños, 220–21
saying "no" and, 228
saying "yes" and, 228
sexism and, 25–26
socioeconomic status and, 225
stereotypes of, 225
Sureños, 222
terminology for, 219
therapy strategies for, 235–36
time concepts of, 229
tradition and, 226
women, 325–26
Hispanos, 219–20. *See also* Hispanics
HIV
 ageism and, 24
 discrimination and, 28–29
Hmong, 279, 283–84. *See also* Asian Americans

Holidays/celebrations
 African American, 111–12
 Arab American, 191–93
 Jewish, 206–9
 Ramadan, 191–93, 199–200
Homelessness, 27–28, 305
 access to health care and, 305
 health care needs and, 302
 poverty and, 296–97
 pregnancy and, 299
Homophobia, 22–23, 28–29, 359, 364
Homosexuals. *See* Lesbians, gays, bisexuals, and transgender (LGBT) people
Horizon of significance, 70
Howe, Neil, 346
Huffington Center on Aging, 344
Hungarians, 81–82, 96
Hunger, 301–2. *See also* Nutrition/eating habits
Hussein, Saddam, 196
Hypertension, 303

I

Identity
 gender, 313, 359, 360
 LBGT, 365–66
 sexual, 358–59
Identity confusion, 370
Immigration
 Arab American, 184–88
 Chinese, 156
 European American, 75
 Filipino, 166–67
 gender and, 336–37
 Hispanic, 219–22, 224
 Japanese, 163
 Jewish, 204
 Korean, 172
 Micronesian, 254–55
 Polynesian, 250–51
 poverty and, 299–300
 Vietnamese, 169–71
Income
 of African Americans, 106
 aging and, 353
 Hispanic, 221
 women and, 298–99
Independence
 beneficence and, 64–65
 Pacific Islanders and, 258
 paternalism and, 350–51
 as rehabilitation goal, 4

Indians. *See* Asian Indians; Native
  Americans
Individualism, 7
  client/patient autonomy and,
    68–70
  collectivism vs., 62–63
  ethics and, 60–62, 63–64
  European American value of,
    75–76
  expressive, 111
  paternalism and, 350–51
  in rehabilitation, 63–64
  in Western culture, 61–62
Individuals with Disabilities
    Education Act (IDEA), 297–98
Infancy, 314–17
Infanticide, 284, 314–15
Information disclosure, 65–66
Informed consent
  Asian Americans and, 155, 175
Ingstad, B., 275
Institute of Medicine, 20–21
Institutional discrimination, 19
Institutionalized cultural
    competence, 6
Insurance
  groups without, 307–8
  number of people without, 302
  poverty and, 26
  uninsured children and, 297
Integrative approach to practice,
    142–46
  contextual considerations in,
    144–45
  experiential considerations in,
    145
  philosophical considerations in,
    144
  pragmatic considerations in, 145
Intercultural diversity, 275
Internal continuity, 352–54
Interpreters
  working with, 97
  working without, 97
Interruptions, 42
Intersexed people, 360, 362–63
Intersex Society of North America
    (ISNA), 363
Interview techniques, 287–88
Intracultural diversity, 275
Iraq, 196–97
Irish, 89–91, 96
Isaza, M. H., 225
Italians, 86–87, 96

J

Jamaican beliefs about disability,
    277–78, 280, 281–83
James, S., 145
Japanese Americans, 163–66. *See
    also* Asian Americans
Jenkins, Cynthia, 103–30
Jennings, B., 2, 3–4
Jewish Americans, 203–17
  aging and, 214
  family and, 213–14
  health beliefs/practices of,
    214–15
  health risk factors of, 215
  holidays of, 206–9
  immigration of, 204
  Judaism and, 206–12
  language/communication of, 205
  life-cycle events of, 209–12
Juneteenth, 112
Justice, 66–67

K

Kaddish, 211–12
Kane, C. A., 350
Katha literature, 161
Klinefelter's syndrome, 362–63
Koreans, 172–74
  communication rules of, 42
Kosher laws, 209–10
Kosrae, 251–52
Kurds, 197
Kuwait, 194–96
Kwanzaa, 112

L

Ladino, 205
Language loss, 44, 48
Languages
  African American, 108–9, 116
  Arab American, 183
  Asian Americans and, 155
  Chinese, 156
  context and, 48
  French, 94
  German, 88
  Greek, 84
  Hispanic, 225
  Hungarian, 81
  interpreters and, 97
  Irish, 90

  Italian, 86
  Japanese, 163–64
  Jewish American, 205
  limited English proficiency, 44,
    47–48
  Pacific Islander, 248–49, 252–53
  Polish, 78
  Romanian, 83
  United Kingdom, 92
  Vietnamese, 170
Latinos. *See* Hispanics
Leadership, 121
Leavitt, Ronnie Linda, 274–92, 280,
    285–86, 288–89
Lebanon, 197–98
Lesbians, gays, bisexuals, and
    transgender (LGBT) people
  aging, 366–68
  attitudes toward, 371–72
  closeted, 366–68, 368–69
  coming out by, 370–71
  community among, 368–69
  cultural complications facing, 371
  guidelines for working with, 372
  medical history taking with,
    363–64
  need for understanding, 364–65
  perceived discrimination
    against, 18–19
  terminology and, 358–63
  transgender people, 360–62
Lesbians, gays, bisexuals, and
    transgender people, 357–76
  heterosexism and, 20, 22–23
  HIV and, 28–29
Life expectancy, 331, 344
Linguistic variables, 39
Lost Generation, 346
Love
  in adolescence, 323
  in childhood, 318–19
  in the elderly, 335
  in infancy, 315
  in middle adulthood, 329
  in older adulthood, 332
  in young adulthood, 325–26
Lower-middle class, 294–95
Lower-upper class, 294

M

Machismo, 229
Macroallocation, 66–67
Madans, 197

Mal de ojo, 231
Mannheim, K., 346
Manzolini, Anna Morandi, 313
Marianas Islands, 251
Marshall Islands, 252
Martin Luther King Day, 112
Maslow, Abraham, 313, 314, 321
Materialism, 7
Mazlish, B., 61–62
Medicaid/Medicare
    African Americans and, 115
    children in, 297
    contraception and, 299
    poverty and, 302
Medical history taking, 363–64
Medicine wheels, 140–41
Melanesia, 245–46. *See also* Pacific
    Islanders
Meningitis, 266
Menopause, 327
Mental illness
    African American, 118–20
    Asian Americans and, 154–55
    gender and, 326–27, 330
    German beliefs about, 89
    Greek beliefs about, 86
    the homeless and, 28
    homelessness and, 302
    homophobia and, 22–23
    Irish beliefs about, 91
    Japanese, 166
    Koreans and, 174
    Native American views of,
      132–33
    Vietnamese and, 171–72
Metabolism, 334
Microallocation, 66–67
Micronesia, 245, 251–55. *See also*
    Pacific Islanders
Middle adulthood, 327–30
Middle class, 294
Millennials, 346
Minorities. *See also individual*
    minorities
    children of, 23–24
    poverty and, 26
    sexual, 357–76
    violence and, 296
Mismatches, communication, 43
Mocumba, Pascoul, 322
Model minority theory, 152
Moralistic orientation, 8
Morgan, D. L., 345
Mortuary games, 137–38

Movement, 111
Muhammad, 194–95
Multilingualism, 44

N

NAFTA (North American Free
    Trade Act), 220
Nakasato, J., 271–72
Narration formats, 40–41
National Council for Culture, Arts,
    and Letters, 196
National Food Consumption
    Survey, 117
National Gay and Lesbian Task
    Force, 367
Native Americans, 131–50
    arts among, 138–39
    beliefs about disability of, 279
    ceremonies/rituals of, 141–42
    characteristics of, 135–37
    health beliefs of, 139
    history of, 133–34
    integrative practice for, 142–46
    natural environment of, 134–35
    number of, 132
    poverty among, 295
    rehabilitation assumptions and,
      132–33
    sport among, 137–38
    traditional healing among,
      140–41
    transsexuals among, 360
Nauru, 254
Neurogenic trauma, 43
New England Journal of
    Medicine, 303
New Shape of Old Island Cultures,
    The (Hezel), 271
Niemann-Pick disease, 79
Nonverbal communication, 39–40
    African American, 109, 119–20
    Greek, 84
    Hispanic, 226–27, 233–35
    Irish, 90
    Italian, 86
    Pacific Islander, 263–64
    Vietnamese, 170
Null, G., 140
Nurturance, 372
Nutrition/eating habits
    African American, 116–18
    Arab American, 191–93
    Asian Indian, 159–60

    Chinese, 156
    effects of poor, 301–2
    elderly and, 334
    Filipino, 167
    Hispanic, 229–30, 236
    Japanese, 164
    Jewish, 209–10
    Pacific Island, 266
    poverty and, 301–2
    Vietnamese, 170

O

Ohio Longitudinal Study of Aging
    and Adaptation (OLSAA),
    352–54
Older adulthood, 331–33
Omnibus Budget Reconciliation
    Act of 1990, 303
Openness
    as U.S. value, 9
Orality, 111
Orderly Departure Program, 170
Organization of Petroleum
    Exporting Countries (OPEC),
    194
Orientation, 358
Otitis media, 266
Overt discrimination, 19–20

P

Pacific Islanders, 242–73
    background of, 244–47
    communication of, 263–64,
      270–71
    cultural competence for, 244
    cultural practices of, 255–69
    education of, 261–62
    family and, 255–57, 269
    health beliefs/practices of,
      264–69
    lifestyle of, 260–61
    Micronesians, 251–55
    Polynesians, 247–51
    religions of, 259–60, 270
    social structure of, 257–59,
      269–70
    time concepts of, 262–63, 270
    useful references about, 271–72
    working with, 269–71
Pacific Nations and Territories
    (Ridgell), 271
Palanca, 229

Palau, 254
Pansexuals, 359
Parents, Family and Friends of
    Lesbians and Gays (PFLAG),
    358
Parsons, E. C., 111
Passover, 208–9, 210
Paternalism, 350–51
Patients' bills of rights, 60–61
Pediatric Evaluation Disability
    Inventory, 287
Perceived discrimination, 18–19
Perez-Arce, P., 154–55
Personal esteem
    in adolescence, 323–24
    childhood and, 319–20
    in the elderly, 335–36
    infancy and, 316
    in middle adulthood, 329–30
    in older adulthood, 332
    in young adulthood, 326–27
Personalismo, 227
Personal Responsibility and Work
    Opportunity and
    Reconciliation Act of 1996
    (PRWORA), 300–301
Personal space, 41
    African American, 108
    European American beliefs
        about, 77
Phenylketonuria (PKU), 79, 91
Philanthropy, 333
Philippines, 166–69
Philosophical considerations, 144
Physician-patient relationships
    Jewish Americans and, 214–15
Physiological needs
    in adolescence, 321
    in the elderly, 334
    in childhood, 317
    in infancy, 314–15
    in middle adulthood, 328
    in older adulthood, 331
    in young adulthood, 324–25
Pipe ceremonies, 141
Pity, 371–72
Pohnpei, 251–52
Polish Americans, 77–79, 96
Polynesia, 245, 247–51. *See also*
    Pacific Islanders
PoMosexuality, 359
Posttraumatic stress disorder
    (PTSD), 80, 318
Pot liquor, 117

Poverty, 293–311
    African Americans in, 106
    discrimination and, 26–28
    the elderly in, 299
    health care needs and, 302–3
    health risks of, 26–27
    homelessness and, 27–28
    hunger and, 301–2
    immigrants in, 299–300
    insurance and, 307–8
    legislation on, 303–4
    rate of in the U.S., 295
    rehabilitation issues and, 304–6
    rural, 295
    social problems and, 296–300
    socioeconomic class and,
        294–96
    urban, 296
    welfare reform and, 300–301
    women in, 298–99
Pragmatic considerations, 145
Prenatal screening, 287–88
Present time orientation, 107–8
Preventive care
    Hispanics and, 300
    the homeless and, 28
    homophobia and, 23
    poverty and, 26–27
    racism and, 21
Prilleltensky, I., 145
Primary sex characteristics, 313
Privacy
    European American values of,
        76
Professional autonomy, 67–69
Progress, as value, 7
Puerto Riqueños, 220–21. *See also*
    Hispanics
Purification ceremonies, 142

Q

Queen, Carol, 359
Queer, 358, 359
Questions
    direct vs. indirect, 41
Qur'an, 189

R

Racism, 20–22
    attitudinal, 19
Ramadan, 191–93, 199–200
Ratliffe, Katherine, 242–73

Real discrimination, 18
Reconstructionism, 213
Reform Judaism, 212
Rehabilitation
    African American attitudes
        toward, 110–11
    ageism in, 24
    assumptions about, 2, 63–70
    beneficence in, 64–65
    communication disorders and,
        43–44
    cultural competence in, 4
    discrimination and, 17–36
    ethical decision making in, 70
    ethics of culture in, 59–73
    family involvement in, 120–22
    independence as goal in, 4
    integrative approach to, 142–46
    justice in, 66–67
    Native Americans and, 139
    Pacific Islanders and, 267–69
    poverty and, 303–6
    professional autonomy and,
        67–69
    purpose of, 3–4
    veracity in, 65–66
Rehabilitation Services
    Administration (RSA), 303–4
Rehabilitation Training Program,
    304
Related Services Assistant (RSA)
    program, 268
Religion
    African American, 107, 114–15,
        117
    Arab American, 183, 184,
        199–200
    Asian Indian, 160, 161
    beliefs about disability and,
        278–79
    Chinese, 156–57
    Croatian, 80
    elderly and, 336
    Filipino, 167
    French, 93
    German, 88
    Greek, 85
    Hispanic, 227, 232–33
    Hungarian, 81
    in Iraq, 197
    Irish, 90
    Italian, 86
    Japanese, 164
    Judaism, 203–17

Korean, 172–73
Lebanese, 198
Pacific Island, 259–60, 270
Pacific Islander, 253
Polish American, 78
professional vs. individual
    autonomy and, 68–69
Romanian, 83
self-actualization and, 327
United Kingdom, 92
Vietnamese, 171
women as leaders in, 330
Religions
Judaism, 203–17
Reproduction, 321
Repulsion, 371
Retirement, 332
Reynolds, S., 275
Rhoades, D. A., 139
Rhoades, E. R., 139
Riddle, Dorothy, 371–72
Rider, N. B., 346
Ridgell, R., 271
Robin, Suzann, 357–76
Rodriguez, Paul, 219
Romanians, 83–84, 96
Rosh Hashanah, 207
Royeen, Matin, 1–16, 131–50,
    181–202
Rural poverty, 295
Russell, C., 351

S

Safety clause, 351
Safety/security needs
    in adolescence, 322–23
    in childhood, 317–18
    in the elderly, 335
    in infancy, 315
    in middle adulthood, 328
    in older adulthood, 331
    in young adulthood, 325
Samoa, 245, 248. *See also* Pacific
    Islanders
Santeria, 232–33
Saudi Arabia, 199–200
School lunch programs, 304–5
Scientific orientation, 6–7
Secondary sex characteristics, 313
Seders, 208–9
Self
    Asian Americans and, 175

mental health tools and, 154–55
    rehabilitation and, 2
Self-actualization
    in adolescence, 324
    in childhood, 320
    in the elderly, 336
    in infancy, 317
    in middle adulthood, 330
    in older adulthood, 333
    in young adulthood, 327
Self-confidence, 352–53
Self-identity, 370
Self-Report Family Inventory, 121
Seung, Hye-Kyeung, 37–58
Sex-change operations, 360
Sex Information and Education
    Council of the United States
    (SIECUS), 359
Sexism, 25–26
Sex reassignment, 360
Sexual abuse, 317–18
Sexually transmitted diseases
    (STDs), 322
Sexual orientation, 358, 362
Sexual preference, 358
Shaheen, Jack, 185
Shari-ah, 189
Shiva, 211–12
Shortchanging Girls, 319
Silence, 41–42
Silent Generation, 347–48, 351
Smudging ceremonies, 142
Social class, 294–96. *See also*
    Socioeconomic status
Social problems, 296–300
Social supports, 353
Socioeconomic status, 294–96
    African Americans and, 114
    Hispanics and, 225
    mental health and, 118
    Pacific Islander, 269–70
    Pacific Islanders and, 257–59,
    260–61
Socio-temporality, 186–88
Sorenson, J. L., 154–55
Soul food, 117
South Americans. *See* Hispanics;
    Sureños
Space, concepts of
    African American, 108
Speech disorders, 46
*Spirit Catches You and You Fall
    Down, The* (Fadiman), 279
Spirituality, 111

Sport
    Native American, 137–38
    self-actualization and, 320
State Child Health Insurance Plan
    (SCHIP), 297
Stereotypes
    ageism and, 24
    of Arab Americans, 182, 185–86
    cultural competence vs., 49
Stigma
    of disability, 279–80
Stigmata, 279–80
Strauss, William, 346
Subcultures, 9–10
    age as, 342–56
    disability-based, 275–76
Substance abuse
    in Greece, 85
    the homeless and, 27–28
    homelessness and, 302
Success
    in adolescence, 323–24
    in the elderly, 335–36
    infancy and, 316
        childhood and, 319–20
    in middle adulthood, 329–30
    in older adulthood, 332
    in young adulthood, 326–27
Sunnah, 189
Supplemental Security Income
    (SSI), 300
Supportive attitude, 372
Sureños, 222. *See also* Hispanics
Sweat lodge ceremonies, 142

T

Talmud, 205
Taylor, C., 62, 63
Tay-Sachs disease, 79, 215
Teen pregnancies, 297, 300–301,
    366
Thalassemia, 85, 87
Thompson, Toni, 218–41
Thompson, W., 133–34
Time orientation
    African American, 107–8
    Arab American, 186–88
    European American beliefs
        about, 76–77
    Hispanic, 229
    Japanese, 164
    Pacific Islander, 262–63, 270
    U.S., 8

Tolerance, 372
Topic selection, 40
Torah, 205
Touching, 41
    European American beliefs
        about, 77
    Hispanics and, 226–27
Transgender, 360–62
Transitional Aid to Needy Families
    (TANF), 300
Transportation, 353. *See also*
    Access to health care
Transsexuals, 360
Transvestites, 360
Truth telling, 65–66
Tuberculosis (TB), 79, 300
    Asian Americans and, 154
    drug-resistant, 300
Tubman, Harriet, 313
Tzitzit, 213

U

*Unequal Treatment: Confronting
    Racial and Ethnic Disparities
    in Healthcare*, 20–21
United Kingdom, 91–93, 97
United Nations Year of Disabled
    Persons, 286
United States
    African Americans in, 105
    cross-cultural communication
        in, 95
    European Americans in, 74–102

mainstream values in, 6–9
Native Americans in, 131–50
poverty rate in, 295
statistics on, 97
Upper-middle class, 294
Urban Indian Health Program, 295
Urban poverty, 296

V

Values
    American mainstream, 6–9
    cohort theory and, 347–49
    European American, 75–76
    socioeconomic class and, 294
Veracity, 65–66
Verve, 111
Veteran's Administration, 303
Vietnamese, 169–72. *See also* Asian
    Americans
Violence
    poverty and, 296
    sexual orientation and,
        365–66
Vocational Rehabilitation and
    Employment (VR & E)
    program, 303
Voice disorders, 46–47
Voice volume, 41

W

Wallace, G. J., 271–72
War brides, 336

Welfare reform, 300–301
Western civilization
    American mainstream values
        and, 6–9
    definition of, 2–3
    individualism in, 61–62
Women
    anger suppression by, 328
    Asian Indian, 160–61
    in clinical research, 25
    educational inequality and,
        319–20
    in Hispanic culture,
        325–26
    HIV care among, 29
    homelessness among,
        296–97
    poverty and, 298–99
    in religion, 330
    sexism toward, 25–26
    sexual abuse of, 317–18
    U.S. roles of, 9
    violence against, 325
Women, Infants, and Children
    (WIC) program, 301
Worldviews, 105

Y

Yap, 251–52
Ybor, Vicente Martinez, 221
Yiddush, 205
Yom Kippor, 207
Young adulthood, 324–27